Covenantal Biomedical Ethics for Contemporary Medicine

Covenantal Biomedical Ethics for Contemporary Medicine

An Alternative to Principles-Based Ethics

JAMES J. RUSTHOVEN

Foreword by Craig G. Bartholomew

☙PICKWICK *Publications* • Eugene, Oregon

COVENANTAL BIOMEDICAL ETHICS FOR CONTEMPORARY MEDICINE
An Alternative to Principles-Based Ethics

Copyright © 2014 James J. Rusthoven. All rights reserved. Except for brief quotations in critical publications or reviews, no part of this book may be reproduced in any manner without prior written permission from the publisher. Write: Permissions, Wipf and Stock Publishers, 199 W. 8th Ave., Suite 3, Eugene, OR 97401.

Pickwick Publications
An Imprint of Wipf and Stock Publishers
199 W. 8th Ave., Suite 3
Eugene, OR 97401

www.wipfandstock.com

ISBN 13: 978-1-62564-002-4

Cataloguing-in-Publication data:

Rusthoven, James J.

Covenantal biomedical ethics for contemporary medicine : an alternative to principles-based ethics / James J. Rusthoven ; foreword by Craig G. Bartholomew.

xvi + 314 pp. ; 23 cm. Includes bibliographical references and index.

ISBN 13: 978-1-62564-002-4

1. Medical ethics. 2. Medical ethics—Religious aspects. 3. Religion and ethics. 4. Religion and Medicine. I. Bartholomew, Craig G., 1961–. II. Title.

R725.5 .R87 2014

Manufactured in the U.S.A.

To Thea, Nathan, Joel, and Daniel,
for their loving support of my work, and in particular
to my son Joel for his patient linguistic and editorial counsel
during the completion of this work.

Contents

Foreword by Craig G. Bartholomew   ix
Acknowledgments   *xiii*

Introduction   1

PART ONE—*The Rise and Dominance of Principles-Based Biomedical Ethics*

1. The Rise of Principlism in Response to an Ethical Crisis   13

2. Challenges to Principlism   48

3. Perspectives on Principles from Diverse Faith Traditions   68

4. Richness and Depth of Understanding within Faith Traditions   98

PART TWO—*A Modest Proposal for a Biblical Covenantal Biomedical Ethic*

5. Conceptual Support for Covenantal Biomedical Ethics   127

6. Groundwork for a Contemporary Covenantal Ethic   183

7. Envisioning Medicine within a Covenantal Ethic   214

8. The Four Principles Revisited   241

   Epilogue: The End of the Beginning   272

Appendix   279
Bibliography   281
Index   301

Foreword

IT IS CLEAR THAT our Western democracies are in a crisis when it comes to ethics in the public square. This crisis has been evocatively and acutely diagnosed by Alasdair MacIntyre. At the outset of his *After Virtue* he imagines a scenario in which for various reasons the natural sciences suffer a catastrophe.[1] Laboratories are burnt down, books and libraries of science burned, and scientists eliminated from society. Later a reaction sets in and people try to recover science,

> But all they possess are fragments: a knowledge of experiments detached from any knowledge of the theoretical context which gave them significance; parts of theories unrelated either to the other bits and pieces of theory which they possess or to experiment; instruments whose use has been forgotten; half-chapters from books, single pages from articles, not always fully legible because torn and charred.[2]

Nonetheless, the fragments are reassembled and the resulting "body" of knowledge is taught and learned. People continue to use the vocabulary of science but the contexts of such knowledge have been lost so that their use of the reassembled knowledge is arbitrary and random. Essentially we are left with fragments and simply don't know how they fit together anymore. For MacIntyre this is an apt description of the situation of the world today in terms of *morality*:

> The hypothesis which I wish to advance is that in the actual world which we inhabit the language of morality is in the same state of grave disorder as the language of natural science in the imaginary world which I described. What we possess... are the fragments of a conceptual scheme... But we have—very largely, if not entirely—lost our comprehension, both theoretical and practical, of morality.[3]

1. MacIntyre, *After Virtue*, 1–3.
2. Ibid., 1.
3. Ibid., 2.

Foreword

How have we arrived at this grave situation? For MacIntyre the failed attempt by Enlightenment thinkers to furnish a universal account of moral rationality led to the rejection of moral rationality altogether by subsequent thinkers such as Jean-Paul Sartre and Friedrich Nietzsche. For MacIntyre, Nietzsche's repudiation of the possibility of moral rationality embodies the consequence of the Enlightenment's mistaken quest for final and definitive arguments that will settle moral disputes through calculative reason alone and without use of teleology.

Theoretically this is, of course, interesting, but far more serious are the practical implications, and not least in health care and the practice of medicine. Like politics and the food business, the way in which ethics is embodied in medicine affects all of us. Sooner or later we all need the help of the medical profession and it is then, often at our most vulnerable, that we discover the sort of practices that nowadays govern medicine.

In this book Dr. Jim Rusthoven focuses on the dominant model in bioethics today, namely *principlism*. Readers should note that Dr. Rusthoven is particularly well equipped to address this issue. He is a distinguished Canadian oncologist who has combined medical research with years of practice and is also well qualified philosophically and theologically. This book brings to fruition years of practice and reflection.

In an analysis that parallels MacIntyre's excavation of our present crisis, Dr. Rusthoven explores the origins and philosophical background of principlism and enables us to see *how* we have arrived at the situation we now find ourselves in. This in itself is a major contribution. Many of us encounter the problems in medical practice today without any sense of why they occur or whether alternative models are possible. Understanding the ethics informing contemporary medical practice goes a long way towards unveiling the contours of its ethos, for better and for worse.

Dr. Rusthoven is not alone in attending to medicine as a focal point of the crisis of ethics in the West. In his *The Malaise of Modernity*, the distinguished Canadian philosopher Charles Taylor cites medicine as an example of an area of social life in which *instrumental reason* has triumphed.[4] By "instrumental reason" Taylor refers to the sort of rationality that measures success by the maximum economic efficiency. In terms of medicine Taylor notes the over-dependence on technology to provide such success. This is helpful, but how, one wonders, could such a beautiful vocation as medicine even be tempted by such inhuman waters?

---

4. Taylor, *Malaise of Modernity*, 6.

Foreword

Dr. Rusthoven helps us to see that the ethical vacuum embodied in principlism creates the context in which the spirits of the age can easily gain dominance. In his trilogy entitled *Sacred Order / Social Order* the late Philip Rieff rightly noted that culture-making is the turning of *sacred* order into *social* order and that the health of any society depends upon a "vertical in authority," which he abbreviates playfully as a VIA. Alarmingly Rieff argues that ours is the first culture to attempt culture-making without a sense of the sacred, without a VIA. That, I think, is precisely what we see in principlism. Apart from a sacred grounding for ethics one is left with an ethical lowest common denominator vulnerable to all sorts of abuse at both the practitioner and patient ends of the spectrum. One is left with ethical shards and fragments ungrounded in a rich tradition.

A major strength of this book is that Dr. Rusthoven not only enables us to see the problem but he proposes a solution. Working within the Judeo-Christian tradition he proposes and fleshes out in considerable detail a *covenantal bioethic* that makes relationship, both vertical and horizontal, central. Lest readers wonder, Dr. Rusthoven is well aware of the pluralistic nature of contemporary Western culture and develops his covenantal model so as to make it maximally attractive and beneficial for those of other traditions. What he does not do, and rightly so, is to seek some neutral, common ground, where all deep commitments are abandoned and we seek a lowest common denominator for bioethics. Such an approach leads us right back into the scenario diagnosed by MacIntyre. Dr. Rusthoven's work consciously takes with utmost seriousness the particularity of the traditions that constitute our pluralistic culture, opening the way for a fertile dialogue with those rooted in alternative traditions. It is through similar work to Dr. Rusthoven's in other traditions that a dialogue could and should emerge, which would enable us to develop a rich, thick bioethics for today.

This is an important and creative work. My hope is that it will be widely read and spark a dialogue that will benefit us all.

Craig G. Bartholomew
Easter 2013

Acknowledgments

THE SEEDS OF THIS book were sown forty-four years ago in a first-year philosophy course taught by Dr. Calvin Seerveld at Trinity Christian College, Palos Heights, Illinois. Despite being raised in a faith community that claimed to have roots in the neo-Calvinist tradition, I had been largely unaware of the true richness of that tradition for Christian living and working. Mentored by philosophy professors Seerveld, Peter Steen, and Richard Russell, historian C. T. McIntire, sociologist Martin Vrieze, and theologian Arnold De Graaf, I began to see the life-encompassing importance of living a Christian life whose entire scope is pervaded by the redemptive story of Scripture. When I felt the Spirit-led calling toward a vocation in the biological sciences, professors Harry Cook and Arie Leegwater, as well as Dean Robert Vander Vennen, began to expose for me the foundations of modern scientific thought. Increasingly aware of the violations of creational norms within the modernist worldview which was cracking under postmodern critique, I started to see the pressing need for an in-depth Christian critique and alternative view of created reality through the natural sciences.

Upon entry into medical school, plans to develop a Christian philosophical understanding of biology in general and medicine specifically were left to gestate as I engaged in the day-and-night life of medical training. I give thanks to the supporting community in Toronto that kept me aware of a life outside of medical training, particularly my church and the Christian academic community that is the Institute for Christian Studies. I also thank Drs. Edmund Pellegrino and H. Tristram Engelhardt for their inaugural leadership in editing the informative and often-inspiring articles that made up the then newly born *Journal of Medicine and Philosophy* of the mid-1970s. The journal provided a refreshing look at medicine beyond the nitty-gritty of daily sleuthing through differential diagnoses and therapeutic decision-making. The journal opened up the multifaceted expressions—the sociological, psychological, political,

Acknowledgments

juridical, spiritual, and other aspects—that together comprise the medical enterprise. Two mentors were particularly formative in showing me the importance of developing teaching methods and sensitivity for the needs of medical trainees and patients at all levels of education and understanding. Dr. George Jackson taught me the importance of showing medical students that they are valued for their views and for their commitment to patients. Dr. David Sackett exemplified the clinician-scientist who applies scientific rigor to clinical research and practice while staying in touch with the nuances of the patient narrative in his clinical teaching.

After twenty years of oncology training, practice, teaching, and clinical research, I felt called to better understand the linguistic and conceptual complexities that are contemporary biomedical ethics. During my first years of course instruction at the Joint Centre for Bioethics, University of Toronto, I was energized by the wisdom and intellectual versatility of Professor Ross Upshur. His inspiration and expertise as a teacher of clinical studies methodology and his knowledge of hermeneutics reintroduced me to the importance of a philosophical understanding of one's calling and discipline, including medicine. As well, I am particularly grateful to Edmund Pellegrino for the hours of engaging and enriching discussions during my visit to the Center for Clinical Ethics at Georgetown University in 2003. His commitment to sharing the wisdom of his Christian tradition with students of biomedical ethics and his unashamed profession of the faith in which his scholarship is rooted has been an inspiration to me in my struggle to articulate the influence of my own faith. I am also beholden to the faculty of the McMaster Divinity College for their patient instruction in theology and Greek, foreign territory for a biologist-physician who sought cross-disciplinary training in order to carry forward Christian scholarship in biomedical ethics.

I would also like to thank Dr. Gerrit Glas and Dr. Andrew Goddard for their encouraging support and conceptual suggestions while supervising the PhD dissertation that has led to this volume. Perhaps the single most influential force in the development of the perspective presented in this book was provided by the primary mentor of that dissertation, Dr. Craig Bartholomew. Philosopher, theologian, and Anglican priest with an irrepressible passion for teaching and writing, he revitalized my aspirations to see medicine and biomedical ethics through Reformed Christian spectacles and nurtured the latent seedling that became this book. He encouraged me to think creatively and taught me the continued importance of seeing medicine as an integral part of my relational

Acknowledgments

life in my daily walk with God. Underpinning all of this reflection and experience has been the continued encouragement of Dr. Cal Seerveld, one of the sowers of the seed whose commitment to a full-bodied biblical worldview has been a deep thread of inspiration through the last forty-five years. His ageless wisdom continues to infect even the most street-savvy contemporary student with inspiring awe and humility.

Finally, I would like to acknowledge the never-failing encouragement and support of my family—my wife Thea, and sons Nathan, Joel, and Daniel—for their constant encouragement and patience. I wish particularly to thank my son Joel, whose long-suffering reviews of the dissertation that preceded this book incalculably improved the linguistic versatility by which I have expressed my thoughts and insights.

In recognizing these human companions, I also acknowledge that they were instruments of the gracious love and support of my God, who is revealed in the Christian Scriptures and for whose kingdom I labored in this work.

Introduction

DURING MUCH OF ITS relatively short life as a distinct discipline, biomedical ethics has been dominated by principles-based ethics. This ethical framework was born out of a perceived need to identify societally acceptable principles for guiding ethical behavior among investigators who were supervising clinical studies involving human subjects. It took many hours of deliberation over four years by many expert consultants in bioethics for the principles of respect for persons, beneficence, and justice to be distilled by the Belmont commission into its 1978 report. Within a year, two participants in these deliberations, James Childress and Tom Beauchamp, published their *Principles of Biomedical Ethics*. Adding a fourth principle, nonmaleficence, they promoted the expanded application of these four principles into many facets of medical research and practice. Today, medical school curricula and postgraduate training programs include courses in medical ethics based largely on the principles-based approach of Beauchamp and Childress.

I began this project out of frustration with a perceived disinterest of numerous bioethicists in exploring the core beliefs that underscore the expression of biomedical ethics today. While the simplicity of the principles-based bioethical framework quickly made it popular among practicing bioethicists and practitioners of medicine, a growing number of scholars engaging the discipline expressed dissatisfaction with the insular focus on these principles at the expense of moral content rooted in philosophical or religious traditions. Moral content takes a back seat to process in large part because the diversity of fundamental beliefs in Western pluralistic society is considered by many to be an impediment to the development of societal standards of bioethical policy and decision-making.

Despite its staying power for over thirty years, principles-based ethics has been widely criticized. Some of the earliest critics, such as K. Danner Clouser and Bernard Gert,[1] argue that the principles have become

---

1. Clouser and Gert, "Critique of Priniciplism," 219.

a mantra, functioning as mere reminders of basic moral tenets, with no substantive moral content, grounding, or justification. These critics coined the term *principlism* to highlight an overemphasis on principles in moral deliberations and decision-making in principles-base ethics. While they seem to use the term in reference to all principles-based ethical frameworks, the term will be used in this book to refer to the principles-based ethical framework promoted by Beauchamp and Childress, unless stated otherwise. Other critics have appealed for a return to the study of moral philosophy, looking for fresh or reconstituted moral theories that could provide moral guidance in addressing moral and societal issues brought about by the consequences of new biotechnologies.[2] However, critics often seem to be caught in a dialogical tension between focusing primarily on procedural approaches to moral situations that rely on rules created by past precedents versus finding moral theories that best serve specific situations. Principlism seems determined to avoid this dialogical stalemate tension, floating above the fray as a mid-level default framework, seemingly independent of moral theories or basic moral beliefs. It tries to procedurally sort out specific situations by adapting a casuistic approach in order to establish moral solutions through reflective equilibrium. Principlism is built on common, albeit minimal, universal beliefs that can be articulated by a common language of ethical reflection. Backed up by the faith in rationality that underlies common morality, principlism relies on the moral authority of consensus, derived through iterative moral discourse among morally serious persons, in order to resolve moral quandaries.[3]

While principlism has gained popularity as a "neutral" way to work out moral dilemmas, the expression of theological voices has gradually waned. In the decades before the Belmont Report, prominent Protestant, Roman Catholic, and Jewish bioethicists wielded formative influence within the newly forming field. Pioneers Paul Ramsey and Richard McCormick wrestled publically over pressing issues of the day, most notably the recruitment of children and adolescents into research and the debates over the moral status of the unborn.[4] But with the formal advent of principlism, fewer theologians seemed willing to risk entering a field that increasingly considered religiously grounded moral views to be outmoded or obstructive to the formation of moral consensus. Even within religious traditions, criticism was sometimes raised against theologians who did

---

2. Green, "Method in Bioethics," 182.
3. Beauchamp and Childress, *Principles of Biomedical Ethics*, 4th ed., 397–405.
4. Smith, "On Paul Ramsey," 24.

Introduction

not overtly and unashamedly declare the influence of their faith on their bioethical positions. Stanley Hauerwas, for one, chided fellow Protestant Paul Ramsey for not being more forthright beyond the preface of his books about the influence of his faith on his positions.[5] Similarly, Leon Kass bemoaned the loss of expression of religious reasons for bioethical positions and suggested that fear over the loss of academic credibility or promotion could be playing an important role.[6]

In this state of diminishing theological expression and increasing reliance on rational discourse alone, I pursued graduate studies in biomedical ethics following eighteen years as a teacher, researcher, and clinical practitioner of cancer care. In a short time, I learned that biomedical ethics had evolved into a process-driven discipline. That is, much of bioethical reflection involved choosing among the various methods available to approach biomedical ethical problems, while little time was devoted to exploring the basic beliefs behind moral positions. As a Christian beginning in the field, it also became clear to me that basic moral beliefs did not arise in classroom discussions or within the context of clinical ethics consultations. Such beliefs were considered private, and not necessarily helpful, to the larger discussion among those in the consultation process.

Given this experienced reality within the discipline, I began exploring the history and theoretical basis of principles-based ethics. Proponents of principlism note that sidelining expressed beliefs in moral authority outside of rational deliberation is key to the utilitarian success of principlism toward moral consensus. Such success is considered inevitable if everyone discusses cases and their moral issues using their common reasoning facility. Still, some critics have insisted that principlism is poor in moral substance. Others suggest returning to moral philosophy, while still others advocate revisiting theological traditions for moral guidance. However, what has been lacking in all expressed concerns is an in-depth critique that explores the worldview and philosophical roots of principlism. Such a critique is required in order to fully understand principlism in its contemporary historical and societal context. Such a critique is necessary for developing a morally richer ethical framework through which these principles can be understood in a more meaningful way.

In light of these concerns about the inadequacies of principlism, this book offers a critical appraisal that explores the worldview and philosophical roots of principlism and its components. Following this critique,

5. Hauerwas, "Christian Ethics," 15–16.
6. Kass, "Practicing Ethics," 6–7.

these principles will be refocused within a bioethical framework that is grounded in the concept of covenant as expressed in the Christian Scriptures. As I hope to persuasively show, this covenantal ethical framework is particular in its fullest meaning but generalizable for all of humankind in practice. That is, the concept of covenant can be articulated and implemented within non-Christian traditions as well. The idea of covenantal relationality has been raised by a variety of medical caregivers in contemporary medical literature.[7] Some ground their appeals in the pagan Greek medical tradition or ancient Eastern traditions, while some give either glancing or direct reference to roots in the Judeo-Christian tradition. It is my contention that the most meaningful expression of covenant is appreciated through the covenant theme which is revealed by God through the Christian Scriptures. However, the basic features of such a covenantal theme as a relational model for all human relationships can be a common starting point for ethical reflection that focuses on human relationships as the core of medical practice, medical research, and medicine in general.

This book is divided into two main parts. The first part exposes the crisis that led to the development and dominance of principles-based ethics and unpacks the major criticisms that followed up to the present. Chapter 1 presents the historical circumstances leading up to the entrance of principles-based ethics into biomedical ethics. Subsequently, the ethical crisis generated by the revelation of unethical conduct in research involving human subjects in the late 1960s resulted in the creation of the Belmont Commission by the United States Congress in 1974. Major conceptual contributions by commission members and their invited consultants were distilled into three principles of respect of persons, beneficence, and justice, all meant to guide the ethical conduct of research investigators engaged in research involving human subjects. The report quickly became a catalyst for developing a more comprehensive application of these and other ethical principles to biomedical ethics. The most widely adopted of these applications is the principles-based ethical framework developed and promoted by James Childress and Tom Beauchamp. These prior consultants to the Commission added a fourth principle of nonmaleficence. While many bioethicists consider the latter to be an implied companion of beneficence, I will argue in chapter 8 that nonmaleficence must be a free-standing principle within principlism because it forms the core of ethical common ground for the common morality on which principlism

---

7. Cassel, "Physician-Patient Covenant," 604; Nisker, "Covenantal Model," 502; Li, "Patient-Physician Relationship," 918; Coffey, "Nurse-Patient Relationship," 308, 309; Brothers, "Covenant and Vulnerable Other," 1133.

is founded. The last section of the chapter 1 reviews philosophical predecessors of principlism, such as W. D. Ross, William Frankena, and John Rawls, points out some ideological borrowing from natural law theory, and presents the primary focus of the principle of justice within principlism as the fair allocation of limited resources.

The next three chapters focus on a decades-long series of responses to principlism, ranging from rather scathing critiques to constructive suggestions for improvement. It is partly in response to these criticisms and suggestions that Beauchamp and Childress have produced the subsequent editions of *Principles*. Chapter 2 presents critiques from three early, formative critics, K. Danner Clouser, Bernard Gert, and Robert Veatch. As secular perspectives in bioethics became more dominant, some bioethicists who overtly spoke from particular religious traditions, like Christian bioethicist James Gustafson and Jewish bioethicist Leon Kass, openly lamented the fading of theological voices and the concomitant loss of their insights within the discipline. Such diminution of theological influence is thought to be due in part to fewer theologians entering the field but also to an unwillingness by many to openly express the influence of their faith on their bioethical reflections. Some like John H. Evans accuse many theologians of capitulating to procedural bioethics and its preoccupation with autonomy, particular as expressed in debates regarding informed consent. Evans and Gilbert Meilaender go so far as to propose a conspiratorial element, led by those who wish to preserve scientific progress by minimizing bioethical objections through the professionalization and insulation of bioethical concerns. Chapter 3 relates the diversity of responses to principlism of formative bioethicists across major faith traditions. Some of these responses come from Christian bioethicists who indeed have boldly disclosed the impact of their religious beliefs on their bioethical views, including those on principles-based ethics. Edmund Pellegrino, H. Tristram Engelhardt, and Paul Ramsey have been chosen as leading bioethicists who speak directly or indirectly on principlism from Roman Catholic, Eastern Orthodox, and Protestant perspectives, respectively. Further views are presented by Islamic and Jewish critics, showing the wide scope of concern and attempts to reconcile principles to specific faith traditions.

Chapter 4 presents the wider variety of Christian views within specific denominational traditions that directly address the strengths and weaknesses of principlism, showing the richness of responses and global impact of principlism on theological reflections. In the last section of chapter 4, I outline my own critique of principlism from a Reformed Christian perspective. Distinct from other critiques presented, it exposes the worldview and philosophical roots of principlism, showing the modernist and postmodern elements that joust for position through the common-morality motif. This lays the groundwork for an alternative ethical framework with roots anchored in a biblical notion of moral authority, justification, and covenantal relationality.

The second part of the book rolls out a more relationally focused, covenantal ethical framework. It is based on the theme of covenant derived from that taught in the Christian Scriptures. Chapter 5 presents an in-depth justification for a covenantal biomedical ethic, tracing covenantal concepts in Christian and non-Christian traditions. The biblical theme of covenant as interpreted in the history of the Christian church is explored, as is the relationship between the covenant theme and other biblical themes. The appropriation of this theme as a major component of bioethical frameworks of earlier Protestant bioethicists such as Paul Ramsey and William F. May is presented, along with less comprehensive allusions to the covenant theme by other Christian ethicists. The chapter concludes with an argument regarding the importance of firm Christian theological and philosophical foundations for a biblical covenantal ethic.

Chapter 6 presents the components of a biblical covenantal biomedical ethic, articulating three key elements of a biblical ethical framework: 1) development of a biblically grounded worldview, philosophy, and theology, 2) incorporation of a biblical anthropology based on the relationship between human beings and God and on the limits of human authority and responsibility, and 3) demonstration of the importance of structural and directional normativity for human relationships. Like its companion theme (i.e., God's kingdom) in Scripture, the covenant theme weaves through the redemptive story like a golden thread.[8] It similarly weaves through Reformed Christian worldview, philosophy, and theology, whose meaning and direction are anchored in that redemptive story. The interpretive current of the Reformed Christian worldview is particularly well suited for developing a covenantal relational ethic, drawing from the insights and wisdom of John Calvin, Abraham Kuyper, Herman Bavinck, Herman Dooyeweerd, Gordon Spykman, Albert Wolters, Craig Bartholomew, and others. In this chapter, the anthropological foundations of a biblical covenantal ethic are also discussed. The created status of human beings as image-bearers of God in a covenantal relationship with God is articulated, with attention being given to the particularly formative and resonating views of Reformed theologian

---

8. Spykman, *Reformational Theology*, 11.

Bavinck and Jewish contemporary rabbi and scholar David Novak.[9] For these men of faith, covenant and the image of God are intertwined motifs that provide the basis for the covenantal relationship of all human beings with God. It is through this relationship that the ethical unity of humankind is defined and grounded.

Chapter 7 presents the relational reality of medical practice, the insights that can be gained, and the normative expression maintained by way of a covenantal ethical framework for understanding those relationships. In this context, the Christian social philosophy of Dutch philosopher Herman Dooyeweerd is introduced, and arguments are put forward which suggest that this philosophy of social structures is applicable to normative medical practice and that it is complementary to a covenantal ethic for medicine.[10] The biblical teaching regarding the treatment of strangers is introduced as a dimension of covenantal ethical expression that holds particular meaning in the context of medical practice. Such ethical expression has a universal attraction for human beings regardless of their basic moral beliefs.

Chapter 8 revisits the four principles of principlism in light of the covenantal ethical framework just presented. The first section contrasts principlism and covenantal ethics, highlighting the key critical voices of Pellegrino and William F. May from Roman Catholic and Reformed Protestant traditions, respectively. While Pellegrino tries to rework the principles in terms of appropriate moral weight from a virtue ethics perspective, May develops a covenantal ethic beyond Ramsey's initial concepts, describing the covenantal relationship as a gratuitous, growing edge that goes beyond the planned, self-interested limits of a contractual relationship. In breaking with more authoritarian or paternalistic relational models, the notion of a physician as a contractor has its attractions. These include legalizing relationships, encouraging collaboration, promoting self-interest, and advocating full respect for the dignity of patients.[11] However, May's concept of patient autonomy is defined within the relational context, its responsibility and accountability being within the relational matrix of medical practice. In short, in going beyond a contractual model, a covenantal relationship can be transformational by probing into and addressing a patient's deeper needs.[12]

9. Bavinck, *Reformed Dogmatics*, 554–55; Novak, *Human Person*, 48.

10. Dooyeweerd, *New Critique*, vol. 3, 157–781; Chaplin, *Herman Dooyeweerd*, 5–138.

11. May, "Code, Covenant," 33.

12. May, *Physician's Covenant*, 119–20; May, *Testing the Medical Covenant*, 68–70.

In common-morality language, according to Beauchamp and Childress, there are private moralities with distinct basic religious beliefs that lie outside of the common morality; yet these must be compatible with the latter in order to be considered part of a global moral enterprise. However, the argument is made in chapter 8 that the common morality is itself just another private morality. Its claim to "common" status is based on the hope that it will gain the voluntary moral agreement of a majority of morally serious persons by means of minimal moral claims and requirements. In this context, the claim is made and argued that the addition of nonmaleficence as a principle distinct from beneficence (a distinction not made in the Belmont Report) is an attempt by Beauchamp and Childress to gather supporters of the common morality. They argue that adherents to the common morality cannot be expected to show beneficence beyond their own personal desires. Furthermore, since an upper limit of beneficent expectation cannot be readily established, the addition of a distinct principle of nonmaleficence formally allows for a lower limit of beneficent expectation that is reduced simply to the phrase "doing no harm." This is not a biblical understanding of beneficent expectations toward fellow human beings and is incompatible with covenantal love within a covenantal ethical framework grounded in the Word of God.

In a biblical covenantal ethical framework, autonomy is not the dominant principle expressed in the cultural setting of western individualism. Individuals are important, but personhood is only meaningful in the context of relationships with God, other human beings, and the created reality in which we live. Personal accountability to God defines the importance of the individual; one's community or church gives comfort and support in life, but ultimately each person is accountable to God for living obediently or disobediently to the covenantal obligations laid out in the new covenant, that made possible by the death and resurrection of Christ. Pellegrino repudiates the dominance of autonomy and, along with Oliver O'Donovan, declares the love-command of God to be the overarching principle that guides the normative role of other principles in situations. However, Pellegrino's Thomistic elevation of rationality is challenged by O'Donovan's caution that the rationalist tradition tends to move toward a reductive immanentism and premature eschatological fulfillment.

As the exception, Robert Veatch (*Theory of Medical Ethics*, 118–21) considers covenant to be a subtype of contract, exposing the contractual nature of the humanly constructed relationships in his triple contract theory.

Introduction

From the perspective of a covenantal ethic, autonomy is a false autonomy unless considered in a relational context. As Charles Taylor notes, suffering is minimized, even reviled, in modern notions of autonomy. By contrast, the biblical notion of suffering is that of an accepted if not a necessary expression of the human condition under sin. Suffering provides learning and fosters patience and perseverance while Christians wait for the perfect renewal of this world promised at Christ's return. The inherent power struggle between empowered caregivers and the vulnerable needy that characterizes the contemporary notion of autonomy instead becomes caring concern for healing and comfort.

For Pellegrino, beneficence as care is at the core of his philosophy of medicine and should replace autonomy as the most dominant of the four principles. He also calls this beneficence-in-trust. However, like the other three principles, beneficence is given meaning in specific situations through the oversight of love. Still, Pellegrino's distinction between beneficence and love is not always clear; for example, he applies the term *ordering principle* to beneficence in some contexts while applying it to love in others. Looked at within a biblical covenantal ethic, beneficence can be understood as a normative aspect of the created order when understood as the qualifying ethical aspect of medicine within Dooyeweerd's Christian social philosophy. Love is understood as the core element for relating to the whole of created reality, and thus it takes on a philosophical and cosmic dimension. Nonmaleficence, on the other hand, has no status as a moral principle within a covenantal ethic. To do no harm is an empty default that has negative, codal connotations. Providing active assistance at some risk to the benefactor, on the other hand, has a positive, covenantal meaning. To act with nonmaleficence but without beneficence rings hollow, given a biblical covenantal idea of human relating and interhuman obligation. Expressions of beneficence in a covenantal ethic, such as care for the unborn and for the incapacitated, exemplify a concept of personhood wherein all human beings, regardless of capability, have moral worth and dignity by virtue of their created status as image-bearers of God.

Beauchamp and Childress promote the principle of justice by means of a qualified egalitarianism in which unequal treatment may be considered in the interest of serving those in greater need than others. This egalitarianism prompts them to propose a fair system of health care rationing that offers acceptable minimal care to all citizens. However, they avoid recommending solutions to health care injustice, leaving such recommendations to the moral judgments of societal consensus. Unfortunately, in

American society, faith in individualism impedes progress toward sacrifice and selflessness inherent in a covenantal ethical framework of societal justice. In the Christian tradition, justice has many interpretations, and commonly held views are articulated in this chapter. Within a covenantal ethic, the inherent rights of human beings are grounded in our ontic status as image-bearers of God *and* by virtue of our relationship with God. In a covenantal ethical framework, justice demands prioritizing need into discrete levels and fully informing patients in such levels of need why they may or may not receive care at a particular time.

A biblical covenantal ethical framework provides a common thread of human relational aspiration in an imperfect world distorted by self-interest. Once the delusion of the common morality is exposed as simply another private morality whose moral authority rests on the shaky ground of the facility to reason, a covenantal ethic rooted in the relation with transcendent God, established at the creation of the cosmos, takes on deep meaning. It acknowledges the human yearning for human companionship based on trust and support rather than on self-preservation and legal security.

I would like to add one final note regarding the use of several key terms. Throughout this book, I will concentrate on *biomedical ethics*, a subdiscipline of *bioethics*.[13] Environmental ethics and other areas subsumed under bioethics will not be discussed. As well, the term *principle* will be used extensively. It is derived from the Latin word *principium* (a beginning or starting place), meaning a statement that takes primacy in a discourse. Its meaning and use have varied among prominent bioethicists. Ramsey often uses it in the same context as moral rules. As the core of various ethical frameworks, principles are often considered generalizations that aid in incorporating details of a problem into a thought process and/or in relating those details back to a fundamental belief. Albert Jonsen likens principles to hooks on a lattice.[14] "At the highest level," he argues, principles have equal importance, but when applied to circumstances, "the circumstances, the facts of the case, are weighed in the balance or scales of the principles."[15] In my view, such principles are more analogous to the lattice itself, given that without them a principles-based ethical framework would collapse.

---

13. The term *bioethics* was reportedly first coined in 1970 by Van Rensselaer Potter, a biochemist whose 1971 book *Bioethics: Bridge to the Future* introduced ethical concerns in the area of environmental conservation and stewardship.

14. Jonsen, "Clinical Ethics," 16.

15. Ibid., 20.

Part One

The Rise and Dominance of Principles-Based Biomedical Ethics

1

The Rise of Principlism in Response to an Ethical Crisis

My conscience is clear, but that does not make me innocent. It is the Lord who judges me. Therefore, judge nothing before the appointed time; wait till the Lord comes. He will bring to light what is hidden in darkness and will expose the motive of people's hearts. At that time, each will receive his praise from God.

—1 Cor 4:4–5 (Today's NIV)

HISTORICAL BACKDROP TO PRINCIPLISM

Development of Natural Law, Casuistry, and Moral Certainty

To understand the philosophical and worldview roots of principlism, it is important to understand a few highlights of the history of ethics that have influenced bioethical thinking and practice. In early medieval times, neither systematic ethics nor formal ethical theory existed. Ethics was taught by clergy, particularly monks who taught using stories about the virtues and actions of saints. Sources of ethical authority included Scripture, the patristic writings, and Latin fragments of classical texts.

By the thirteenth century, ethics had become entrenched in the discipline of rhetoric, as practiced within the new universities arising throughout Europe. As such, scholars such as Roger Bacon and Abelard systematized ethical concepts, bringing together church teachings and pagan traditions. Bacon attempted to merge, on the one hand, Aristotle's ideas of virtues, gleaned in part from the latter's *Nicomachean Ethics* ("rediscovered" in 1245) and Stoic teachings with, on the other hand, Christian doctrine and Scriptural interpretations of the day.[1]

In the same period, some scholars began to consider the post-Fall vestigial remnant of humanity's moral law. For many, natural law represented simple obligations to do no harm while also actively doing good for others. Over time, ethicists—and, later, bioethicists of various faith persuasions—looked to natural law as a justification for moral decisions. Noting that the scholastic concept of natural law was formulated from Scripture, reason, and nature, Jean Porter agrees with Richard Horsley regarding the significance of Stoic influence on the medieval scholastic idea of natural law, particularly the influence of Cicero and the Roman jurists under Justinian. For Stoics, humanity is under one universal law of justice within a single commonwealth.[2] In stark departure from Aristotle, the natural equality of all persons manifests as an equal capacity to practice virtue, providing a basis for egalitarian arguments for common-morality theory today.[3] To these Stoic concepts was added the notion of a transcendent deity as divine legislator. With reason and nature grounded in, and reflective of, a transcendent reality, the law of nature could be understood as an expression of the will of a divine legislator.[4]

Porter points out that theologians of the scholastic period understand natural law as precepts. For them, moral discernment derives its strength from fundamental norms, basic principles, or axioms of natural law that are starting points for rendering moral judgments. The canon lawyers, on the other hand, see natural law as a capacity for judgment. Neither group understands natural law as specific moral rules but neither do they clarify the relationship between these precepts (principles) and the capacity to make judgments and specific moral rules.[5]

Thomas Aquinas tries to link these concepts by relating Jesus's summary of the law with the Ten Commandments. For Aquinas, the overarching

---

1. Jonsen and Toulmin, *Abuse of Casuistry*, 123–24, 130.

2. Horsley, "Law of Nature," 39; Colish, *Stoicism*, 358–59. The Roman jurist Ulpian broke with the Stoics in that the Stoics distanced human rational behavior, and with it morality, from animal behavior, while Ulpian taught that the law of nature was common to human beings and all animals. In so doing, he ensured that reason itself was not the basis of the concept of natural law.

3. Porter, *Natural and Divine Law*, 68.

4. Ibid., 69.

5. Ibid., 90–91.

The Rise of Principlism in Response to an Ethical Crisis

commands to love God and neighbor that summarize the Decalogue are self-evident principles of natural law knowable to all persons, requiring some reflection of which all humans are capable.[6] He proposes natural law to be the form of "general processes" by which all creatures participate in God's eternal law. However, only human beings as rational creatures can follow natural law rationally and virtuously.[7] Acknowledging conflicting interpretations of the relative importance of reason among scholastic thinkers, Porter suggests that their idea of reason is neither the autonomous, self-legislating practical reason of Kant nor equivalent to a newer formulation of natural law.[8] Aquinas, himself, identifies a first principle of practical reason: that is, pursing good and avoiding evil. However, how he assigns self-evident principles is not always clear. In some of his writings, practical reason is self-evident and the most fundamental precept of natural law, whereas in other writings, Jesus's summary of the law is called a self-evident principle.[9]

For Aquinas, principles derived from primary principles of natural law are natural inclinations, expressed during moral deliberations and decisions, directed toward the moral good. They may also become evident from common conclusions derived from first principles. Other principles arise as human persons move toward their proper end; for the Christian, this is death, followed by the final judgment day. Either way, principle-associated obligations may fail to apply or be adhered to in unusual situations, due to unrevealed or unappreciated aspects of a situation "deformed by passion or poor education or poor habits."[10]

Casuistry arose in the medieval period out of established traditions regarding rabbinic Judaism and early Christian decision-making. According to Jonsen and Toulmin, the moral challenges and perceived moral paradoxes of some of Jesus' ethical teachings promote casuistic methods

---

6. Ibid., 92.

7. Ibid., 163–64. Aquinas suggests here that, while all creatures participate in some way in God's eternal law, human beings uniquely do so by way of reason and virtue.

8. Ibid., 68, and George, "Natural Law Ethics," 460–65.

9. Porter, *Natural and Divine Law*, 92–93; Jonsen and Toulmin, *Abuse of Casuistry*, 126. As I will show in chapter 3, this provides justification for Edmund Pellegrino's claim that the principle of beneficence, expressed as care, is at the core of medical practice. It is interesting that for Aquinas, "do no harm" and "doing good for others" are one principle, implying that to "do no harm" alone has no moral meaning. However, the inclination to do good that is provided by natural law requires virtue in order to act on such inclinations.

10. Jonsen and Toulmin, *Abuse of Casuistry*, 126.

PART ONE: The Rise and Dominance of Principles-Based Biomedical Ethics

that were later developed and practiced in the church.[11] For instance, Jesus teaches using various methods, including reinterpretations of familiar rules or laws in order to teach moral behavior beyond the letter of the law. In Acts and 1 Corinthians, situations arise among Christians that require reflection on previous practices, teachings, and laws, all of which may be interpreted differently in light of particular situations. Ultimately, decisions are made and carried out after an invocation for assistance from the Holy Spirit. For example, in Acts 15, a problem arises regarding the observance by Gentile converts of Judaic rituals and moral obligations. In 1 Corinthians 8, 10, and 11, the church debates what constitutes appropriate associations with pagans. After the apostolic period, church authorities wrote about specific cases that they were asked to adjudicate. After the persecutions under emperor Dacia (c. 250), Cyprian published a treatise concerning cases of Christians who chose to renounce their faith rather than flee to avoid persecution. From Clement of Alexandria onward, numerous attempts were made to apply Stoic teachings to Christian ethics.[12] In light of these challenges in the early church, means for interpreting Scripture were sought to better understand the wishes of the Holy Spirit in specific situations of uncertainly.

In the struggle to put concepts of the Holy Trinity into humanly understandable terms, the concept of personhood evolved. The Western, Latin-speaking church spoke of *persona* through its known association with ancient theatre and law courts, while the eastern, Greek-speaking church understood personhood as *hypostatis*, a substantive reality underlying all expressed qualities and characteristics. Personhood attains a rationalistic flavor already with Boethius in the early sixth century and later, more substantively, with the Enlightenment philosophers.[13] After Boethius, there appears to be greater concern for the relationship of the individual person to God. Books appear that give advice to clergy and laypersons regarding appropriate penance for confessed sins. While these initial *Penitentials* are mainly lists of transgressions and appropriate penitent responses, later works are more nuanced in their understanding of expressions of sinful actions. For instance, degrees of seriousness and punishment are translated into monetary penalties or contributions to the church.[14]

11. Ibid., 91–92.
12. Ibid., 93–95.
13. O'Donovan, *Begotten or Made?*, 52–59; O'Donovan, *Resurrection and Moral Order*, 237–39; Rusthoven, "Are Human Embryos."
14. Jonsen and Toulmin, *Abuse of Casuistry*, 99.

The Rise of Principlism in Response to an Ethical Crisis

Because of the more systematic understanding of natural law under Albert the Great and Thomas Aquinas, casuistic practices become formalized and are accepted as normative methods for addressing individual cases of repentance and penance. In addition, conscience becomes a primary defense for using casuistry in moral deliberation. In Romans 2:16, Paul talks about the consciences of unbelievers bearing witness to the law and about their conflicting thoughts accusing and excusing them. Later, St. Jerome considers the conscience to be the fourth part of the soul, while *synderesis* refers to the spark of the conscience that is dominant over the other three parts of the Platonic soul (the rational, emotional, and appetitive). By the thirteenth century, Philip the Chancellor distinguishes *conscientia* from *synderesis* in Jerome's texts. Here, *synderesis* refers to the power of perfect discernment that cannot err, while *conscientia* is associated with free choice. This link allows for the possibility for *conscientia* to err and provides the basis of the medieval doctrine of conscience.[15]

With Aquinas, *synderesis* becomes synonymous with the intellect's grasp of the first principles of practical reason; it is considered "a natural disposition concerned with the basic principles of behavior, which are the general principles of natural law."[16] Alternatively, *conscientia* can determine what needs to be done in a particular situation but can also reflect back and test whether the action was done rightly, thus allowing error in judgment to be recognized. Using the justification of *conscientia*, Aquinas could excuse a sinful error based on ignorance of the situation. While prudence is taken up as a key virtue by Albert the Great, it is further developed by Aquinas as correct reasoning about what ought to be done. Thus, according to Aquinas, prudent, circumspective reflection of circumstances leads to the selection of good and evil human action possibilities.[17]

During the time of high casuistry, another method of moral deliberation develops that tries to justify moral choice on the basis of *probable certitude*. Promoted initially by Bartholomew Medina, a Dominican theologian from Salamanca, Spain, moral probablism teaches that opinions or decisions could be acceptable if considered probable, even if another opinion or decision is more probable.[18] Traditionally, it had been considered sinful to act while in doubt, so resolution might be sought through investigation, prayer, and recourse to wise and prudent experts and advisors.

---

15. Ibid., 127–28.
16. Aquinas, *Quaestiones Disputatae de Veritate*, Qq. 16–17, 122–36.
17. Jonsen and Toulmin, *Abuse of Casuistry*, 131.
18. Jones, *Soul and the Embryo*, 188–91.

Part One: The Rise and Dominance of Principles-Based Biomedical Ethics

A distinction is also made between doubt and opinion; opinion constitutes probable certitude, usually, but not always, leading to truth. By the sixteenth century, this distinction becomes less clear; "probable" connotes plausibility or possible truth. Therefore, according to this way of thinking, a point of view or opinion with any degree of probable or possible doubt becomes acceptable.[19] In the seventeenth century, Blaise Pascal leads a scathing critique of this relativistic tendency in moral deliberation. Pascal wanted certainty, and he objected strongly to the moral skepticism that resulted from nearly any opinion being considered as good as another.[20]

This blending of a conscience-directed, prudentially contextualized natural law with casuistic thinking became the historical and conceptual footing for contemporary bioethical deliberative method, albeit detached from its transcendental, presuppositional foundations. Such thinking foreshadows the postmodern, minimalist thinking of contemporary moral ethics and bioethics, given that it accepts views as morally valid that have any hint of leading to a morally acceptable position, even if the likelihood is low. Such an approach lacks guidance with regard to justifying a choice between a number of more-or-less probable opinions. In short, if there is no obligation to reject one action over another, either one could be judged acceptable. In the next section, I will show how natural law and casuistry have been transformed in secular circles, being stripped of their traditional teleological connection with God as the good toward which all decisions are directed. Their influence on contemporary biomedical ethics is reflected in the minimalist, common-morality basis of principlism.

Contemporary bioethics has developed from these moral traditions, but the struggle for moral certainty has played out in the clash between foundationalism and its detractors. The natural law tradition sees principles or precepts on several levels; some are immutable and self-evident, such as the principle to avoid evil and to do good. Principles derived from first, self-evident principles are subject to error, due to unrevealed or unappreciated aspects of a situation that might be deformed by passion, poor education, or poor habits.[21] Casuistry, though traditionally focused on the particulars of a given situation, looks to the natural law idea to provide justification for choosing one opinion or view over another when both were deemed possibly feasible or not without doubt.

19. Ibid., By concentrating on law and liberty of conscience, probablism drifted toward laxism, wherein virtually all views could be acceptable as truth on the slimmest of evidence.

20. Pascal, *Provincial Letters*, 81 (letter 5).

21. Jonsen and Toulmin, *Abuse of Casuistry*, 126.

Foundationalism, Anti-Foundationalism, and the Concept of Truth

By the early 1970s, these aspects of moral deliberation and decision-making intensified by means of the struggle between foundationalism and anti-foundationalism. Foundationalism in its classical sense holds that some propositions are properly basic or *self*-evident, while others can be rationally accepted only on the basis of evidence.[22] For the foundationalist, human beings conform to norms, duties, or obligations through being and acting rationally. These are derived from *noetic structures*, defined as a set of propositions that are beliefs and epistemic relations involving the knower and these propositions. Some of these beliefs are basic; others are based on prior beliefs. Within noetic structures are degrees of belief wherein some beliefs may be alterable and revisable based on additional evidence.

Alvin Plantinga argues that the concept of self-evidence is often presented as a visual metaphor, with an epistemic and a phenomenological component.[23] For instance, Aquinas holds a proposition to be basic if it is self-evident or evidenced by the senses.[24] However, Plantinga shows that properly basic beliefs, such as belief in the existence of God, do not require the criteria of classical foundationalism, which include self-evidence or sensory-derived evidence. Drawing support from Herman Bavinck, John Calvin, and Karl Barth, he exposes the fallacy that belief in the existence of God must be established by proofs or arguments, a position taken by Aquinas and Scotus and, later, Descartes and Leibniz.[25] Rather, belief in God can be grounded in observational circumstances that justify belief in God's existence.[26] Everyone, Plantinga argues persuasively, has a tendency to apprehend God's existence and something of his nature. This belief is as much one of the "deliverances of reason" and a "part of our natural noetic equipment" as are other beliefs, such as truths of the past and truths about other minds.[27]

As a reaction to foundationalism, antifoundationalism denies absolutely secure insights that ground our knowledge. Instead, all that we

---

22. Plantinga, "Reason and Belief," 48.
23. Ibid., 57.
24. Ibid., 55–58.
25. Ibid., 64.
26. Ibid., 78–82.
27. Ibid., 89–90.

Part One: The Rise and Dominance of Principles-Based Biomedical Ethics

can know comes from purely subjective, contingent experience.[28] Sissela Bok critiques "the scatter shot" manner of antifoundationalist critique and its habit of making Nietzschean-style leaps, from the denial of divinely ordained moral laws or values to the conclusion that there are, thus, no secure foundations for morality. Bok blames this in large part on the tendency to define "foundation" as an unequivocal, rock-bottom basis of justification, which she traces to a misinterpretation of the foundation metaphor of John Locke. Locke tries to convey through this metaphor the prevalent problem of finding some support for all qualities that we find in reality. Denis Diderot reapplies this metaphor to connote the uselessness of a hypothesis that tries to explain incomprehensible aspects of nature by way of the concept of a similarly incomprehensible deity.[29]

Nonetheless, Bok seems empathetic to antifoundationalist attempts to invalidate absolutist claims of religious groups that are based on a divine origin of morality. She feels that such claims are unfair to those with less firm convictions. She suggests an approach to morality that does not discard the concept of foundations ("with all of its metaphorical baggage") but that prefers a broader concept of *grounds*.[30] Bok favors exploring some basis of common moral ground that would foster dialogue, debate, and accommodation more than she does striving for absolute certainty. Her minimalist, common-morality approach rests on the need to survive, a motive that drives communities to work out mechanisms of support and respect through the identification of minimal basic values and common ground for moral discourse.[31]

A recent exchange between Richard Rorty, Alvin Plantinga, and Nicholas Wolterstorff highlights the main antagonists in this debate, the core of which involves a debate over the concept of truth. Discussing the perceived role of religious belief in the work of academia, these scholars discuss matters relating to the invalidity of foundationalism and current efforts to find common ground for addressing ethical questions. On the importance of rationality in forming the basis of primary belief, all three agree that persons with either religious or non-religious core beliefs can be *fully rational* in maintaining those beliefs. Furthermore, Wolterstorff and Rorty agree that classical liberalism is mistaken in assuming that only reason can present a body of moral truths that would provide an operative

---

28. Bok, *Common Values*, 69.
29. Ibid., 72–73.
30. Ibid., 74.
31. Ibid., 79–80.

The Rise of Principlism in Response to an Ethical Crisis

framework for polity and economy. As an atheist, Rorty limits the designation "religious" to indicate belief in a non-human power. Denying such power, he considers it more courageous to "rely on ourselves, on *our group efforts*" than on a non-human power.[32] Rorty's inferences point toward a need for consensus as the basis of truth; however, Plantinga follows by challenging Rorty's statement that truth is what one's peers allow one to get away with. Rorty's atheistic moral equivalent of religion is a utopian dream that social hope can be achieved by all in a globally prosperous, democratic, and tolerant human community.[33]

Thus far in this section, I have highlighted the historical development of themes and methods of moral reflection that are important for a robust critique of the basic roots of principlism. The contemporary exchange of basic ideas of truth and moral certitude between Rorty, Plantinga, and Wolterstorff is rooted in that history. Wolterstorff notes that he and Rorty both oppose foundationalism and liberalism, but Rorty does so based on a philosophical stance of *coherentist* anti-realism, while Wolterstorff adheres to a realist approach.[34] The latter's concept of moral truth is realized in God's revelation through creation and Scripture. It is contextualized within, and has influence on, culture and history but is not solely contingent on them. Rorty's approach is grounded in faith in rational consensus through culturally conditioned moral truth that is self-evident. Such a consensus-driven, coherentist pursuit of culturally and historically contingent common moral values is at the core of principlism today.

Search for a Common Ethical Framework

Another important conceptual dilemma in principlism, and in biomedical ethics in general, is the development of a dialectic tendency to pit theories and principles against the particulars of cases and situation. This dialectic is often played out in the distinction between *applied* and *theoretical* ethics. Robert Holmes approaches this issue by reflecting on recent claims concerning the nature of moral philosophy in bioethics. He draws a parallel between the contemporary search for practical value in analytical bioethical thought and Aristotle's criticism of his mentor Plato's account of the good having little impact on moral conduct. Through this analogy, Holmes

---

32. Louthan, "On Religion," 179 (emphasis mine).

33. Such hope could be interpreted as an eschatological substitute for an elusive common morality.

34. Louthan, "On Religion," 183.

Part One: The Rise and Dominance of Principles-Based Biomedical Ethics

describes the shift away from metaethics, which addresses theories of the nature, concepts, and analyses of moral judgments, among contemporary philosophers when addressing practical ethical problems. In the early part of the twentieth century, G. E. Moore convinced many ethicists that metaethical problems needed to be addressed and adequately resolved before work could move forward in normative and applied ethics. As bioethics developed, however, such top-down approaches were replaced by greater attention to the preeminence of the particulars in bioethical problems.[35] This methodologic dialectic is an expression of the struggle over the relative importance of metaethics, normative ethics, and applied ethics.

There is now a conventional acceptance that moral judgments can be adequately made without metaethical expertise, with less concern about what justifies calling any decision and action "right." The nature of metaethical discussions has shifted to concerns about proper methods for analyzing moral dilemmas, at times questioning whether or not these dilemmas are simply false, thus requiring no solutions! However, some philosophers, such as Richard M. Hare, continue to advocate for metaethical reflection in the form of a *principle of universalizability*.[36] Such a principle would justify the relevance of particular moral judgments over others by ensuring that moral judgments are consistently made across similar situations.

Holmes tries to show the circular process that occurs when trying to apply normative theories to specific problems. Without metaethical justification, one may choose a normative theory, such as deontological or utilitarian theory, simply to suit desired solutions for particular problems and to provide a consistency of judgments within one's preferred normative theory. He uses the example of a person who is pro-choice but holds a Kantian belief that persons should be treated as ends rather than means. While Kant might conclude that abortion is morally unacceptable, a pro-choice Kantian might justify abortion by the belief that, while a fetus should be treated as an end, in the final analysis it is simply not a person.

Preoccupation with analytical method and process has thus become the focus of much bioethical decision-making. However, Holmes shows that attempts to construct so-called *neutral* analyses still lead to problems when applying theories to practice. In cases in which principles or theories that apply to apparently similar cases do not fit a particular circumstance,

---

35. Holmes, "Limited Relevance," 144.

36. Ibid., 147–48. The reader should note from above that Childress discusses this as a formal principle in his contributions to the Belmont Commission deliberations.

moral correctness independent of principles or theories must come from within the character of the act itself.[37] Thus, Holmes acknowledges that personal moral beliefs may affect our bioethical decisions more than absolutist adherence to a particular theory. He proposes that the cultivation of moral character is more important than analytical skills and should be developed to give validity to the use of philosophical analysis.[38]

Holmes exposes the tension inherent in the failure to ground normative ethical theory within concepts of right and good. In an effort to avoid this decision-making dialectic, he turns instead to a care ethic that redirects the focus from moral decision-making to the welfare of the patient. However, in my view this fails to escape the dialectic. The same moral issues arise, thus requiring the same moral justification for decisions of care, such as moral identity, end-of-life decisions, normative caregiver-patient relationships, etc. What is lacking is authoritative moral grounding for moral positions beyond rationality alone.

Loretta Kopelman has analyzed whether or not applied ethics can be considered derivative of ethical theories. She takes the anti-foundationalist position that theories or previously considered judgments are not *epistemically privileged*—that is, they do not resist change as a result of their application to particular cases. Kopelman challenges those who claim that ethical principles are normative and self-justifying (or known by intuition) because they have nonempirical and independent properties.[39] She notes that agreement among informed persons of goodwill is more likely if moral theories have epistemically privileged foundations in principles. Intuitionism, she argues, does not help us to determine *why* principles might motivate us to use them as guides for moral action rather than as statements ascribing properties to things. However, a weaker version of intuitionism allows for revision of what we believe to be self-evident principles based on new scientific revelations or discoveries, and this possibility of revision undermines this version's status as epistemically privileged. Kopelman concludes that principles are not epistemically privileged and, therefore, that applied fields are not considered to be derived from them.[40]

37. Ibid., 156.

38. Ibid., 157.

39. Kopelman, "What is Applied," 202–3. W. D. Ross states that principles of common morality are recognized by intuitive induction. For Beauchamp and Childress, two or more nonabsolute principles form a set of moral norms agreed upon by all morally serious persons. Thus, the common morality is a morality by consensus.

40. Kopelman ("What is Applied," 204–18) goes on to show that specific judgments and moral theories also fail the test of epistemic privilege, thereby debunking foundationalism.

Part One: The Rise and Dominance of Principles-Based Biomedical Ethics

Holmes and Kopelman expose major insufficiencies in contemporary bioethical thinking. Holmes shows the "willy-nilly" nature of choosing theories to fit the situation and acknowledges the importance of personal moral belief. Nevertheless, he cannot find the grounding he seeks through care ethics because it also rests on a theory that lacks presuppositional and morally authoritative grounding. Like Rorty and Wolterstorff, Kopelman rejects foundationalism while also showing the groundless nature of intuitionism. However, neither Holmes nor Kopelman offers a normative alternative. Both fail to show the importance of pretheoretical beliefs as directional starting points from which theorizing and resultant theories can be justified and subsequently applied. They lack the recognition that control beliefs discern the theories that are compatible with their presuppositional beliefs, the latter being religious in nature.[41] Theory, and acting based on theory are real aspects of bioethics. Both reflect created structures of reality whose normative appreciation can only be fully understood and acted upon when biblically directed. In chapter 7, I will re-examine theorizing and acting in medicine in light of a Christian philosophical understanding of social relationships for medical practice.

If applied fields such as bioethics are not formally and derivatively linked to principles or background theories, how can moral decisions be justified in bioethics? Ronald M. Green provides an excellent analysis of foundations and methods of moral deliberation, starting with acknowledging the contemporary preoccupation with methods of bioethical deliberation and decision-making. Influential bioethical scholars such as Edmund Pellegrino, Robert Veatch, LeRoy Walters, Beauchamp, and Childress have advocated for the application of general theories or principles to specific cases or problems in medicine and biological research.[42] Green responds to three possible disclaimers to the view that biomedical ethics is a form of applied ethics aligned with moral philosophy. These include counter-

---

41. Wolterstorff, *Until Justice and Peace Embrace*, 69–75ff. Wolterstorff argues that Christian scholars should devise and weigh the importance of theories on the basis of control beliefs and religious beliefs ought to function as control beliefs. Such beliefs help Christian scholars to devise theories as well as to reject or accept existing theories based on what it is important to have theories about. Such control beliefs should reflect the belief content of their authentic Christian commitment regarding how Christ-following ought to be actualized.

42. Green, "Method in Bioethics," 180–81; Clouser, "Bioethics," 116. Clouser argues that bioethical principles as defined by Beauchamp and Childress are not theoretical foundations for biomedical ethics. However, he argues that historical theories of ethics are sufficient to deal with bioethical concerns, "peculiar in its realm of concerns" as such concerns may be.

claims that 1) bioethics cannot be truly aligned with moral philosophy because it is multidisciplinary, and thus multiple methods of analysis are employed, 2) religious beliefs act as confounders in public bioethical discourse, and 3) the growing interdisciplinary complexity and novel nature of many new questions require a new kind of ethics to accommodate these developments.

He responds that ethics and moral philosophy act as the indispensable foci of bioethical inquiry regardless of the nature of the underlying field of investigation.[43] Also, agreeing with Clouser, Green does not believe that a new ethics with new principles or foundations is evolving or is needed. Rather, there should be more effort "to squeeze out all the relevant implications from the ones it already has."[44] Finally, he believes that religious beliefs do influence moral positions. However, when expressed outside of the moral communities from which they originate, proponents may not articulate their religious reasons.[45] Such reservation of expression may be due to fear of being unpersuasive to those not sharing such a perspective or of being discounted altogether.[46] Other proponents from faith-based communities believe that basic conceptual and ethical issues beyond particular religious communities should be the basis of reasoned ethical analysis in a pluralistic society.[47]

However, Green is more concerned with a tendency in bioethics toward the identification and rote application of principles and concepts that drifts away from ongoing, self-critical testing of its theoretical foundations.[48] He particularly bemoans contemporary attention to the identification and application of moral principles at the explicit exclusion of "the essential work of deriving basis, meaning, and scope of these principles."[49] Cited as an exception, Robert Veatch is lauded for his attempt to develop a new theory of medical ethics. In his theory, greater theoretical consider-

---

43. Green, "Method in Bioethics," 182.

44. Clouser, "Bioethics," 124–27.

45. This position must be distinguished from one that does not permit moral or political views to be accepted if articulated using religious reasons, particularly for policy decision-making. Such a view is promoted by Jürgen Habermas (*Between Naturalism and Religion*, 130–35), whose philosophical influence on principlism and Christian critiques to such a position is further discussed in chapter 4.

46. Ibid., 183–84; Gustafson, *Contributions of Theology*. Green draws support from James Gustafson for this point.

47. Spicker and Engelhardt, *Philosophical Medical Ethics*, 5.

48. Green, "Method in Bioethics," 186.

49. Ibid., 190.

ation is directed to foundational issues than in the approach of identifying and applying principles championed by Beauchamp and Childress.[50] As such, Veatch constructs a social contract theory that he hopes can form a common community of moral discourse, particularly among those who doubt that a universal basis for moral decision-making can be discovered.[51] Green compliments Veatch for his theoretical engagement, his development of a theory of ethics from the ground up, and his skill at adjudicating ethical conflicts with principles derived from that theory.

However, Green qualifies this enthusiasm by expressing his disappointment in Veatch's lapses into intuitionism. The latter considers moral preferences to be intuitively or self-evidently acceptable choices in specific situations, rather than focusing on developing specifications and justifications for appropriate constraints within a contractual arrangement. Indeed, Green is highly critical of "the almost deliberate avoidance of deep engagement with basic theoretical issues in ethical theory."[52] Others, like L. W. Sumner, criticize Veatch's contention that people with very different moral foundational beliefs will usually converge through dialogue toward substantive agreement on principles.[53] This process, promoted by Beauchamp and Childress, starts with rational reflection. This leads to a reflective equilibrium of moral agreement by way of the cohesion of initially diverse concepts. Such concepts, in turn, are based on previously considered judgments that are agreed-upon, revisable moral convictions.[54]

Green pointedly criticizes Beauchamp and Childress for their conscious decision to relegate metaethics to a secondary role in their ethical framework.[55] He asks: "How . . . when principles are in conflict, is it possible to make progress in normative discussion unless one has at hand some procedure for establishing priorities among principles and how is

50. Beauchamp and Childress, *Principles of Biomedical Ethics*, 5th ed., 12–23; 384–408.

51. Veatch, *Theory of Medical Ethics*, 117–18.

52. Green, "Method in Bioethics," 188.

53. Sumner, "Does Medical Ethics," 38. He also asks why Veatch would go to the trouble of developing an ethical theory that gives no basis for choosing among several options based on certain principles. Sumner is particularly outspoken about his perceived lack of philosophical skill.

54. Beauchamp and Childress, *Principles of Biomedical Ethics*, 5th ed., 398–400.

55. Ibid., 2; Beauchamp and Childress, *Principles of Biomedical Ethics*, 1st ed. In their first edition, they speak of metaethics as the effort to analyze moral reasoning, including the *nature* of moral justification. By their fifth edition they say that metaethics describes terms and characteristics of ethics rather than how ethical decisions are justified.

that procedure defended apart from a more basic understanding of the moral reasoning process?"⁵⁶ Further on he argues "moral analysis cannot be confined to a process of identifying and applying moral principles . . . when the essential work of deriving the basis, meaning, and scope of these principles is left undone."⁵⁷

Green suggests several reasons for this lack of theoretical sophistication and methodological precision, including growing public pressure to develop morally relevant public policy and to take legislative action on rapidly emerging and novel ethical quandaries. This public dimension of bioethics is seen by some as a separate sub-field of bioethics because of certain unique elements. These elements include a greater sense of urgency and social dynamics that influence moral discourse and decision-making.⁵⁸ Green concludes that bioethics at large has adopted an intermediate position between normative ethics and public ethics, resulting in "its disturbing tendency to pass over difficult but vital questions."⁵⁹ He resists calling bioethics an applied ethics and insists on a continued conversation between moral theory and applied ethical work.⁶⁰

I agree with Green's refusal to disengage bioethics from in-depth reflection on the presuppositional grounding of principles and moral decisions. However, it is disappointing that his excellent critique is not followed by an ethical framework that incorporates such grounding and justification in deliberations and decisions regarding moral positions and policies.

It is evident from this historical backdrop that principles-based ethics evolved within a struggle concerning the very nature of biomedical ethics. The rich tradition of moral teaching within the Roman Catholic Church gave rise to casuistic reflection but also to a struggle regarding the nature of moral certainty. In more recent times, such uncertainty has taken the shape of a struggle between foundationalism and antifoundationalist sentiments. The reactive and unsystematic reaction of the latter is captured by Bok's insight into "the scatter shot" nature of antifoundationalist critique and its tendency to leap from denying divinely ordained moral laws or values straight to the conclusion that there are no secure

---

56. Green, "Method in Bioethics," 189.

57. Ibid., 190.

58. Jonsen and Butler, "Public Ethics," 22–24; Callahan, "Emergence of Bioethics," xxvi–xxvii.

59. Green "Method in Bioethics," 190.

60. Ibid., 191.

Part One: The Rise and Dominance of Principles-Based Biomedical Ethics

foundations for morality. One might construe this struggle as a variation on the theme of modernism's search for scientific certainly and postmodernism's retort that truth is in the eye and mind of the beholder. At the same time, pressure was mounting in the mid-twentieth century to find practical solutions to growing ethical concerns in light of new biotechnologies, leading to heightened tension between applied or practical ethics and moral philosophy.

It is from this historical backdrop and within a contemporary climate of fierce debate over the fundamental nature of ethics in a rapidly changing biomedical and biotechnological context that principles-based ethics arose and took root.

AN ETHICAL CRISIS IN HUMAN RESEARCH

The Belmont Commission

Through much of the history of biomedical ethics, perceived unethical human interaction created the urgent ethical need out of which principles-based ethics evolved. Post-World War II revelations of the recruitment of human subjects into experiments without consent under the Nazi regime brought increasing attention to the plight of those recruited and subjected to clinical research. The flashpoint of concern came in 1966, when Henry Beecher, a Harvard University anesthetist, published in the prestigious *New England Journal of Medicine* a report on fifty cases of his era containing examples of questionable or outright unethical practices (in his terms "ethical errors") involving human experimentation.[61] Infractions included lack of consent (forty-eight of fifty cases), withholding effective treatment, and failing to stop administering the drug under study in the face of obvious toxicity. Beecher identified striving for informed consent and "the presence of an intelligent, informed, conscientious, compassionate, responsible investigator" as absolute requirements in research involving human subjects.[62] He concluded that the ethical propriety of an experiment should be judged from its inception and should strive for equal or greater anticipated gains than risks from participation in clinical research.

---

61. Beecher, "Ethics and Clinical Research." Twenty-two of the fifty studies were selected for elaboration in the article. He also refers to an additional 186 "further likely" examples of ethical violations.

62. Ibid., 1360.

Ends, he concluded, do not ethically justify means in research involving humans.

Seven years after Beecher's publication, the United States Congress established the National Commission on the Protection of Human Subjects. Its mandate was "to identify *basic ethical principles* that should underlie the conduct of biomedical and behavioral research involving human subjects."[63] Consisting of lawyers, physicians, two biomedical researchers, a civil-rights leader, and two bioethicists, the Commission deliberated monthly for nearly four years.

Identifying these principles proved to be challenging. Kurt Baier, Alasdair MacIntyre, and James Childress were initially consulted, each providing an assessment of different aspects of the problem.[64] In his consultation essay, Baier reviews various contemporary schools of ethics. These include 1) the ethical theories of G. E. Moore and W. D. Ross, founded on judgments that attribute extraordinary ethical *properties* to things, 2) the ethics of R. M. Hare, for whom reason-derived judgments are ethically based on their prescriptive and universalizable characteristics, and 3) the emotivists and prescriptivists, who view ethics as peculiar *functions of expression*, such as the expressive and the evocative (emotivism) or the imperatival, action-guiding functions (prescriptivism).

Baier considers moral reasoning to be practical, not theoretical, in that it is justificatory and normative in nature. Practical moral reasoning looks for reasons why someone should do something and what beliefs are behind specific moral claims. He discounts as implausible any morality that society recognizes as superior to all others; this includes moralities distinguished by embedded religious beliefs. Instead, Baier favors Hare's version of practical reasoning in which certain principles and rules not only override others but are also *universalizable* and *prescriptive*. Baier

---

63. Emphasis added. Ryan et al., *Belmont Report*; Jonsen, *Birth of Bioethics*, 90–98. This Commission was preceded by the Mondale hearings (1968) and the Kennedy hearings (1974). These hearings revealed the diversity of ideas and high emotions regarding biomedical research, exposing further examples of unethical human research while expressing concerns that rigorous ethical constraints could impede scientific progress.

64. Jonsen, *Birth of Bioethics*, 333. The appendices to the Belmont Report include several sections of consultations addressing ethical issues in human research. The authors of the consultations mentioned in this section constitute the majority of contributors to that section, excluding Alvin R. Feinstein and LeRoy Walters. Their contributions did not address the question of so-called "mid-level principles" but rather that of rules that apply to specific aspects of clinical research. As a result, I do not include their papers in this analysis.

notes, however, that this leaves no room for supererogation, which he does not consider universalizable.⁶⁵ Rules are means for "playing the game" (as he calls the process of ethics) for its own sake, not for attaining pre-existing ends. Consequently, he suggests dropping any requirement for Kantian categories within morality. Rather, morality is a societally created, rationally self-correcting moral and social order whose members are morally equal. Moral problems are rationally adjudicated in light of societal mores and laws. Rational egoism is not tolerated if it favors actions that strive toward achieving only one's own best interests (a position with Stoic *eudaimonian* overtones).⁶⁶ Baier considers principles to be valid only if they are associated with equal and adequate reasons to follow them.

Alasdair MacIntyre begins his appraisal of ethical principles by noting several prevalent meanings of the term "moral." He distinguishes two classes of discernment among reasons for moral action. *Expressions of personal preference* are motivated by relationships with others. Their authoritative force is dependent on the context of their spoken expressions. *Evaluative expressions*, on the other hand, are expressions of moral concepts such as "good" and "right" and of virtues such as "generous," "just," or "valid." Evaluative expressions reflect standards of value or authority rather than the attitudes of expressers or listeners.⁶⁷

MacIntyre notes that some moral philosophers, like Hare, see universalizability and/or prescriptiveness as necessary components of moral judgments. Moral rules and principles hold varying levels of status; some are of primary justificatory importance, others are of overriding importance, and still others are content-laden for identifying particular benefits and harms. He shows that moral decisions in our culture are often made using inferences from premises. However, a method for weighing the merits of equally attractive premises is lacking, a problem due largely to *incommensurable* rival premises derived from radically different concepts. For example, in the just-war debate, one position is based on an Aristotelian concept of justice, another on a Machiavellian idea of deterrence and self-interest, and another on a theme of liberation for the poor and oppressed. He links appeals to divergent moral theories and principles with the difficulty of defining morality in general.⁶⁸

---

65. Baier, "Ethical Principles," 3–11.

66. Eudaimonism has its root in ancient Greek philosophical thought and has strong root in contemporary ethical thought.

67. MacIntyre, "How to Identify Ethical Principles," 5–7.

68. Ibid., 10–12.

For MacIntyre, our moral claims are often derived from fragments of moral concepts and systems drawn from philosophical traditions as diverse as those represented by Aristotle and John Locke. His overarching point is that mutually exclusive moral systems can lead to self-evident rights that are rooted in moral contradictions so that attempts to arrive at rational agreement on central issues of morality usually fail.[69] MacIntyre goes on to present the concept of the *good for man* in the classical polis tradition as a rational agreement among community members about what the good of each community should be and how it can be achieved. Virtuous activity is intimately tied to the pursuit of this end. He then contrasts this tradition (within which he includes Christian and Jewish Aristotelians and Platonists) with the modern reliance on the sciences. The latter uses much of the same language as the classical tradition, but the meaning of morality varies according to which of the rival fragments of past moral traditions are believed.

MacIntyre shows that American founding fathers, such as deist Thomas Jefferson, claim to "intuit timeless truths" that protect individuals from interference by others. Thus, the concept of isolated, autonomous individuals disengaged from a polis community became the ideal of contemporary American society. MacIntyre notes that a private-versus-public split in morality is not found in the classical tradition but exists today as a rebirth of the classical tradition alongside modern, rights-based individualism. This in turn leads to very different versions of unethical conduct within the professions, some emphasizing the autonomy of persons and others emphasizing the pursuit of a particular type of good as the *telos* of that profession.

In modern individualism, the idea of human rights becomes a negative, minimalist notion of personal preferences that fills the moral gap left by fragmentation. This notion leads to the alienation of strangers in contemporary society. In ancient Greece, an attitude and expression of hospitality to the stranger outside of the polis existed among members of the polis. By contrast, today societal members are strangers to each other, lacking a sense of community in which a concept of the stranger can draw moral force. In short, to look for commonly agreed-upon, substantive moral principles with firm, justificatory foundations in our morally fragmented cultural setting seems doomed to failure.

---

69. Ibid., 15. For a full discussion of MacIntyre's insights into moral fragmentation in western culture, see MacIntyre, *After Virtue*.

Part One: The Rise and Dominance of Principles-Based Biomedical Ethics

James Childress approaches the problem of principles in a different way.[70] He uses Talcott Parsons's concept of historical differentiation, in which religious beliefs as the common transcendent basis for creating laws and policies are replaced by autonomous institutional ideologies in Western culture.[71] With this backdrop, Childress tries to distinguish moral from amoral reasons and action-guides for decision-making. Drawing from William Frankena, A. D. M. Walker, and Hare, Childress suggests that the formal criteria of morality are prescriptiveness, universalizability, and overriding character that require material content to specify them as moral action-guides.[72]

Childress supports these three formal criteria above, as well as Frankena's "material consideration for others," as collectively necessary and sufficient conditions of morality, but he favors open discourse for accommodating rival moral views rather than any *ultimate authoritativeness*. In claiming a neutral position, he is concerned about accusations of letting the analytical process "do the work" of normative ethics or of choosing sides in a moral debate. However, such neutrality claims ignore the reality that ethical discourse involves reconciling different interests. While he has sympathies with teleological aspects of moral discourse, he favors deontological considerations for purposes of setting limits along the path toward certain ends. As well, while he understands the historical and immediate importance of religion for many in society, he resists associating religious action-guides with supreme or supernatural authoritativeness in an attempt to avoid favoring one religious perspective over another. Instead, he prefers using the concept of *sacredness* as a defining characteristic of religion, appealing to a definition offered by David Little and Sumner Twiss that seems more adaptable, neutral, and less offensive than making reference to specific religions.[73]

In his attempt to rationalize the preservation of the universalizability criterion of morality, Childress reduces religious viewpoints to *qualifiers of morality* that provide different interpretations or evaluative descriptions of the same facts regarding human welfare. Given this, religious interpretations might then infer new derivative duties from basic ones that could be

---

70. Jonsen, *Birth of Bioethics*, 332. Childress is a theologian of Quaker background with an ethical inclination toward rule deontology.

71. Childress, "Identification of Ethical Principles," 2.

72. Ibid., 6–9; Frankena, "Concept of Morality"; Walker and Wallace, "Introduction."

73. Childress, "Identification of Ethical Principles," 26; Little and Twiss, "Basic Terms," 62–67.

The Rise of Principlism in Response to an Ethical Crisis

commonly acknowledged. As a result, universally agreed-upon principles could form the moral core of basic moral agreement as well as of a common moral language for fresh interpretations of different viewpoints. One can see here his early formulation of a common morality from which he claims his subsequent principles-based ethical framework is intuitively and rationally derived.

Childress hopes that excluding supreme moral authority will more likely lead to moral reconciliation and consensus. Such consensus is more likely, he surmises, through ethical discourse and decision-making that incorporates an allegedly neutral, logical analysis. That is, he hopes that providing ground rules for the debate and determining the weight of different reasons offered for justifying specific judgments will replace the need for substantive grounds for moral choices, somehow resulting in commonly agreed-upon judgments. Furthermore, religious beliefs have to be tempered and limited in their contribution to moral deliberation for the sake of moral consensus.[74]

Undaunted by the initial failure to arrive at a consensus with regard to ethical principles, the Belmont Commission consulted three more bioethics scholars, namely Tom Beauchamp, H. Tristram Engelhardt, and LeRoy Walters, to help identify such principles.[75] Contributions of the first two scholars will be discussed here because of their impact on the final report of the Commission. Beauchamp addresses the question of distributive justice, focusing on comparative justice involving competing claims between a person and others when determining what that person deserves. Like Childress, his concept of justice emerges from a framework of formal and material principles; he accepts the Aristotelian principle of formal justice, which declares that equals ought to be treated equally and unequals unequally.[76] He complements this with principles of material justice based on notions of equal sharing, individual need and effort, merit, and societal contribution. Theories of distributive justice spin off from one or more such material principles. The viability of such theories depends on the quality of the moral argument, supporting the premise that one or more associated material principles should be given priority over others.

---

74. Childress, "Identification of Ethical Principles," 33. Much of the foundation of principlism is laid out here.

75. Jonsen, *Birth of Bioethics*, 332.

76. Beauchamp, "Distributive Justice," 4.

Beauchamp argues that properties defining distributive justice are fixed and independent of moral arguments and decisions. Their relevance is determined by basic principles of morality, which he assumes are not arbitrary or changeable by individual preferences.[77] He offers a principle of respect for persons, including human autonomy, as an example, inferring the primacy of this principle. When moral claims and principles conflict, the weight of moral arguments and moral standards of fairness determine what criteria are relevant for a just distribution of resources. He provides no grounds or justification for the determination of material relevance other than the strength of the moral argument (that is, persuasion). In concluding, Beauchamp admits that he does not attempt to work out the "right" theory of distributive justice but rather an ethical framework for understanding the implications of any theory.

Unlike his consulting peers, Engelhardt immediately distinguishes philosophical ethics from theological ethics. The former looks for general principles through a process of *disinterested reflection*. He sees disinterestedness as a regulative ideal from which objective moral judgments can be made. In the context of human experimentation, he focuses on questions regarding the moral agent who deserves respect, and he questions pursuing the path toward desired goods and values.[78]

Engelhardt contends that serious consideration of ethical principles can only be made if all persons undertaking particular moral actions believe in the presuppositions that individuals have a sense of moral responsibility and are free from outside influence. From these assumptions, a moral community is formed, held together by *mutual respect*, which is his first ethical principle regarding human experimentation. His second principle is *support for the best interests of research subjects*. The third is *maximization of societal benefits of participation in research*. This is accomplished by improving human health, maintaining autonomy, increasing knowledge, and satisfying the desire of research subjects to contribute to the larger, common good. By considering duties and the respect of rights, the first principle is deontological. The second and third are more teleological, with their focus on ends such as best interests, goods, and values.

Engelhardt notes that, at that time, these principles appeared in various forms in existing ethical codes, emphasizing that more than one principle may be involved in the same moral question. He suggests that creating procedural maxims can better capture the reality that one human

---

77. Ibid., 6–12.
78. Engelhardt, "Basic Ethical Principles," 1–2.

action may serve more than one purpose. Engelhardt highlights a typology of positions taken by various ethicists based on his principles and procedural maxims. He believes in the potential justification of deception to obtain the most helpful study result but with the assurance of minimal risk to the research subjects. However, he also speaks about coercion as an evil against the freedom of the research subject and consequently against the greater good of society.[79] Engelhardt concludes that basic ethical principles constitute the best attempt to capture and understand the meaning of rights and values for human research subjects.

The Belmont Report: Three Basic Principles

The final report of the commission, the Belmont Report,[80] identifies three basic ethical principles, defined as general judgments "that serve as a basic justification for the many particular ethical prescriptions and evaluations of human actions."[81] These appear to be largely derived from Engelhardt's first two ethical principles—respect for persons and considering the best interest of the research subject (a specific application of beneficence)—as well as Beauchamp's principle of justice. According to the report, these judgments are considered "among those generally accepted in our cultural tradition."[82] The nature of these principles is explained in the report as follows.

Respect for persons incorporates at least two distinct ethical convictions: persons should be treated as autonomous agents, and those with diminished autonomy should be entitled to protection. Disregarding a person's decisions, denying that person the freedom to act on those decisions, and withholding information necessary to make such decisions are considered disrespectful actions. For the physically or cognitively incapacitated and for the developing immature human being, protection from harm should be exercised. This principle addresses the need for informed consent, one of the most pressing ethical issues of that time. The report reflects a backdrop of overriding concern that subjects should be free to

---

79. Engelhardt, *Foundations of Christian Bioethics*. This is particularly interesting given that after his later conversion to the Antiochean Orthodox faith, he provides justification for coercion on confessional grounds. That it, coercion is acceptable or even desired if it leads the coerced individual closer to union with God.

80. Ryan, *Belmont Report*.

81. Ibid., 4.

82. Jonsen, *Birth of Bioethics*, 103.

decide, for their own reasons, whether or not to participate in a research study. *Autonomous choice* is the specific context in which autonomy was conceived under the mandate of the commission.

Beneficence refers to an obligation of helpfulness rather than to its more popular meaning of kindness or charity. Beneficence is further understood as the rule for maximizing the chances of benefits while also minimizing the chances of imposing harm. Specifically, investigators should carefully weigh the likelihood of benefits against that of harm to research subjects during participation in research studies. However, as is the case with respect for persons, when the principle of beneficence is interpreted through different ethical frameworks from which investigators and study subjects derive their basic beliefs and values, the ratio of benefits to risk can vary considerably. Which benefits are more important or carry more weight than others? How does physical harm compare in importance to psychological harm? How do short-term benefits weigh against the risk of long-term harm?

Justice is understood in the sense of what is deserved and what is fair in the distribution of services or resources. The report distinguishes individual versus collective entitlements. It would be unjust, for example, to deny an entitled benefit or to impose a burden for which a good reason could not be provided. Justice is considered a principle of Aristotelian derivations—that is, of equals being treated as equals. Social justice in the clinical research context justly discriminates between which groups of subjects would be most suited for which research studies. Social justice has also been invoked in the debate concerning the ability of teenagers to give truly informed consent independent of parental judgment. Positions have appealed to principles of justice and of respect for persons in the debate.[83]

Justice should also involve fairness in subject selection for research studies. Selection should be made on the basis of subject characteristics or factors directly related to the study question or problem, while exclusion on the basis of gender, race, minority status, etc. requires justification. The commission acknowledged that different interpretations and applications of justice reflect different underlying ethical theories. For example, according to an egalitarian perspective, each person should receive an equal share of commodities or services, whereas a care ethic may support his or

---

83. Harrison et al., "Bioethics for Clinicians," 827–28. See also Levi and Drotar, "Health-related Quality," 58–64.

her distribution more directly according to need. Libertarian perspectives tend to favor distribution on the basis of merit.

ETHICS BEYOND HUMAN RESEARCH: THE FOUR PRINCIPLES AND PRINCIPLISM

Moral Philosophy, Theory, and Situations: Early Tensions

As alluded to earlier, the Belmont Commission and its consulting bioethicists were undoubtedly influenced by the earlier works of Frankena, Jonsen (who served on the commission), and Ross. Ross believes that moral convictions, like sense perceptions in science, are data to be accepted as true or rejected as illusions. He distinguishes right or wrong acts from good or bad character and motivations.[84] His starting point is the moral beliefs of thoughtful, ordinary persons. Ross identifies irreducible moral principles and their associated obligations. These include promises that create obligations of fidelity, expressions of generosity that produce obligations of gratitude, and obligations of reparation for wrongful actions. Other obligations include self-improvement, justice, beneficence, and non-maleficence. Yet, no single overarching ethical principle links these obligations. Rather, Ross considers principles to be the product of *intuitive inductions* implied in previous judgments already rendered on particular acts.[85] He considers the awareness of such principles as knowledge, not just opinion. When obligations conflict and judgments need to be weighed and balanced, the situation must be reflected upon until a *considered opinion* is reached.[86]

Several decades later, Frankena presented an ethical framework based on principles of beneficence and justice.[87] He derived these from David Hume's postulates that beneficence and justice are the two major principles of morality. Hume distinguishes the public point of view of humanity from the private interests or partial judgments of the individual. The former has common language and sentiments and is driven by some universal principle. The latter expresses the language of self-love with person-specific sentiments arising from particular situations. In both cases,

---

84. Ross, *Right and the Good*, 41.
85. Ross, *Foundations of Ethics*, 169–70.
86. Ross, *Right and the Good*, 19. See this influence in the submissions of Beauchamp and Childress to the Belmont Commission noted above.
87. Frankena, *Ethics*.

morality is seen as a sentiment culminating from reasoning, comparing, examining, discriminating, etc. Hume sees practical rationality as beyond the caring of morality. He respects reason for its ideals of consistency and integrity. It determines no preferences and holds beliefs in matters of facts or relations of ideas.

For Frankena, the moral point of view consists of caring about persons at the level of imaginative realization beyond one's self, not at the level of benevolence, love, or even sympathy. This caring does not necessarily concern the good or even the welfare of others but rather concentrates on nonindifference.[88] However, it is unclear whether Frankena's moral points of view—short of, but leading to, ultimate rationality—are corrections of self-interest or are equal alternatives that are iteratively and reflectively worked out using reason.[89] Frankena divides beneficence into four general obligations, listed in order from greatest to least precedence: 1) to not inflict evil or harm, 2) to prevent harm and evil, 3) to remove evil or harm, and 4) to do or promote good.[90] The first general obligation is an intentional refrain from doing harm. The other three require action to be implemented. Some moral philosophers consider such action to be moral ideals rather than general obligations, resulting in a principle of nonmaleficence distinguished from a principle of beneficence.[91]

In the 1973 inaugural issue of the *Hastings Center Studies*, Daniel Callahan presents a vision for bioethics. This fledgling discipline, he argues, should use traditional modes of philosophical analysis, be sensitive to feelings and emotions, and factor in political and social influences in order to reach reasonably specific and clear decisions in medicine and science. Callahan cautions against *disciplinary reductionism*, practiced at that time by representatives of distinct disciplines beginning to engage in the new discipline of bioethics. In response to this, he suggests a more populist approach to bioethics, exhorting bioethicists to stay in touch with the ordinary language and thought processes of those whose bioethical

---

88. Baier, "Frankena and Hume," 352. Frankena believes, however, that such caring through non-indifference will likely manifest as benevolence rather than malevolence.

89. Ibid., 357. Baier suggests that this focus on seeing ourselves as part of humankind through our care may be the "inverse equivalent for religion which is needed if a secular morality is not to degenerate into self-indulgent license or its bleak aftermath." This suggests more emphasis on *who are cared for* than on *those who care*, what Baier calls *an asymmetry of care* rather than necessary reciprocity.

90. Frankena, *Ethics*, 47; Clouser and Gert, "Critique of Principlism," 224.

91. Beauchamp and Childress, *Principles of Biomedical Ethics*, 5th ed., 114–19.

problems are being addressed. In fact, they need "unfettered imagination" to appreciate fully the ethical moments anxiously experienced by the persons involved.

A bioethicist must be skilled at knowing and applying normative and metaethical theories. But Callahan encourages focusing on the human dimensions of specific cases, keeping alive "a tension-ridden dialectic" between physicians and scientists on the one side and philosophers and theologians on the other.[92] In his view, discussion among those with diverse academic languages forces an accommodation of terms, thoughts, and beliefs. Already in Callahan's day, theological language had been tempered when concepts such as sanctity of life entered the public morality lexicon. It was a time when philosophers attempted to enter a world of non-philosophical moral discourse, moving outside of the "rarified air of deontological and teleological theory."[93] Foreshadowing the formation of the Belmont Commission a year or two later, Callahan mourns the absence of ethical systems such as the Roman Catholic scholastic and Jewish *responsa* traditions, which he feels are now untenable because the worldview and cultural conditions of those systems no longer exist. As a result, he declares "it has become absolutely urgent that the search for a philosophically viable normative ethic, which can presuppose some commonly shared principles, go forward with all haste."[94]

Jonsen points out that moral ethicists have traditionally been more casual with their use of the term "theory" than have philosophers of science, who generally see theories in terms of hypotheses, observations, and data. For example, Richard Brandt considers ethical theory to be a set of ethical principles from which all true ethical statements could be deduced.[95] For George Kerner, ethical theory is an exploration of modes of reasoning and meanings of terms used to discuss moral issues in practice through the logical analysis of ordinary moral language.[96] For John Rawls, theory is formulated using intellectual capacity through which a reasoning skill is acquired in order to judge matters as just or unjust, right or wrong. As this capacity matures, a set of principles is formulated as a framework that joins one's beliefs, knowledge of circumstances, and

---

92. Callahan, "Bioethics as a Discipline," 68–73. This dialectic parallels the methodological dialectic championed by the same parties and will be discussed later in this chapter.

93. Jonsen, *Birth of Bioethics*, 326.

94. Callahan, "Bioethics as a Discipline," 72.

95. Brandt, *Ethical Theory*, 5.

96. Kerner, *Revolution in Ethical Theory*, 2.

PART ONE: The Rise and Dominance of Principles-Based Biomedical Ethics

supporting reasons for judgments.[97] Like Callahan, K. Danner Clouser sees bioethics as new applications of standard ethical theories for new problems in medicine. He sees no need for new principles or rules and no need for special methods. Thus, despite the novel problems arising from new biomedical technologies, the basic rules of traditional ethics should suffice. The traditional deontological and teleological theories are building blocks for creating structures that isolate concepts and specify conflicting principles that need clarification. Good reasoning and the full participation of all concerned remain critical.[98]

During the early 1970s, various bioethical theories, structures, and frameworks were proposed, leading to a flurry of critiques and suggestions for improvement. For example, Paul Ramsey responds to the proposal of Jonsen and Hellegers for a new comprehensive umbrella theory encompassing three "subtheories" by criticizing their failure to order, rank, or prioritize their theories of virtue, duty, and justice.[99] In chapter 3, I will show how Edmund Pellegrino addresses this problem within principlism by proposing that love should function as an overarching principle that serves a mediating function when other principles conflict.[100]

Principles-based Common Morality Ethics

In 1979, within a year of the publication of the Belmont Report, Tom Beauchamp and James Childress published their first edition of *Principles of Biomedical Ethics*.[101] Adding a fourth principle to those in the Report, their formulation of the four moral principles of the autonomy of persons, beneficence, nonmaleficence, and justice became the most systematic effort to develop a principles-based bioethical framework with no basis in moral theory or presuppositions. Answering the exhortation of Callahan in 1973, the authors were driven by the growing perception that bioethics needed a *useful* method. They were less concerned with right or wrong solutions than were their predecessors in moral philosophy. For these

97. Rawls, *Theory of Justice*, 46–53.
98. Clouser, "Medical Ethics," 384–87.
99. Ramsey, "Indignity," 23.
100. Pellegrino and Thomasma, *Christian Virtues*, 74.

101. Beauchamp and Childress have subsequently published seven editions. Most of the citations from their book in this volume come from the 2001 edition. Citations from the 2009 edition are made to identify new information not present in the earlier edition or to highlight meaningful changes or expansions of concepts presented in the 2009 edition.

authors, the role and purpose of biomedical ethics was to make practical decisions that are useful to persons or groups who may be from diverse backgrounds with diverse moral beliefs.[102] They acknowledged the central role of beneficence and nonmaleficence in the history of medical ethics as asserted by Thomas Percival already in the early nineteenth century. However, they also acknowledged the emergence of other principles in response to events and reflections leading up to the Belmont Report.[103]

The principles-based framework of Beauchamp and Childress, or principlism, has two key assumptions: 1) a set of norms exists that all morally serious persons share, and this constitutes a common morality, and 2) four clusters of moral principles can be identified that can function individually as guidelines and collectively as an analytic framework expressing the general values underlying rules in a common morality.[104] Historically, while principles of beneficence and nonmaleficence have often been combined, the authors feel that important distinctions are obscured in doing so.[105] I will argue later in chapter 8 why this distinction is a necessary, minimalist requirement for their common morality.

Beauchamp and Childress present different theories regarding common morality, including those of Ross and Frankena. However, they all have the same starting point in the ordinary, shared moral beliefs of rational, morally serious persons. Beauchamp and Childress claim that their common morality is a universally shared product of human experience and history. The principles reputedly stand on their own, requiring no grounding or appeal to pure reason, rationality, or natural law. Beauchamp and Childress call these shared moral beliefs *pre-theoretical common sense moral judgments* with which any common-morality theory should be consistent.[106]

They also acknowledge the existence of private moralities. Often distinguished by religious groups for whom moral justification is grounded in a transcendent being, these private moralities also often adhere to moral ideals. By contrast, universal moral claims based on a common morality

---

102. Iltis, "Bioethics," 273.

103. Beauchamp and Childress, *Principles of Biomedical Ethics*, 5th ed., 12.

104. Ibid. For Beauchamp and Childress, terms such as *norms, values, rules,* and *principles* often lack precision and distinctiveness. While they refer to each of the four principles as a cluster of principles, these "principles" are said to express general *values* that they also call *norms*. Respect of autonomy and nonmaleficence, for example, are each called single norms while beneficence and justice constitute groups of norms.

105. Ibid., 114; Frankena, *Ethics*, 47.

106. Beauchamp and Childress, *Principles of Biomedical Ethics*, 5th ed., 403.

might not be claimed by those with certain religious presuppositions.[107] While Beauchamp and Childress try to portray the common morality *alongside* other moral viewpoints that reside within the greater morality of humankind, they ultimately exclude those with particular moral points of view that clash with components of the common morality. However, they never reveal who has the authority to decide what components constitute the common morality and by what criteria and method opinions from outside of the common morality can be judged as conforming to that morality.

Beauchamp and Childress consider the origin of the norms of the common morality to be "no different in principle" from those of a particular morality—that is, all are learned and transmitted in communities. Particular moralities are defined as distinct moral communities with their own moral ideals, such as those of religious commonality. Most importantly, Beauchamp and Childress distinguish particular moralities on the basis of cultural differences, whereas the common morality *transcends* such individual and cultural differences.[108] Curiously, however, they concede that the common morality may not have *total* authoritative moral force. They admit that some ethicists make false claims that do not have the backing (or, in their terms, "moral force") of the common (universal) morality. Unfortunately, Beauchamp and Childress again fail to provide guidance regarding who determines which claims are "false" and, if considered false, why they should be considered of lesser moral worth. However, they admit that they cannot necessarily claim the authority of the common morality for everything built on that morality.[109] This curious statement seems to lay claim to different sources of moral authority, the most basic and primary source being the common morality, but it supports the split of morality into public and private components, an idea rooted in the Enlightenment tradition.

In my view, the common-morality idea has its roots in natural law, which historically appeals to Scripture. But the idea of a basic humanity

---

107. Ibid., 3–4.

108. Ibid.

109. Ibid., 5. On this point, Beauchamp and Childress waiver on the issue of a universal moral authority of the common morality: "To say that we build on the common morality is not to say that we can validly claim this authority for everything we build." They seem to imply that moral claims founded on religious beliefs can completely diverge from common morality claims and can validly claim their authority outside of the common morality. However, this risks completely severing public from private moral authority and thus practices.

The Rise of Principlism in Response to an Ethical Crisis

retained after the Fall into sin, as understood by medievalists, was transformed into a secular formulation during the Enlightenment. MacIntyre argues that the period from 1630 to 1850 saw the transformation of morality in Western culture, from human moral behavior based on God-revealed laws of nature and Scripture to rules of conduct based on rational justification alone. During and since that time, Western society has lost *a shared vision of the good* for humankind and has no way to weigh various moral claims by way of human reason alone. Among existing moral theories, there are no standards or any rational justification for choosing one theory over another.[110]

For Beauchamp and Childress, such choosing is unnecessary. What is needed is rational consensus among morally serious persons.[111] Such consensus exists as a reflective equilibrium as conceptualized by Rawls. It is never a final moral position but is always contingent upon new insights over time. Their ethical framework rests on *coherence theory*, which teaches that, starting with considered judgments from the past, the addition of information about current cases will somehow lead to the convergence of past and current ideas with some degree of moral resolution.[112] As a postmodern construct, reflective equilibrium is never immune to revi-

---

110. MacIntyre, *After Virtue*, 19, 236, 270.

111. Ronald Preston ("The Four Principles," 25–26) sees the common morality movement as a way to redeem some aspects of morality through rationality. Rather than restricting contributors of the common morality as morally serious persons, he sees it evolve from the common discussions of the neighborhood pub where he believes there is a substratum of common ground, an element of populist objectivity to which people of otherwise diverse beliefs tend to gravitate during moral debates. Preston portrays religious faith and belief as superimposed on common principles that are hidden from sight behind such beliefs unless one looks carefully. From this stance, he sees the four principles as based on a concept of rational personhood.

112. Beauchamp and Childress, *Principles of Biomedical Ethics*, 5th ed., 398–401; Rawls, *Political Liberalism*, 384–85. In his model of coherence theory, John Rawls distinguishes between narrow reflective equilibrium (consideration only of considered judgments) and wide reflective equilibrium. The latter involves particular judgments, first principles, and general convictions of multiple citizens and is considered a full, reflective equilibrium. Rawls claims that reflective equilibrium resembles the test of moral truth or validity that Habermas (*Between Naturalism and Religion*, 47–52) defines as fully rational agreement in the situation of ideal discourse. That is, both processes can never be fully or ideally realized as ultimate truth because further discussion and infusion of ideas lead to more reasonable conclusions that rationally surpass the previous position. This unstable equilibrium is admittedly intersubjective, but the more citizens that are involved and the more that reflective time and elements are committed, the closer one comes to the truth (though, like infinity, theoretically it cannot be reached).

sion; rather, revision will occur with reflection on new information and perspectives.[113] Their ethic rests on the conviction that reasoned deliberation will overcome differences based on moral theory as long as participants believe in, and remain focused on, the universal moral principles of the common morality. For MacIntyre, however, there is no hope of moral consensus in the fragmentation of Western morality. Virtues and the idea of common good embedded in the Judeo-Christian tradition have been largely lost from society at large but are retained with some integrity in smaller communities.[114] The common morality represents a loss rather than gain of moral content, while the "private moralities" of faith-based communities represent the residual remnants of moral virtue and good previously accepted by a larger segment of society at large.

Beauchamp and Childress expanded the applicability of the principles in the Belmont Report into medical practice. The meaning of respect for persons developed from obtaining uncoerced consent of research subjects to engage in research to including medical decision-making by caregivers, patients, and supporting relatives or neighbors. However, their primary focus remains on patient consent, with only a passing allusion to relational autonomy in the broader sense, as introduced by feminist and care bioethicists.[115] Elements of patient consent, including disclosure, understanding, capacity, competence, and voluntariness, are all discussed with the emphasis put on patient empowerment and protection. As well, issues of surrogacy are addressed through a typology of surrogate roles and duties. Their discussions tend to concentrate on measures to protect the perceived preferences and beliefs of the patient against those of others, including surrogate decision makers, rather than on the potential help that relatives and friends can provide.

Nonmaleficence was introduced by Beauchamp and Childress as a principle distinguished from beneficence. In the Belmont Report, the Hippocratic maxim "do no harm" is interpreted as a complementary expression of beneficence.[116] However, in qualifying this, the report notes that in the Hippocratic tradition, physicians are required to benefit their patients, acknowledging that this may require exposure to risk. Nowhere does the report suggest that the meaning of "do no harm" in that tradition was meant to simply avoid harming someone. Rather, it provides the cau-

---

113. Beauchamp and Childress, *Principles of Biomedical Ethics*, 5th ed., 406–8.
114. MacIntyre, *After Virtue*, 252.
115. Beauchamp and Childress, *Principles of Biomedical Ethics*, 5th ed., 61.
116. Ryan, *Belmont Report*.

tion that, in fulfilling the encouraged action to be helpful, one should do so reflectively and in a way that minimizes risk while offering assistance or treatment. Beauchamp and Childress try to justify isolating nonmaleficence as a separate principle by appealing to situations in which doing no harm should override being beneficent.[117] However, I will argue in chapter 8 that a covenantal ethic does not separate nonmaleficence from beneficence because the overarching love-command render nonmaleficence meaningless apart from beneficence.

For post-Enlightenment figure David Hume, beneficence is at the centre of common-morality theories.[118] W. D. Ross believes that positive obligations to help others are human moral requirements, that these obligations "rest on the mere fact that there are other beings in the world whose condition we can make better."[119] To him, helping others is a self-evident universal moral truth. I agree with Charles Taylor that any attempt to universalize beneficence in a common morality reflects a proceduralist ethic that gives special status to such principles "by segregating them from any considerations about the good." This is rooted in the tradition of Enlightenment naturalism and falls in line with Bentham's love of humankind and agnostic commitment to progress.[120]

Beauchamp and Childress devote considerable discussion to the nuances of beneficence. However, in the context of a common morality, they cannot be seen to impose any moral obligation to be beneficent based on that morality.[121] They cannot specify limits to obligations of beneficence, fearing such limits would "both sharpen and alter the common morality, which is not sufficiently refined to supply an answer."[122] However, in their preoccupation with avoiding distinguishing levels of obligatory beneficence, they provide no guidance at all! As I will show in chapters 7 and 8, having no overriding principle, such as love, they are unable to give moral privilege to helping others, particularly strangers, because such help often involves risk to the benefactor. In an effort to justify beneficence at all,

---

117. Beauchamp and Childress, *Principles of Biomedical Ethics*, 5th ed., 115.

118. Later, Jeremy Bentham and W. D. Ross agreed that obligations to help others are human moral requirements.

119. Ross, *Right and the Good*, 21.

120. Taylor, *Sources of the Self*, 496.

121. Beauchamp and Childress, *Principles of Biomedical Ethics*, 5th ed., 173. "No doubt more precise limits of obligatory beneficence can be drawn, but it is certain to be a revisionary line in the sense that it will draw a sharper boundary for our obligations than exists in the common morality."

122. Ibid.

they appeal to a reciprocity-based justification and cite William F. May, who suggests that the beneficent care of patients is rooted in a "reciprocity of giving and receiving" that creates an obligation of beneficence.[123] Although I will show that I agree with much of May's development of a covenantal ethic for medicine, I disagree with this proviso as a requirement within a biblical covenantal ethic.

Regarding justice, Beauchamp and Childress clearly favor the theory of justice developed by John Rawls and adapted to health policy by Norman Daniels.[124] This theory concentrates on justice at the societal level. Theirs is a qualified egalitarianism wherein some basic equalities are required among individuals but in which inequalities are permitted if they benefit the least advantaged. "Fairness" is the core concept, even to the point of forcing beneficence on citizens who do not believe that the needy have a moral right to health care.[125] In this sense, they offer a notion of justice that favors the weak and vulnerable, at least to the point of supporting their access to a decent minimum or adequate level of care.[126] While not divulging the basic underlying beliefs that justify such a notion of fairness, it resonates with biblical teaching regarding God's love for the needy and his expectations of such love on the part of his human covenantal partners.

Beauchamp and Childress struggle admirably with difficult issues of resource allocation. On the level of the individual patient, they argue for attention to prioritization according to need; if the need is deemed equal, however, they allocate according either to chance or to "first come, first served." They decry the unfairness of the health insurance system in the United States as morally shameful, blaming insurers and legislators for failing in their civic responsibility.[127] Others such as Harry Stopes-Roe take a humanist position in the struggle between individual and communal ethical responsibility in health care allocation. Like Beauchamp and Childress, he believes that collective morality is distinct from individual morality, suggesting that allowance for selfishness in helping others may be less justifiably tolerated in collective morality because of its communal nature. Extending this to health care, he bemoans the inadequate

---

123. May, "Code, Covenant," 33.

124. Beauchamp and Childress, *Principles of Biomedical Ethics*, 5th ed., 234; Rawls, *Theory of Justice*; Daniels and Sabin, *Setting Limits Fairly*.

125. Beauchamp and Childress, *Principles of Biomedical Ethics*, 5th ed., 243.

126. Ibid., 244, 272. This, they argue further, should be in a framework of allocation that incorporated both utilitarian and egalitarian standards, though the reason for this needed balance is not given.

127. Ibid., 240, 242.

responses of individual physicians to their responsibilities to the health care system when making individual patient decisions. For Stopes-Roe, a physician cannot be solely or even primarily an advocate for her or his own patients but must also consider the needs of the collective of other patients in the health care system.[128] Unfortunately, Stopes-Roe does not provide guidance for giving priority to patients; perceptions for degrees and urgency of need are often influenced by an inherent bias to serve one's own patients preferentially. As I will show in chapter 8, I think his idea of justice in the appropriation of medical care approaches one that is consistent with a covenantal ethic.

128. Stopes-Roe, "Principles and Life Stances," 117–33.

2

Challenges to Principlism

> Throughout the land, arising from the throngs of converts to bioethics awareness, there can be heard a mantra "... beneficence ... autonomy ... justice ..." It is this ritual incantation in the face of biomedical dilemmas that beckons our inquiry.... We believe that the "principles of biomedical ethics" approach (hereinafter referred to as "principlism") is mistaken ... about the nature of morality and misleading as to the foundations of ethics.... Our quarrel is not so much with the content of the various "principles" as it is with the use of "principles" at all.[1]
>
> —CLOUSER AND GERT (1990)

VEATCH, CLOUSER, AND GERT

Since the appearance of principlism on the contemporary stage, its common-morality core has created a tendency to distil the basis of moral truth and the justification for moral decisions and policies into a few simple concepts to which few can object. Consensus by reasoned persuasion is its primary method; underlying religious beliefs are necessarily relegated to private moral considerations. This section will focus on the variety and depth of direct responses by formative bioethicists to principlism, keeping in mind the background tension between ethical theory and practice introduced in the previous chapter. The bioethicists discussed in this chapter

---

1. Clouser and Gert, "Critique of Principlism," 220.

are either clearly secular in their basic moral beliefs, or they profess some affiliation to a Christian tradition but do not overly express their Christian faith in their bioethical reflections. In the next chapter, I will present the views of Christian bioethicists who overtly express the influence of their Christian commitment on their views regarding principlism. The purpose of this distinction is to highlight the impact of various basic beliefs on one's bioethical perspectives.

From its earliest years, the importance and usefulness of the four principles of principlism have been challenged. Through the spectacles of his Enlightenment-rooted, triple-contract theory, Veatch analyzes the principles of beneficence, autonomy, and justice. In Rawlsian fashion, Veatch begins with *an original moral position* that all persons are equal, stripped of the characteristics that made them unequal. From this moral vantage point, those interested in contracting with others create the moral content of their ethical system. This system consists of basic ethical principles for their contracted community, principles that are identified by invention, discovery, or some revelatory mechanism.[2] This activity is done within a covenantal context, though for Veatch a covenant is a type of contract rather than something to be contrasted against it. He makes no reference to a biblical basis for such a concept.

Veatch also offers his own set of principles: promise keeping, honesty, protection of life, striving for equality, respect for the autonomy of others within the moral community, and producing good for each other.[3] Veatch suggests that contracts be struck at several levels, such as those between society and specific professions, between expert professionals within professions, and between professionals and their clients or patients (part of his triple-contract theory). He seeks to create a system through which those who derive their personal ethical theories from absolute moral precepts and beliefs can use reason and/or moral sentiments to arrive at basic moral agreement.

One of the most persistent challenges to principles-based ethics comes from K. Danner Clouser and Bernard Gert. They were the first to attach the word *principlism* to "the practice of using 'principles' to replace

---

2. Veatch, "Models for Ethical Medicine," 118–21; 137–38. In his attempt to synthesize contract theories into a social contract theory for bioethics, he tries to minimize, if not eliminate, the distinction between covenant and contract, preferring to consider the Judeo-Christian tradition to be contractarian rather than covenantal. This risks the loss of the richness that a biblical teaching of covenant offers, a point that will be expanded on in chapter 5.

3. Ibid., 327–29.

both moral theory and particular moral rules and ideals in dealing with the moral problems that arise in medical practice."[4] For Clouser and Gert, principles are embodiments of one or more moral theories from which they arose, functioning as meaningful moral directives for action that can stand alone without conflicting with other principles. They vigorously challenge the use of, and the initial meanings given to, the concept of principles by Frankena[5] and subsequently by Beauchamp and Childress.

Clouser and Gert declare that principlism "is mistaken about the nature of morality and is misleading as to the foundations of ethics."[6] Its principles act more like checklists that *remind* bioethicists about issues; however, they fail to guide moral reasoning, and they misuse moral theory. While the *language* of principlism implies firm moral justification, the term "principle" lacks precision. In reality, the moral agent weighs multiple diverse moral considerations that are under the heading of a particular principle. Clouser and Gert suggest that each principle might be construed as an attractive, potential surrogate for a particular moral theory. For example, they link the utilitarianism of Mill with beneficence, the deontology of Kant with autonomy, the minimalist theory of Gert with nonmaleficence, and Rawls's theory of justice with justice.[7]

Clouser and Gert are particularly critical of the unsystematic, disconnected methods by which Beauchamp and Childress identify the conditions necessary to denote a duty of beneficence toward someone else.[8] They criticize the failure to distinguish requirements, duties, and obligations from ideal and supererogatory acts, as well as their explanation of the relationships between these concepts.[9] To Clouser and Gert, a unified and

---

4. Clouser and Gert, "Critique of Principlism," 219–21. They focus their critique on the principles-based ethics of Beauchamp and Childress, since their version is the most widely used. However, they identify the ethical approach of Frankena as the progenitor of principlism.

5. Frankena, *Ethics*.

6. Clouser and Gert, "Critique of Principlism," 220.

7. Ibid., 222–23.

8. Ibid., 228.

9. Beauchamp and Childress (*Principles of Biomedical Ethics*, 5th ed., 167) do give examples of beneficent acts that, in their judgment, exceed the basic requirements of generosity that should be expected under the principles of the common morality and thus should be considered ideals. But their post-Belmont Report identification of nonmaleficence as a principle distinct from beneficence secures a minimal requirement to "do no harm" and probably reflects the anticipated difficulty of getting consensus on the obligatory degree of generosity and risk that should be required of adherents to the common morality.

comprehensive moral theory is needed. Drawing from Mill, they suggest either that one self-evident principle be at the root of all morality or that a self-evident rule be recognized that resolves conflicts among principles.[10] The suggestion of such an overarching principle conceptually resonates with the unifying principle of love articulated by Pellegrino and Oliver O'Donovan that will be discussed in chapters 3 and 5.[11] However, unlike Pellegrino and O'Donovan, whose overarching principle is grounded in Scripture, Clouser and Gert give no reference to the nature of moral grounding for their suggested, self-evident principle.

Principlism's groundless nature, claim Clouser and Gert, leads to a relativistic method of moral deliberation and decision-making wherein bioethicists pick and choose bits of theories on an *ad hoc* basis. Their solution is an articulated moral system based on a single moral theory, revisable like scientific theories that can systematically deal with aspects of each principle when making moral judgments.[12] In the end, however, Clouser and Gert conclude that there are no moral principles. Five years later, Clouser again addresses the inadequacies of principlism but now as a reluctant critic with an assigned role. He almost apologetically offers that his previous criticism of principlism might be perceived as "picayune concern over some abstract points."[13] In what he calls a partial critique of principlism, Clouser reiterates that Beauchamp and Childress are misleading in their suggestion that specific ethical theories underlie the validity of their principles. However, now he describes principles as signposts to ethical values rather than just reminders that need to be factored into ethical deliberations.[14] Still, he remains convinced that principles are "*ad hoc* constructions" that give rise to what he and Gert call the *anthology syndrome*. That is, readers of principles-based texts are presented with an anthology of bioethical theories and are asked to pick and choose which theory/theories fit a particular case.[15]

---

10. Clouser and Gert, "Critique of Principlism," 236. Mill (*Utilitarianism*, 3) also believes that for those who invoke principles, one principle or one rule should have the authority to decide between conflicting, mid-level principles.

11. Pellegrino and Thomasma, *Christian Virtues*, 109; O'Donovan, *Resurrection and Moral Order*, 199–202.

12. Clouser and Gert, "Critique of Principlism," 232.

13. Clouser, "Common Morality," 222.

14. Clouser and Gert, "Critique of Principlism," 220. This idea is in contrast to their earlier description of principles as merely checklists.

15. Ibid., 230.

Part One: The Rise and Dominance of Principles-Based Biomedical Ethics

As an alternative to principlism, Clouser and Gert advocate for a complex system of ethical inquiry that includes moral rules, moral ideals, the morally relevant details of each situation, and a detailed process for adjudicating conflicts. Permission to violate a rule can be justified on the basis of *public allowability*. That is, if *every rational, impartial person* finds the violation to be acceptable in similar morally relevant situations, then the violation is permissible. The basis of justification lies in the rational ability of such persons to come to consensus.[16] For Clouser, moral theory arises from a need to justify *common moral intuitions* that, in turn, result from moral experience.[17]

Disappointingly, Clouser and Gert do not provide the foundational basis for principles that they claim is lacking in principlism. They simply move away from principles as a starting point for bioethical reflection toward the level of the case or situation wherein the moral experience lies. From the accumulation of such cases and situations, moral rules can be discovered that are "embedded in the features of human nature."[18] In my view, this so-called alternative to principlism sounds like a version of casuistry or situationalism. Moral instincts and innately embedded moral rules initiate and structure the new moral process of their alternative complex system of ethical inquiry. The justification of moral choices is based on both public consensus and rational, unbiased buy-in. They provide no better justification for this schema than do Beauchamp and Childress, against whose framework Clouser and Gert object so strongly as a means of making normative moral judgments and decisions. In my view, the basic moral premises of their alternative ethical system are very similar, if not identical, to those of principlism. Both ethical frameworks are fundamentally variations of the theme of common rational consensus as the grounding for moral truth. As well, both pairs of bioethicists ignore any supratemporal authority in which to ground moral decisions and policies.

---

16. Louthan, "On Religion," 180. One can recall, at a more fundamental philosophical level, Plantinga's earlier challenge to Rorty that truth for Rorty seems to become a matter of persuasiveness leading to consensus among peers.

17. Clouser, "Common Morality," 230. Taking the avoidance of harm as an example, Clouser states, "harms share a universal aspect, namely, they are harms that all rational persons, by virtue of their rationality alone, would want to avoid, unless they had an adequate reason not to."

18. Ibid., 235.

EFFORTS TO IMPROVE PRINCIPLISM: SPECIFICATION, CASUISTRY, AND HEURISTIC TOOLS

Referring to principles as *ethical norms*, Henry Richardson has proposed *specification* in order to the guide the process of resolving conflicting principles. In this process, norms are brought to bear on cases. When specification is appropriately carried out in a given context, "it will be sufficiently obvious what ought to be done," and a morally acceptable solution to the problem will simply become evident.[19] David DeGrazia declares that this *specified principlism* is the most promising model yet devised for the bioethical deliberative process.[20] In the 1994 edition of their *The Principles of Biomedical Ethics*, Beauchamp and Childress confidently endorse the specification of principles as a necessary first step in the deliberation process in order to "specify unclarities and problems away."[21]

In its contemporary applications, casuistry is a method that provides more detail and relevance to specific cases and situations. It is, firstly, a hermeneutical method, using analogies and paradigms to formulate particular moral obligations. These, in turn, are framed in general heuristic rules rather than with universal principles. Thus, a notion of the good is only certain when considered under the conditions of a specific agent involved in particular circumstances of action.[22] Jonsen identifies three key components of the casuistic method that relate casuistry to rhetorical reasoning and the interpretation of cases: 1) the perception of form and structure, such as the interplay of circumstances and rules within a case perceived through moral argument and reasoning; 2) the ordering of cases into types defined by paradigm features that provide the moral context and weight to perceptions of rightness and wrongness; and 3) kinetics as practical wisdom or prudence that should govern the process.[23] Prudence is considered *common sense joined with experience*, linked to ideals that make good judgment possible.[24]

---

19. Richardson, "Specifying Norms," 294.

20. DeGrazia, "Moving Forward," 512.

21. Beauchamp and Childress, *Principles of Biomedical Ethics*, 4th ed., 29. In their fifth edition (17–18), they are more tempered in their enthusiasm, noting the limits of specification.

22. Jonsen, "Casuistry as Methodology," 297.

23. Ibid., 302.

24. Ibid., 306.

Part One: The Rise and Dominance of Principles-Based Biomedical Ethics

Carson Strong proposes a form of casuistry in which ethical principles are important features. He dismisses Richardson's specification method as insufficient for providing details of the case or situation, criticizing two major inadequacies in the specification process: 1) the way one chooses to specify principles is affected by prior choices when assigning priority to principles that conflict, and 2) assigning priorities to principles is better accomplished with casuistic methods. For Strong, casuistry could be considered a pre-requisite to specified principlism.[25] Indeed, he argues that casuistry can provide coherence among the norms or principles.

Both Richardson and Strong try to give particular applicability to principles, either by claiming greater sensitivity to particular cases (Richardson) or by proposing that casuistry is a forerunner of specific principlism (Strong). In either case, their iterations of principlism do not address the fundamental problems of a lack of moral authority and of a failure to anchor their ethic in a moral principle or theme that can give guidance in addressing competing moral claims.

In their insightful critique of principlism, Eric Meslin and colleagues assess the relevance and usefulness of principlism in its original context: clinical research and, specifically, the ethical appraisal of clinical trials through research ethics boards. They begin by proposing meta-criteria "to assess the principle-based source of ethical appraisal that currently provided the foundation for the specific criteria used for ethical review of clinical trials."[26] In so doing, they assess whether these principles themselves possess ethical authority. Following others who have identified such criteria, they use effective guidance, coherence, completeness, simplicity, and reconcilability as basic criteria. The authors believe that principlism is not meant to function as a theory but rather as an action guide in bioethics. They proceed to examine whether or not the four principles are a secure appraisal source to satisfy their meta-criteria, which they consider "indicators for judging the rigor of a way of thinking that has *normative force*." In addition, they require justification that is even more convincing if these principles are to be considered standards on which the criteria for research ethics review are based.[27]

Meslin and colleagues define principles as *heuristic devices* that can "reduce complex tasks of assessing probabilities and predicting values to

---

25. Strong, "Specified Principlism," 330.
26. Meslin et al., "Principlism," 401.
27. Ibid., 403.

simpler judgmental operations."[28] Consciously avoiding the controversy over the relationship between moral theory and principles, they nonetheless note that there has never been a formal assessment of the philosophic justification for the principles from which guidelines and policies for assessing the ethics of clinical studies can be generated.[29] Despite this, they favor adopting the four principles as practical tools with which research ethics board members can iteratively compare ethical aspects of clinical-trial protocol constituents using principles and vice versa.

They attempt to show that, as heuristic tools, principles go beyond the function of prompts or checklists as suggested by Clouser and Gert. Rather, principles can be part of "an internalized strategy that can be imposed on a set of facts to facilitate ordered decision-making."[30] However, their attempt to transform principles into heuristic devices becomes a variation of principlism rather than a demonstration of internal moral justification. Instead of being the core of the language of moral deliberation within the process of reflective equilibrium, principles become tools to reduce complex problems to "simpler judgmental operations" through a dialectical process. Ironically, their preference for a casuistic approach and their concluding description of heuristics as cognitive prompts sound very much like the earlier critique offered by Clouser and Gert.[31] Regrettably, they provide little additional insight into the underlying nature of principles, while maintaining an emphasis on deliberative process. Thus, they fail to show that utilizing principles functions as a test of rational rigor or of moral justification.

DIALECTICAL TENSIONS

Principles and the Question of Moral Grounding

Historically, medical ethicists were concerned primarily with social and relational aspects of medicine involving physician disposition and behavior.[32] But revelations in the late 1960s about unethical conduct involving human subjects in clinical studies created an *atmosphere of urgency* to regulate the treatment of human subjects. At the same time, in light of

28. Tversky and Kahneman, "Judgment under Uncertainty," 1124.
29. Meslin et al., "Principlism," 410.
30. Ibid., 413.
31. Clouser and Gert, "Critique of Principlism," 220–23.
32. Jonsen, *Birth of Bioethics*, 3.

Part One: The Rise and Dominance of Principles-Based Biomedical Ethics

recent biotechnologies that have raised new and complex ethical issues, there has been a clamor by concerned segments of society, including religious groups, to urgently address these issues. Confronted with a pluralistic society, and increasingly doubtful that any one ethical theory could become universally accepted by all, bioethics has moved away from both foundational beliefs and ethical theories. Mid-level principles have been considered more malleable than foundational principles, such as Hare's universalizability principle, in the face of moral pluralism.[33] Ana Smith Iltis insightfully notes that both specification and principlism are in fact *theories without theories*. That is, they lack a universally accepted background theory that tells us *how* to specify and *how* to choose between conflicting specifications.[34]

Thus, in principlism, validating the justification for identifying certain principles over others and justifying their nature and scope has no morally authoritative grounding. Beauchamp and Childress claim that their principles are derived from shared moral beliefs, which they also call pre-theoretical common-sense moral judgments.[35] Like Ronald Green,[36] Baruch Brody criticizes their failure to deal with the origins of their principles. From which fundamental ethical tradition(s) should one ground a particular principle? He cites Alan Donagan, who argues that the principle of non-maleficence, as applied to the impermissibility of mutilating oneself, is based on the fundamental Kantian claim that all human creatures should respect others and themselves as rational creatures.[37] By *what moral authority*, Brody asks, does Donagan justify such a claim?

Unfortunately, like Green, Brody too has no solution for establishing groundings to justify the principles. He emphasizes high-quality scholarship, the means by which one establishes the theoretical foundations of mid-level principles (which would include the four principles) and the path along which one could go in order to get from the foundations to the principles.[38] For Brody, good scholarship consists of *awareness, sensitivity, and good effort* in adopting some way of dealing with principles using the reflective equilibrium method proposed by Rawls. Brody sees the prob-

---

33. That is, principles that are more specific than moral theories but less specific than moral particularities of individual situations.

34. Iltis, "Bioethics," 273–74.

35. Beauchamp and Childress, *Principles of Biomedical Ethics*, 5th ed., 403.

36. Green, "Method in Bioethics," 180–89 (see chapter 1).

37. Donagan, *Theory of Morality*, 76–81.

38. Brody, "Quality of Scholarship," 168–69.

lem as the missing link between foundational theoretical grounding and so-called mid-level principles. He argues that the nature of fundamental moral theory needs to be resolved before a firm grounding of principles is possible.[39]

Processes of Moral Analysis

Brody insightfully identifies a dialectic between the upwards-down and the downwards-up models that specify the direction of analysis between foundations of moral theory, mid-level principles, and empirical investigations. Both models fall short of providing either the foundations or the path that links them with principles. Bioethics scholarship itself seems caught in a *reflective equilibrium ad infinitum*, see-sawing back and forth between methods as situations arise.[40] But reflective equilibrium needs a starting point, perhaps from pre-equilibrium insights or intuitions about a particular case and relevant fundamental truths.[41] The moral fragmentation articulated by MacIntyre creates doubt and confusion regarding that starting point, and bioethics has become trapped in a *dialectic of methodologies* by the exclusion of core, basic beliefs. Both the top-down and bottom-up approaches suffer from a lack of grounds for justifying moral choices.

Raymond Devettere has made the point that the dialectic involving general principles and particular judgments is an underdeveloped claim of Beauchamp and Childress. He argues that principles and rules are but one component of applied normative ethics. In other words, normative principles and particular normative judgments are complementary, and overemphasizing one at the expense of the other "misreads what ethics has always been in the best of both our religious and philosophical traditions."[42] Both rigid adherence to moral principles or rules and a tyranny of unfounded particular judgments can create moral victims. Extending this perspective further, the process of ethical consideration is iterative, with both normative principles and particular normative judgments included in each

---

39. Ibid.,

40. Ibid., 172. Brody states, "Actual scholarship in bioethics often seems to be moving in both directions at the same time—sometimes using fundamental or mid-level principles to argue for detailed and practical conclusions, and sometimes using the practical implications to argue for or against mid-level or fundamental principles."

41. Ibid., 173.

42. Devettere, "Principled Approach," 44.

iteration. The issue is not which direction the thinking or discourse should take but rather to consider the support of rules and principles by the particulars of a situation and the compatibility, or lack thereof, of rules and principles with those particulars. Such iterative reflection leads to moral discernment, analogous to clinical discernment in medical practice. However, to keep this coherent, structurally and morally, such deliberations need a founding principle. For the Greeks, he suggests, this was living well and striving for the good life.[43] For Christians, this is the principle of love of God and love of fellow human beings, a principle grounded in, and given justification by, the Word of God.

Neither faith in rationality, substantiated by human experience, nor faith in intuitive conclusions after iterative reflections fed by multiple moral views has resulted in common moral satisfaction. Unfortunately, no religious perspectives such as those of Islamic, Jewish, or Christian faith traditions have been able to release bioethics from this dialectical oscillation. Rather, bioethicists from these broad traditions have varied in their depth of critique regarding the importance of the principles in bioethical decision-making. Roman Catholic perspectives, for example, generally affirm principlism through a reason/faith dualism. Faith is often added as a modulating or illuminating factor to rationally perceived and deliberated principles that flow from a natural-law theology. For some, the importance of principles founded on natural law may even transcend that of faith belief.[44] Such preferential reliance on rationality has recently been criticized in favor of a properly basic and entirely rational belief in God.[45] Diversity among Roman Catholic bioethicists will be addressed in more detail in chapters 3 and 4.

---

43. Ibid., 44–45.

44. Preston (1994, 25–29) seems to accept this dialectical oscillation as normative deliberation in bioethics, though he clearly gives more weigh to casuistic method in this process: "Those involved [in cases in medical ethics] have found that principles and the case data react reciprocally on one another. It has, for example, been a fairly common experience that agreement could be reached regarding what it was best to do in a particular case by those who had difficulty agreeing on the precise statement of principles."

45. Plantinga, "Reason and Belief," 72.

WANING OF THEOLOGICAL VOICES
THE SECULARIZATION OF BIOMEDICAL ETHICS

Whose Moral Common Ground?

In ancient times, bioethical issues were addressed by religiously diverse groups, from pagan philosophers to the prophets and leaders of the children of Israel. Later, early Christians provided insight into how to live life rightly under the new covenant in Christ. As the post-Constantinian church became a more powerful force in society, its leaders focused more on the particulars of how to lead the Christian life. Casuistic methods were developed for judging measures of penance for confessed sins. At the same time, moral philosophy developed in parallel with teaching manuals that addressed the moral expectations of living in a right covenant relationship with God. As a result of the Protestant Reformation, Reformers and their followers rejected the monopoly on scriptural interpretation by the ecclesiastical hierarchy, promoting greater responsibility by members of the church to understand God's revelation for leading the righteous life. With the Enlightenment came moral fragmentation under the influence of new philosophical movements.[46] A transcendent God was replaced by the human capacity to reason as the ultimate source of moral authority.

Since the dawn of the distinct discipline of bioethics in the mid-twentieth century, those entering the field have spoken with varying degrees of forthrightness and articulation regarding the basic presuppositional beliefs in which their perspectives are rooted. Christian bioethicists, most being theologians, have also contributed their perspectives alongside colleagues of Jewish, Islamic, and secular faiths. Over the last fifty years, as Roman Catholic theologians have reassessed central moral doctrines, such as double effect, Protestant theologians have debated the appropriate application of general moral rules or principles to particular moral situations. These discussions over the relative importance of such particularity and the method by which such particularity is considered in moral deliberation have been called the "norm versus context" debates.[47] Since the rapprochement of Vatican II, dialogue has increased among Ro-

---

46. MacIntyre, *After Virtue*.

47. Jonsen, *Birth of Bioethics*, 40; Woodward, *Doctrine of Double Effect*. Also known as the rule of double effect or double effect reasoning, the doctrine of double effect is summarized with the claim that sometimes it is permissible to bring about, as a merely foreseen side effect, a harmful event that would be impermissible to bring about intentionally.

PART ONE: The Rise and Dominance of Principles-Based Biomedical Ethics

man Catholic theologians and between Catholics and Protestants. Jonsen suggests that engagement in such discussions does not take place just for participants to understand each other's positions but for them to search for moral common ground.

It is also interesting that secular bioethicists have been searching for moral common ground but one of a very different nature. For Christians, belief in God as the final authority for moral justification binds those who search for common doctrinal ground in order that they may overcome differences of biblical interpretation and/or specific historical barriers.[48] By contrast, many secular bioethicists search for common moral consensus by way of rational discourse, grounded in faith in the inherent intuitive or anthropocentric authority of basic, minimal moral principles. Principles emanating from a minimalist common morality are the core of principlism, and its single source of authority is faith in rationality alone.[49]

Daniel Callahan has chronicled the influence of theologians in the field of biomedical ethics.[50] Entering the field in the mid-1960s, he witnessed what LeRoy Walters calls the "renaissance of bioethics."[51] Through the following decade, religious traditions, particularly Christian and Judaic, were drawn into bioethical discourse over emerging contemporary issues such as organ transplantation, renal dialysis, prenatal diagnosis, and definitions of death. Some theologians unabashedly expressed the theological basis of their bioethical views. Callahan notes particularly the voice of Paul Ramsey, who professes to be "a Christian ethicist, and not some hypothetical common denominator."[52] Others who stand out include Gilbert Meilaender, James Gustafson, Stanley Hauerwas, Allen Verhey, and William F. May from Protestant traditions; Richard McCormick, Germain Grisez, and Bernard Haring from the Roman Catholic tradition; and Immanuel Jakobovits, Ronald Green, David Novak, Leon Kass, and J. David Bleich of the Jewish tradition. Martin Marty suggests that these theolo-

---

48. This issue of common ties among Christian traditions is raised in a discussion of Christian worldview in chapter 6.

49. Beauchamp and Childress, *Principles of Biomedical Ethics*, 6th ed., 3. The common morality, according to Beauchamp and Childress, is "the set of norms shared by all persons committed to morality . . . applicable to all persons in all places, and we rightly judge all human conduct by its standards."

50. Callahan, "Religion," 2-4.

51. Walters, "Religion and the Renaissance," 3-16.

52. Ramsey, "Commentary," 47-62; Hauerwas, "How Christian Ethics," 15. Nonetheless Hauerwas, referring to this declaration, states that "I am not . . . convinced that his execution matched his candor."

gians have in common an openness to talk about God as the focus of their theological perspective, despite their theological differences regarding God's relationship to human beings and the rest of the cosmos.[53]

Over the two decades prior to the publication of Callahan's short history, the field "moved from one dominated by religious and medical traditions to one now increasingly shaped by philosophical and legal concepts."[54] This "enlightenment" of bioethics grew out of eighteenth-century roots, anchored in the suspicion of particular traditions and the celebration of individual autonomy over and against the authority of priests, magistrates, and, more recently, physicians.[55]

Theological Silence, Rationalistic Universalism, and Professionalization of Ethics

The responses of Christian bioethicists to this development expose the substantial differences among them regarding contemporary bioethical issues. One of the most illustrative comparisons is that between James Childress and Stanley Hauerwas. Childress directly contributed to the work of the Belmont Commission, and his Quaker background may explain his comfort in contributing to the search for a consensus-derived universal set of moral beliefs or principles. Noting Childress's "universalist impulse," Marty quips that to some critics "he looked quite like a secular rationalist with a reminiscent Quaker piety."[56] Courtney Campbell wryly summarizes this Quaker influence: "As in Childress's case, there may be *theological* reasons for not doing medical ethics theologically" (emphasis in original).[57] Childress's principles of nonmaleficence and beneficence orient action in such a way as to achieve optimum consequences or ends, while justice and autonomy place moral constraints on the means to achieve those results.

---

53. Marty, "Medical Ethics," 243–52.

54. Callahan, "Religion," 2.

55. Verhey and Lammers, "Introduction," 3.

56. Marty, "Medical Ethics," 248.

57. Campbell, "On James F. Childress," 127–32. As an example, Campbell states Childress believes that the principle of nonmaleficence is independent of theological premises as a bedrock of human morality and social interaction. Campbell also argues that Childress's own moral framework has important distinctions from that developed in his collaborative framework with Beauchamp in *Principles of Biomedical Ethics*. For example, Childress gives theological grounds for claims around the principle of respect for persons including the Quaker notion that *imago Dei* expresses that of God in every person (136).

Part One: The Rise and Dominance of Principles-Based Biomedical Ethics

However, while Childress regularly ties his principles (Marty calls them "themes") with *agape* love, justice and autonomy can conflict with *agape* in certain circumstances.[58] In addition, his minimalist requirements for beneficent action in a common-morality framework have no semblance to a biblical concept of *agape*. Yet, despite such allusions to *agape* love, Childress provides little insight into his anthropology of human destiny and the good that human beings should pursue. In this regard, Courtney notes that Childress's reliance on a common morality limits the scope of his appreciation for the influence of theologically particular moral communities on the moral meaning and significance of the principles.[59]

Campbell further notes that Childress makes correlations between the plurality of the divine nature in the Trinity and an ethical method that draws from multiple moral principles. Childress perceives these principles to be independent of, rather than derived from, a single norm, such as love. Theology illuminates relevant moral obligations that are already accepted by non-believers on non-theological grounds, a position reminiscent of Richard McCormick's natural law idea.[60] According to him, the idea of common moral obligations and a natural law are the same for all human beings and, along with moral law, are not dependent on faith or revelation. Rather, the latter provide *motivation* for fulfilling universal moral commitments.[61] For both Childress, the Quaker, and McCormick, the Roman Catholic, reason provides the mechanism for discovery. Along with Charles Curran, McCormick says, "From the viewpoint of moral theology

---

58. Ibid., 131; Ramsey, *Basic Christian Ethics*, 14, 89. Campbell notes that Childress and Ramsey disagree here in that Ramsey considers justice as a second-order derivative of love, yet both justice and love are rooted in Scripture. Ramsey's principle of justice is "To each according to the measure of his real need, not because of anything human reason can discern inherent in the need but because his need alone is the measure of God's righteousness towards him" (14). Love goes beyond this: "Everything is lawful, absolutely everything is permitted which love permits, everything without a single exception" (89).

59. Campbell, "On James F. Childress," 152.

60. Ibid., 135; Childress, *Priorities*, 102ff.; Childress, "Scripture and Christian Ethics," 279ff. Childress makes a curious link between the *prima facie* status of his principles and the interaction of the three persons of the Trinity. However, as Campbell points out, there is a limit to this analogical link, exemplified in that the inseparability of the persons of the Trinity has no counterpart in Childress's principlism. In addition, moral principles are not necessarily derived from a single overarching norm such as love. Here again he departs significantly from Ramsey, who believes moral principles and rules are derived from *agape* love.

61. Cahill, "On Richard McCormick," 88. Cahill feels that McCormick ties his ideas more integrally with biblical texts than many of his Catholic peers.

or Christian ethics anyone who admits human reason as a source of moral wisdom adopts a natural law perspective."[62]

By contrast, Hauerwas rejects natural law and abandons the search for a universally agreed-upon morality. To him this idea is an illusion and a manifestation of liberalism, with its language of the larger society that supersedes distinct sub-communities of faith.[63] Rather than being an illuminator or motivator of substantive moral principles discoverable through reason, the Christian faith encompasses a particular morality distinctive in its commitments to God based on his covenant with human beings.[64] Morality should focus on character, not on decision-making, if its purpose is to instruct people about who they are and might become.[65] To practice Christian ethics, says Hauerwas, one must acknowledge that we are sinners sustained by the moral resources given to us by God. The moral life path is a meta-narrative of stories that forms a community, and Christian ethics must assist the community in the task of being truthful.[66] A major consequence of secularization is the mode of public discourse that engages secular themes within a culture of individualism, themes such as universal rights, individual self-direction, procedural justice, and a systematic denial of either an overarching good or a transcendent individual good. This secularization was aided in the 1970s by the redirection of theological institutions to issues of poverty, economic justice, and racial equality. The few theologians who entered the field seemed more comfortable framing the issues in secular and philosophical rather than theological terms, while philosophers and lawyers teamed up with physicians to become the leaders in the new field of bioethics.[67]

Gustafson laments that due to their increasing theological silence, theologians have been failing those in religious communities who want to live out their lives in faith "not just with impartial rationality."[68] This

---

62. Porter, *Natural and Divine Law*, 31; Curran and McCormick, *Natural Law and Theology*, 1.

63. Hauerwas, *Against the Nations*, 18; Lammers, "On Stanley Hauerwas," 58. For Hauerwas, liberalism is an impulse derived from the Enlightenment to free people from their historical particularity in the name of freedom.

64. Lammers, "On Stanley Hauerwas," 58–59.

65. Ibid., 60.

66. Ibid., 63. For a more contemporary discussion of the importance of narrative for understanding Scripture as a grand story, see Bartholomew and Goheen, *The Drama of Scripture*.

67. Verhey and Lammers, "Introduction," 3.

68. Verhey, "On James Gustafson," 30.

amounts to theologians abandoning their responsibility to do Christian ethics theologically. Scholarly Jewish voices such as Leon Kass also complain that religious ethicists are leaving their special insights at the door.[69] Asking if the Western world lives in the morally fragmented world as portrayed by MacIntyre, Hauerwas protests, why should secular rationality become the privileged mode that gains a monopoly on moral standards?[70] Some theologians seem to fear revealing their deepest convictions at conferences, preferring to talk the common language, or what Jeffrey Stout calls the *moral Esperanto*,[71] in order to be accepted. Leading Christian ethicists like Edmund Pellegrino admire principlism as one attempt to establish a common language even while criticizing its lack of genuine moral content and authority.[72]

Very recently, Christian sociologist John H. Evans observes that public debates about human cloning served to consolidate the formal rationality of bioethics and to establish autonomy as an unexamined end in itself. At the same time, the tendency remains for theologians to capitulate to a procedural bioethics that reduces substantive moral values to autonomy and informed consent.[73] Gilbert Meilaender supports Evans's thesis that government commissions are not constituted in response to a desire to achieve overlapping consensus in an increasingly pluralistic society. Rather, they are created to preserve research from public oversight by designating professional bioethicists from a wide diversity of traditions and disciplines to do the job.[74] This, Evans proposes, represents the desire of the scientific community to avoid formal regulation of their work in genetics.

---

69. Kass, "Practicing Ethics," 6–7; Marty, "Medical Ethics," 246–47.

70. Lammers, "On Stanley Hauerwas," 59.

71. Stout, *Ethics After Babel*, 5–6, 60–81, 294. On page 5, Stout suggests that moral Esperanto arises when philosophy aspires to universality. It becomes the moral language and its rules become the deep structure of morality. Nonconformity with those rules becomes a sign of viciousness or irrationality and the diversity of moral languages ceases to matter.

72. Pellegrino, "Four Principles," 360. He has praised principlism for providing a *lingua franca* for communication among doctors and ethicists "whose moral presuppositions might otherwise have been incommensurable with one another." According to his perspective, the simple use of a common moral Esperanto still lacks the moral authority to override or neutralize fundamental moral beliefs as the basis for moral positions.

73. Evans, *Playing God?*, 158–65.

74. Meilaender, "Comments of Gilbert Meilaender," 192.

Because such commissions found considerable difficulty arriving at moral agreement, substantive modes of argument gave way to more formal and process-oriented ones. As a result, the content of arguments and their justifications "thinned" as consensus was sought. This process began during deliberations about human experimentation by the Belmont Commission but soon became the basic method for moral thinking in bioethics in general. Meilaender suggests that advisory commissions may best serve the public when they are not pressured to forge lowest-common-denominator recommendations (i.e., those that inevitably marginalize the deepest concerns of religious believers) but rather when they are free to play out the arguments.[75] In fact, Jeffrey Stout presents the view that commissions, by nature, are modern equivalents to feudal councils that actually insulate policy-making from a wider context of public deliberation.[76] In my view, Evans, Stout, and Meilaender touch on an important conspiratorial element wherein societal leaders seek to preserve scientific progress by professionalizing and insulating bioethical concerns and to debate rather than confront the ethical and societal implications of such "progress."

One objective of consensus agreement within principlism is the "neutralizing" of positions in order to avoid justificatory associations with basic beliefs that could conflict and thwart consensus. Lisa Cahill, however, argues that public discourse is not value neutral but possesses its own core values of individualism, faith in science and technology, profits and markets, etc. She challenges theologians to recover their religiously distinctive prophetic voices and enter public policy debates as energetic adversaries of the liberal consensus. To accomplish this, they must "remain unapologetically theological in orientation, while still seeking common cause and building a common language with all who are similarly committed to health care justice."[77]

Callahan also expresses a sense of disillusionment and discontent with the detached neutrality and rationalistic universalism reflected in the Belmont Report. This universalism is played out in attempts to find consensus through the pursuit of common moral judgments, in turn sought through iterative debate toward reflective equilibrium; these are all central tenets of principlism. He complains that the *principles movement* draws as

75. Ibid., 192, 193, 195.
76. Stout, "Comments of Jeffrey Stout," 190.
77. Cahill, *Theological Bioethics*, 18. Reformed philosopher Roy Clouser (*Myth of Religious Neutrality*, 185–233) agrees that religious neutrality is a myth. Theoretical thinking is not autonomous; all theories are unavoidably formed and regulated by some type of religious belief.

Part One: The Rise and Dominance of Principles-Based Biomedical Ethics

much from "unfettered imagination" (a quality that he previously lauded) as it does from logic.[78] The rules of the language of common morality deny the particulars and irregularities of real communities, discourage vision and speculation about goals and meaning, and promulgate the discourse of wary strangers preoccupied with rights as the preferred mode of daily relations.[79]

Another important debate regarding principlism is *the relationship between the principles.* Jonsen notes that there is a surprising paucity of references to respect for persons or respect of autonomy in modern moral philosophy and in early bioethical literature.[80] The Belmont Commission's special emphasis on the right of research subjects to autonomously choose to participate in research puts the priority for bioethical scholarship squarely on the human research subject and away from foundational matters. Engelhardt's essay for the Commission elevates respect for the freedom of persons as *the* value that forms the basis of the human sense of moral responsibility, an idea admittedly arising from the Kantian ideal of freedom as a presupposition for claims to morality.[81] Elsewhere, Engelhardt declares that autonomy is a basic presupposition for secular ethics.[82]

In this chapter, we have examined challenges to principlism within the moral disquiet of fragmented morality in Western culture. This problem of moral fragmentation is compounded by the dominant reliance on rationality as the source of understanding and knowledge at the explicit exclusion of the religious basic beliefs. This leads to a search for conceptual and justificatory stability through certain moral principles that cannot (or will not) be grounded on transcendent, presuppositional truth or ideals. The result is an oscillating movement of conceptual importance from principles to case and back again, with a concomitant lack of justification for making specific moral choices.

Based on this assessment, it is my contention that there is a need to return to an ethical framework that provides firm and reliable

78. Callahan, "Religion," 3; Jonsen, *Birth of Bioethics,* 329.
79. Callahan, "Religion," 4.
80. Jonsen, *Birth of Bioethics,* 334.

81. Engelhardt, "Basic Ethical Principles," 2. Citing Kant, he holds the proposition that persons, being free, must be presupposed in any discussion about human morality.

82. Engelhardt, *Foundations of Bioethics,* 43–46; Veatch, *Theory of Medical Ethics,* 193–95. Veatch and Rawls promote this prominent position for autonomy as a basis for their theories of contract.

authoritative grounding and justification for moral choices and policies. The principles themselves have validity as concepts that connote moral values or rights, which, in turn, retain some normativity despite the distortion of human relationships and actions arising from sin. However, the principles require recontexualization within an ethical framework grounded on moral authority and justification outside of rational consensus alone. In the next two chapters, I will review the voices of bioethicists from various broad and diverse faith traditions who express a wide variety of responses to principles-based ethics. In the next chapter, I will present perspectives of representative figures from major Christian traditions, as well as views from Islamic and Jewish traditions. In chapter 4, I will show how diverse the responses to principlism have been within some traditions, as exemplified by views within Roman Catholic and Anglican traditions. In addition, as the end of chapter 4, I will provide my own perspective and insights into the basic beliefs and worldviews that have shaped principlism from my Reformed Christian tradition. Only with such an in-depth understanding of principlism can a more substantive ethical framework be developed that gives greater moral meaning and relational relevance to biomedical ethics.

3

Perspectives on Principles from Diverse Faith Traditions

Ramsey, in spite of his strong declarations to be working as a Christian ethicist, prepared the way for the developments that Gustafson laments—that is, the subordination of theological ethics to medical ethics ... in many ways, the more orthodox Ramsey prepared the way for the Christian ethicist to become a medical ethicist with a difference, the difference being the vague theological presumptions that do no serious intellectual work other than explaining, perhaps, the motivations of the ethicist. As a result, Christian ethicists continue to leave the world as they found it.[1]

—STANLEY HAUERWAS ON PAUL RAMSEY (1995)

DIVERSITY ACROSS CHRISTIAN TRADITIONS: PELLEGRINO, ENGELHARDT, AND RAMSEY

IN THE LAST CHAPTER, I highlighted an overview of major movements in Christian moral thinking, beginning with the church prior to the Protestant Reformation, the influence of that movement, and the subsequent influence of the Enlightenment. In this chapter, I will illustrate the diversity of perspectives across different faith traditions concerning the role of principles in biomedical ethics. I will begin with a review of the perspectives of three influential Christian bioethicists who represent bioethical

1. Hauerwas, "How Christian Ethics," 25–26.

thinking that comes out of major distinctive Christian traditions. I will then present several views on principlism from Islamic and Jewish faith traditions.

I will begin by highlighting the contributions of key representatives of three major Christian faith groups: Edmund Pellegrino, a Roman Catholic; H. Tristram Engelhardt, representing an Eastern Orthodox perspective; and Paul Ramsey, one of the most prolific and formative writers within the Protestant tradition.

All three leaders have at various times explicitly expressed the faith beliefs of their respective Christian traditions and have been widely recognized for examining and articulating fundamental issues within bioethics through those beliefs. For instance, Pellegrino finds the four principles helpful, but he reconceptualizes them in his philosophy of medicine. For Engelhardt, by contrast, the four principles are a secular necessity for maintaining minimal moral order among moral strangers in a pluralistic society. However, they represent, he says, a hollow triumph. Substantive moral content and meaning are found in particular communities of specific faith commitments, the most meaningful of which is that of the Eastern Orthodox Church. Lastly, Ramsey struggles to find the normative place of principles and rules within a context of covenantal fidelity in medical relationships. The principles serve as instruments for serving others under the ultimate norm of love. Unfortunately, his covenantal ethic was developed only incompletely toward the latter part of his career. However, his incomplete ethical framework has been further developed by William F. May. Working out of that Reformed Christian tradition, I continue their efforts more systematically, as I will show in part two, which explores a robust covenantal ethical framework for the web of medical relationships.

Edmund Pellegrino: Leading Persistent Roman Catholic Voices

Christian theologians from various traditions began to address a growing number of bioethical issues in medicine in the 1960s. This interest came out of a long tradition of Christian concerns for the value of human life at all stages of development and function. The church addressed moral issues of the unborn as early as the first century in the *Didache (Teaching of the Twelve Apostles)*.[2] However, specific references to medical ethics only appeared around the sixteenth century. In the Roman Catholic tradition that emerged after the Reformation, moral theology began to focus more

---

2. Jones, *Soul and the Embryo*, 57.

PART ONE: The Rise and Dominance of Principles-Based Biomedical Ethics

intensely on issues of biomedical ethics, particularly from the nineteenth century onward, in the form of treatises and practical guides for pastors ministering to the sick in Catholic hospitals. David Kelly documents the development of Roman Catholic moral theology in biomedical ethics, outlining the dominant method of identifying moral principles from natural law and Scripture using casuistic analyses of specific medical topics.[3]

Direct papal interest in matters of biomedical ethics increased markedly in the 1950s, expressed through numerous papal statements by Pope Pius XII. But resistance to magisterial interpretations and reliance on natural law doctrine also increased. Catholic scholars such as Richard McCormick, Charles Curran, and Bernard Haring have advocated for moving away from the physicalism of natural-law doctrine toward a greater attention to direct biblical teaching on pastoral matters of moral living. Abortion and contraception have also been flashpoints of concern among Catholic laity. Traditional moral theology was inadequately addressing increasingly complex biomedical issues brought on by new technologies, and formative lay scholars such as Callahan, Cahill, and others previously mentioned have been helping to revitalize dialogue among church scholars.[4] McCormick has argued that those who dissent from magisterial teaching speak with legitimate voices by teaching through dialogue.[5]

McCormick has sought to make natural law a more experience-based, malleable concept adaptable to contemporary bioethical problems and to draw the natural-law method closer toward an overall Christian commitment to bioethics. Out of this response to traditional church teaching, the method of *proportionalism* challenges the traditional idea of intrinsically evil acts by re-evaluating of the role of "objective" particulars within individual moral dilemmas. This approach questions the adequacy of absolute moral rules that label certain acts as sinful when determining right and wrong actions in all situations.[6]

Out of this movement toward relevant moral teaching, Edmund Pellegrino offers a philosophical approach that recontextualizes the four principles within a faithful expression of his Christian tradition. Amidst these struggles within Roman Catholic thought, Pellegrino promotes an understanding of medicine as a distinct expression of human relating through beneficence toward the needy. Unlike McCormick and other

3. Jonsen, *Birth of Bioethics*, 36; Kelly, *Emergence*.
4. Jonsen, *Birth of Bioethics*, 37–38.
5. Cahill, "On Richard McCormick," 84–85.
6. Ibid., 81.

Catholic theologians who are embroiled in the struggle to challenge and re-define normative church teaching, he is a physician with no advanced degree in philosophy or theology. Yet, he is also a former director of the Kennedy Institute of Ethics, founder of the Center for Bioethics at Georgetown University, and founding editor of the *Journal of Medicine and Philosophy*. Pellegrino is boldly committed to teaching the expression of the Christian faith in the practice of medicine:

> Christian physicians fail in their obligations if they do not witness in private and public life to the way the values of the Gospel can and do transform their lives. . . . Then the issue is how, in a pluralistic society, the Christian physician can remain both Christian and a physician, acting charitably toward those who do not share his or her view but simultaneously responding to Christ's invitation: "Come, follow me."[7]

He was a consultant for the Belmont Commission,[8] later praising Beauchamp and Childress for having "skillfully and wisely taken four principles of 'the common morality' as *prima facie* guides to the resolution of practical medical ethical dilemmas."[9] The principles, he says, give order to the process of moral decision-making, increase sensitivities to ethical issues, and provide a common language around the table of moral discourse.[10] However, he then notes that this principles-based ethic has been criticized for its lack of grounding in a moral philosophy.[11]

Pellegrino outlines the cultural and historical circumstances that have led to "the relative poverty of ethical theory in American bioethics."[12] The Enlightenment challenged the presuppositions behind virtue ethics, including a distinct good as the goal of human existence and an authority from which morality could claim its moral force. Through the influence of Immanuel Kant, principles and duties became ends in themselves,

---

7. Pellegrino and Thomasma, *Christian Virtues*, 2. While Pellegrino co-authored several key publications with David Thomasma concerning various aspects of his philosophy of medicine and his critique of principlism, I agree with Daniel Sulmasy ("The Essentialist Medical Ethics," xxvii) that the dominant voice in these publications seems to be that of Pellegrino. Consequently, I will refer primarily to Pellegrino in this section.

8. See chapter 1.

9. Pellegrino, "What the Philosophy," 324.

10. Pellegrino, "Four Principles," 360.

11. Pellegrino, "What the Philosophy," 324; Clouser and Gert, "Critique of Principlism."

12. Jonsen, *Birth of Bioethics*, 379.

PART ONE: The Rise and Dominance of Principles-Based Biomedical Ethics

while the cultivation of character became a secondary moral enterprise. Furthermore, moral authority shifted away from a supratemporal God toward human reason. As a result, people today look for moral guidance through faith in reason rather than through beliefs that bind specific moral communities. Consequently, those with belief in a moral authority other than reason are expected to keep such beliefs private. This is the credo behind the Belmont Report, principlism, and the President's Commission for the Study of Ethical Problems in Medicine and Biomedical and Behavioral Research.[13] Principles are sought that can be commonly accepted and followed and that transcend the beliefs of particular communities.[14] Recently, even reason has come under attack, and moral philosophy has turned to emotivism for solace and meaning. Thus, moral relativism and skepticism have gained normative status in moral philosophy and bioethics.[15] Bioethics has become a *process-oriented ethic*, ostensibly for overcoming obstacles to consensus on substantive ethical issues that are attributed to religious and cultural diversity within a pluralistic society.

Against this backdrop, Pellegrino sets out to develop a philosophy of medicine that is linked to an ethics of medicine and that is grounded in the physician-patient relationship.[16] The *architectonic* that grounds his philosophy is *the good of the patient*. It is the *telos* toward which all patient-care activity is directed.[17] While conclusions derived from such a philosophy may be congruent with principles-based ethics, they are grounded in something more fundamental than common morality. In his philosophy, such conclusions are based on a metaphysic that is, in turn, built upon concepts of ends, goods, rights, dignity, and norms, all of which give meaning to bioethical arguments and choices. Pellegrino notes the influence of the contractual theory of Locke and its premise that human beings have the inherent negative right not to be harmed or coerced by others. This theory subsequently developed into an individualistic egoism most notably articulated by Robert Nozick.[18] Thus, community is transformed from being defined by a notion of the good (often a transcendent God)

---

13. Pellegrino, "Epilogue: Religion," 139–40.

14. Pellegrino and Thomasma, *Christian Virtues*, 8. In the language of neo-Calvinism, the loss of direction has resulted in a distorted recognition of the content of morality due to the loss of a transcendent grounding.

15. Pellegrino, "Epilogue: Religion," 140–41.

16. Pellegrino and Thomasma, *Philosophical Basis*.

17. Pellegrino, "Four Principles," 360, 362.

18. Nozick, *Anarchy, State, and Utopia*.

into being defined by common self-interests.[19] From a Nordic cultural perspective, Hendrik Wulff has voiced similar concerns about individualism ingrained within principlism. He contrasts this individualism with what he calls the "Golden Rule approach" that is pervasive in the Nordic cultures. He cites the 1988 Appleton Consensus Conference on guidelines for foregoing medical treatment as an example of the individualistic and legalistic spirit of principlism with its emphasis on self-determination (i.e., autonomy) at the expense of other principles. This leads to contractual relationships based largely on mutual respect for party rights. By contrast, the Golden Rule approach is more concerned with having an empathic understanding of patients' experiences of illness. In this case, true human autonomy involves duties to others, and human rights are secondary to these duties to others. Wulff argues that the roots of this Golden Rule approach are grounded in the Sermon on the Mount, its moral codex, and the Lutheran faith tradition but with a strong affinity to Kantian moral theory. In comparing the two moral approaches, he concludes that the Golden Rule encompasses the four principles, while the principles, when ranked, are incompatible with the Golden Rule.[20]

Rather than abandoning the four principles, Pellegrino argues that they need linkages with other sources of ethical insight.[21] Virtues of the moral agent must be infused into the concept of principles, which in turn must be grounded in the phenomena of physician-patient relationships.[22] The virtue of charity or love provides guidance regarding how the principles are lived out and applied to specific situations. By contrast, strong paternalism is uncharitable toward patients by denying full freedom to be accountable for one's responsibilities and decisions. Love *informs* the four principles; that is, the virtue of love illuminates a special way of living out the principles and applying them to specific situations. By reflecting on issues such as active euthanasia or assisted suicide, love illuminates autonomy through recognition of the sovereignty of God without which autonomy can erode the communal nature of human beings. However, in a secular context, autonomy often conflicts with beneficence, is the dominant principle in principlism, and thus distorts the relationship between

19. Pellegrino and Thomasma, *Christian Virtues*, 120; Bellah et al., *Habits of the Heart*.

20. Wulff, "Against the Four Principles," 279–86.

21. Pellegrino, "Four Principles," 360.

22. Pellegrino and Thomasma, *Christian Virtues*, 117–24; Pellegrino, "The Four Principles," 362. This "grounding" seems too narrow to me as it excludes other relationships in medical encounters and does not account for other aspects of medicine.

the principles. For Pellegrino, such conflicts must be worked out through love in the spirit of the Beatitudes, which he connects directly to the personhood of Jesus Christ.[23]

To the four principles, Pellegrino wants to give substance and moral authority that is "as much a reality of the moral life as love and cannot be fully disengaged from it."[24] Within the same natural-law tradition as McCormick and other contemporary Catholic theologians,[25] Pellegrino sees the *fours principles as structural realities* that can be ascertained by human reason alone. Religious belief expands their significance and enlightens their meaning.

Pellegrino examines in detail the four principles in the context of the physician-patient relationship. He acknowledges that principlism has dominated bioethics since the late 1960s if one includes the early influence of William Ross.[26] In his reconceptualization, the principles are grounded in the phenomena of human relationships, more specifically in the obligations owed to humans by humans. These obligations, in turn, derive from our status as creatures of God, with whom we are drawn into a relationship through grace.[27] True to his Thomist synthesis tradition, however, he also believes that the traditional Hippocratic model has served medicine well. In the Hippocratic Oath, a covenantal relationship between physicians and their mentors is described, and a code of behavior guides physician and patient relationships.

In principlism, autonomy is perceived as protection against coercion and abuse of physician power and also as the preservation of patient control over medical decisions.[28] Yet, it also provides the impetus for new, consumer-oriented models of physician-patient relations. This leads to the commodification of medical care in consumer terms and to trust in a legalistic contractual model instead of a covenantal one.[29]

---

23. Pellegrino and Thomasma, *Christian Virtues*, 74.

24. Ibid. They go on to say that these principles, along with rules and duties, are chosen or shaped by charity.

25. Cahill, "On Richard McCormick," 89; McCormick, *Critical Calling*, 204; McCormick, "Does Religious Faith," 156; McCormick, "Bioethics in the Public Forum," 124. According to McCormick, it is the Catholic position that reason informed by faith allows the Catholic Christian to share fully in discussions in the public forum. Thus, the Christian community gains access to "a privileged articulation" of "common human experience."

26. Pellegrino and Thomasma, *Christian Virtues*, 117.

27. Ibid., 107.

28. Pellegrino, "Four Principles," 354–55.

29. May, *Physician's Covenant*.

Pellegrino is critical of the distorting dominance of autonomy in the practice of principlism; his solution is the reorientation of autonomy through Thomist virtue ethics. In this ethical framework, obligations to one's community and to God are directed toward the good realized by the community and are fully realized through prudence and love. Autonomy is an inherent capacity of rational human beings and a moral claim for humans to act toward each other so that the capacity to self-govern can be fully realized.[30] However, absolutized autonomy is not compatible with the notion of creation as seen through a Christian worldview.[31] In its place, beneficence is the guiding principle through which caregivers and clinical researchers freely strive for the good of the patient above the values of science through "autonomy of trust."[32]

Pellegrino is also concerned with maintaining the autonomy of the physician, noting a growing trend toward doing the patient's bidding even if the physician's values or views consider such requests incompatible with the patient's best interests. In objecting to this trend, he recognizes a right to autonomy for the physician as a moral agent within the relationship. Justice would dictate that violating a physician's right to exercise decisions based on his or her own values is as much a maleficent act as violating the patient's right to do the same. Consequently, Pellegrino advocates for better formal mechanisms by which physicians and patients can withdraw from their relationship if confronted with irreconcilable differences in values and choice preferences.[33]

On the other hand, he is also worried about physician power leading to abuse of the more vulnerable party, the patient, yet he insists on retaining the protective aspects of that power. This requires an interaction with other principles that guides the physician to exercise beneficence and justice, sometimes requiring that these principles override autonomy if autonomy endangers the patient or others.[34] He also puts surrogate decision makers under the regulation of the four principles in an effort to protect patients from abuse. Indeed, Pellegrino sees the use of principles as helpful

30. Pellegrino and Thomasma, *Christian Virtues*, 121.
31. Ibid., 123.
32. Pellegrino, "Four Principles," 361–64.
33. Ibid., 359. Today, medical colleges and societies are formalizing the terms of dissolution of the relationship. For example, the College of Physicians and Surgeons of Ontario in Canada (College of Physicians Policy) has a policy that specifies situations whereby such dissolution may be appropriate or inappropriate and what specific actions should be used to end the relationship.
34. Ibid., 361.

when assessing if surrogate decisions should be overridden, such as when a surrogate fails to implement an incapacitated patient's previously stated wishes (an expression of the failure to act beneficently and justly).[35] His admiration for principlism, though, is tempered by its lack of relational focus. He predictably brings in natural law as an ethical theory that can bind human beings together in a mutual quest for the good that resides in the natural order of creation. It can restrict human beings from acting according to their nature and thus can protect against individualism that encourages each person to construct a moral law unto himself or herself.[36]

Pellegrino adamantly objects to the suggestion by Beauchamp and McCullough that beneficence should be equated with paternalism.[37] He considers benevolent self-effacement to be the minimum obligation compatible with the virtue of love.[38] True beneficence seeks the *telos* of medicine, the good of the patient. He offers a rich definition of this good as a hierarchy of goods, ascending from the good that heals physical and psychological aspects of the patient toward a community-associated good, culminating in the good for humans as spiritual beings.[39] Using this hierarchy, he associates autonomy with a human good that can allow for the fullest capacity for one to make responsible choices within a life plan. He considers the promotion of this full capacity to be a benevolent act and sees autonomy (as respect for person in this context) as congruent with, rather than antithetical to, beneficence.

Unlike the other principles of principlism, justice is seen as both a virtue and a principle. Justice is considered a prior principle in the sense that it drives action components of the other principles in seeking the right and the good. For instance, justice is behind the obligation to not harm other human beings, to respect their autonomy, and to do good when possible. Today, justice is often overridden by autonomy, as when

---

35. Ibid., 360.

36. Pellegrino and Thomasma, *Christian Virtues*, 118. They are regrettably vague on this distinction and do not develop his natural law idea in this context very well.

37. Beauchamp and McCullough, *Medical Ethics*.

38. Pellegrino and Thomasma, *Christian Virtues*, 75. In this sense, I would contend that nonmaleficence is unnecessary and meaningless as an independent principle. I will discuss this further in chapter 8.

39. Pellegrino, "Four Principles," 357. This hierarchy fits well with his Thomistic theology but risks losing a more wholistic concept of the patient within the medical context.

a patient who carries the human immunodeficiency virus (HIV/AIDS) refuses to disclose this to sexual partners.[40]

Pellegrino proposes a philosophical orientation of medicine around the good of the patient. It is focused on the physician-patient relationship, though some mention is made of patient surrogates as well. Love is considered an informing and illuminating virtue for the application of principles and for assisting in the resolution of conflicting principles. As well, Pellegrino considers beneficence to be the guiding principle that unifies biomedical ethics and keeps physicians and patients in relationship through autonomy of trust. Thus, the obligation of beneficence renders nonmaleficence devoid of moral force. Rather, implicit in the physician-patient relationship is a promise to act in the best interest of the patient over the interests of the physician. In brief, justice is a requisite duty that crosses other principles and embodies the trust put forward in the offer to help, as well as the confidence engendered by the expressed willingness to act beneficently.[41]

Pellegrino attempts to synthesize the principles with an ethic of virtue taken from the systematic work of Thomas Aquinas.[42] In this ethical framework, natural virtues are those ascertainable by reason alone; they include the cardinal virtues of justice, prudence (or wisdom), temperance, and fortitude. By contrast, the theological or supernatural virtues of faith, hope, and love are gifts of God through grace that have a prominent, guiding role for Christians. These virtues can take the natural virtues to levels of perfection. For example, faith perfects nature, while love is the ordering virtue of the Christian life.[43] Pellegrino humbly acknowledges that virtue ethics has its own limitations but believes that *a complete moral philosophy must take into account both a principles-based and a virtue-based system.* The theological virtues reshape both the natural virtues and the philosophical principles. The principles are raised to the level of grace through the operation of love.[44] He does not explain the relationship of principles

---

40. Ibid., 358.
41. Ibid., 363.
42. Pellegrino and Thomasma, *Christian Virtues*, 6–22.
43. Ibid., 19, 21. Roman Catholic philosopher Josef Pieper (*Belief and Faith*, 60) speaks of the virtues as enabling a human being to seek attainment of the full potential of her nature. He explains that such a conception of virtue is only possible with the inclusion of one's relation to God and the acknowledgment of our creatureliness.
44. Ibid., 22–25, 109, 117. Pellegrino exhibits some terminological ambiguities that raise questions about the relationship between love and the four principles. For example, at one point he speaks of beneficence-in-trust as the ordering principle

to the natural virtues except to acknowledge justice as both a principle and a cardinal virtue.

In my view, Pellegrino's attempt at merging the dualistic synthesis of supernatural and natural elements with principlism remains problematic. Christ's command to love God and fellow human beings summarizes God's law under the new covenant. *All* virtues mentioned by Pellegrino are gifts from God, to be used for his glory and as dispositions or goals of the Christian moral agent.

Pellegrino states that the "grounding" of his philosophy of medicine is in the good of the patient. This is very much aligned with Alasdair MacIntyre's suggestion that particular human practices have defined ends that can specify that good objectively.[45] However, Pellegrino's use of the term "grounding" in this context connotes the ultimate goal or purpose of medicine functionally and vocationally as its ultimate source of moral authority, rather than the triune God. In my judgment, this leaves his otherwise helpful analysis of principlism seriously wanting. He encourages more attention to relationality but fails to appreciate the central importance of the biblical theme of covenant in conceptualizing relationships in medicine. The covenant relationship with God provides the true meaning and purpose of seeking the good of patients. It also allows for broader reflection on the other caregiver-patient relationships in medicine that Pellegrino does not address. Such grounding would provide justification for moral dispositions, options, and choices between human caregivers and provide the template for human relational interactions. I also agree with some critics who observe that he concentrates too much on the beliefs, attitudes, actions, and moral duties of the physician and not enough on those of the patient.[46]

---

among these principles ("Four Principles," 363) while at another point he calls love the ordering principle that can resolve conflicts between moral principles and raise each *prima facie* moral principle to the level of grace (Pellegrino and Thomasma, *Christian Virtues*, 109). Oliver O'Donovan (*Resurrection and Moral Order*, 199–202, 226) also speaks of love as the supreme ordering principle that unifies obligations under the moral law and confers unifying order on the moral field and the character of the moral subject. However, his use of love as the single ordering principle can be distinguished from Pellegrino's idea of love elevating each principle to the levels of grace.

45. MacIntyre (*After Virtue*, 272–77) speaks of "goods internal to practices . . . are . . . but excellences specific to those types of practices," (274). For him as with Pellegrino, the exercise of virtues gain point and purpose both for their own sake and through ends or goods that characterize that practice.

46. Sulmasy, "Essentialist Medical Ethics," xxix. Daniel Sulmasy suggests that Pellegrino extends his characterizations of physicians to other health care professionals by implication. I am not convinced of this. If it were true, however, such packaging of

Pellegrino has been criticized for formulating an incomplete philosophy of medicine and for a lack of philosophical rigor in his deductive arguments regarding moral solutions.[47] Daniel Sulmasy suggests that Pellegrino's philosophy is a "bottom-up" approach to bioethics, looking first at the nature, purpose, and meaning of medicine, then building a theory of biomedical ethics from the ground up.[48] Unlike Ramsey, Pellegrino is not seeking to develop rules and principles in this pursuit of the medical encounter and experience. To the latter's credit, he attempts to avoid the contemporary dialectic tension between fitting particulars of moral situations into theories versus deducing solutions from theories.[49] Sulmasy alludes to this when he notes that Pellegrino's attempt to understand "medicine *qua* medicine" first and then work out moral obligations within a philosophical framework is "One way out of the moral cacophony in medical bioethics."[50] In Pellegrino's philosophy, the basis for normative content in biomedical ethics involves established virtues and principles as well as an appeal to the divine, who gives order and meaning to human activities and decisions.

Pellegrino has faith that physicians and patients will achieve a shared understanding of the human essence within the medical encounter through reasoned reflection when they understand the essence of medicine and of being a patient.[51] While at times he seems to slide toward appeal to the common morality, albeit through his belief in natural law, he fights hard to overcome the secular pressure to establish moral standards through intersubjective consensus or to compromise with other beliefs. However, in my view, his dualistic grace/nature framework puts an enlightened gloss— rather than redemptive pervasion—of grace on otherwise free-standing

---

caregiver morality would not do justice to distinctions in professional functioning and to distinctions of character within caregiving.

47. Van Leeuwen and Kimsma, "Philosophy of Medical Practice," 99–112; Sulmasy, "Essentialist Medical Ethics," xxviii.

48. Sulmasy, "Essentialist Medical Ethics," xxii. Beauchamp and Childress (*Principles of Biomedical Ethics*, 5th ed., 301–97) note that the term "bottom-up" is also used to connote methods of bioethical deliberation beginning with particulars of cases and developing more general rules and principles from such particulars.

49. As mentioned in chapter 1, this methodological tension is created by the search for moral meaning and justification and has encouraged the dominance of principlism. Also as discussed in chapter 1, Callahan speaks of a tension-ridden dialectic between physicians and scientists as well as between philosophers and theologians. See Callahan, "Bioethics as a Discipline," 68–73.

50. Sulmasy, "Essentialist Medical Ethics," xxii. I agree with his assessment.

51. Ibid., xxv.

bioethical rules and principles. This, I submit, remains a stumbling block toward a vision of biomedical ethics as wholly redeemed through Christ.[52]

H. Tristram Engelhardt: An Orthodox Voice in the Wilderness

One Christian tradition that claims to avoid this dualism is the Eastern Orthodox tradition. H. Tristram Engelhardt began his career as a philosopher of Kant and Hegel, then obtained an MD degree and moved into biomedical ethics. Jonsen calls him "the *enfant terrible* of bioethics: irrepressible, irreverent, unpredictable, but ever insightful and brilliant."[53] Engelhardt has also spoken from two faith traditions. Between the first and second editions of his book *The Foundations of Bioethics*, he converted from Roman Catholicism to the Antiochian Orthodox fellowship of the Eastern Orthodox faith.[54] This change is reflected in the differences in perspectives expressed in *The Foundations of Bioethics* and in his subsequent book *The Foundations of Christian Bioethics*.[55]

In the former, he agrees with MacIntyre that Western culture has become morally fragmented, but for Engelhardt, the damage to society as a whole is beyond repair. His main contribution to the Belmont Commission is his formulation of respect for persons as free agents, which he sees as a logical condition of morality.[56] Freedom is a Kantian presupposition underlying claims to knowledge and morality among many secular bioethicists. It is the basis for our sense of moral responsibility.[57] In the first edition of *The Foundations of Bioethics*, Engelhardt joins his secular counterparts in addressing the problem of finding common moral ground. The moral authority of foundational principles of respect for autonomy and beneficence can be established by mutual agreement. The latter principle

---

52. Ibid., xxix. As I will show in chapter 7, a view of medicine through the perspective of a covenant-based ethic can allow this foundation to be more fully realized for the physician-patient encounter but also for other medical relationships.

53. Jonsen, *Birth of Bioethics*, 82.

54. Meilaender, "Book Review."

55. Engelhardt, *Foundations of Bioethics*, 1st ed.; Engelhardt, *Foundations of Bioethics*, 2nd ed.; Engelhardt, *Foundations of Christian Bioethics*, xvi and xxi n 17. In the preface to *Foundations of Christian Bioethics*, he takes time to note that he was a "born-again Texan Orthodox Catholic" at the time of the second edition of *Foundations of Bioethics*. In both editions of the latter book he makes distinctions between moral strangers and moral friends.

56. Jonsen, *Birth of Bioethics*, 153.

57. Ibid., 334.

affirms the common community of welfare and sympathies of which morality consists.[58] Abstract concepts of autonomy and beneficence are filled in by continuous efforts to resolve disputes peacefully. This characterizes the minimal moral conditions of secular bioethics that can allow for necessary peace among communities of divergent beliefs in a pluralistic society.[59] There co-exist two concentric moral communities: 1) a larger, secular community with minimal moral conditions to which all can agree and 2) smaller, culturally and religiously distinct communities in which persons can participate in a richer moral life that is founded on their own concept of the good.[60] His vision of morality at that time was uniformly consistent with that proposed in principlism.

In *The Foundations of Christian Bioethics*, Engelhardt draws heavily from the moral strength that comes from his Antiochian Orthodox community.[61] Here, he is highly critical of the Roman Catholic tradition of moral discourse and the contemporary use of casuistry in bioethics. He gives the name of *crisis casuistry* to that which generates dispute and a lack of clarity regarding how to proceed with a case.[62] Contrary to Pellegrino's appreciation for the limited value of the four principles to moral discourse, Engelhardt considers their prominence in bioethics to be a failure of philosophy to justify a content-full ethical system and to be the result of a "theoretically intractable" secular moral pluralism.[63] This leads to individuals presenting themselves to each other as *moral strangers* if they do not share a moral vision that binds moral friends within a particular moral community. Thus, he calls the necessity of secular minimalist ethics among moral strangers a hollow triumph.

Engelhardt describes the religious nature of secular morality using overtly religious language. The claim of a moral vision shared by all persons (i.e., a common morality) is a *canonical secular moral vision* that lacks

58. Ibid., 330; Engelhardt, *Foundations of Bioethics*, 1st ed.

59. Engelhardt, *Foundations of Bioethics*, 2nd ed., xi. However, he says that neither edition was meant to be "a defense of a secular pluralistic ethic" as "Some may wish."

60. Jonsen, *Birth of Bioethics*, 330.

61. In this preface, he says that if one wants to engage in the "thick morality of moral friends" (to which he only superficially alludes in *Foundations of Bioethics*) that goes beyond the spare morality of secular reason that binds moral strangers who are deaf to God, one should join a religion and choose the right one. For Engelhardt (*Foundations of Christian Bioethics*, xvi), Antiochian Orthodoxy is that religion, and its thick morality is that about which he elaborates in *Foundations of Christian Bioethics*.

62. Engelhardt, *Foundations of Christian Bioethics*, 32–33. For a critique of contemporary casuistry from a Roman Catholic perspective, see Wildes, *Moral Acquaintances*.

63. Engelhardt, "Four Principles," 136.

moral content.[64] It gives the illusion of a unified moral understanding as the guide to public policy. However, in reality, the fragmentation of morality into communities of moral friends privatizes both secular and Christian moralities. He considers secular attempts at consensus to be forms of ecumenism that seek social similarities and common influences.[65] He also argues that secular bioethicists function as priests and moral theologians of a secular faith. Claims to a common secular morality embody a false consciousness, designed to hide the moral diversity that underlies its illusion of consensus.[66] The consensus of the common morality is groundless in that it seeks justification and meaning from nature and biological reality. Engelhardt cites Richard Rorty, who, in foregoing any substantive grounding for morality, presents a morality without reference to deeper meaning or transcendence. To Engelhardt, Rorty's morality has a "groundless grounding" not requiring God or even reason. Rather, it is grounded in the contingencies of history, place, and perspective.[67]

The claim of a common morality, says Engelhardt, is:

> morally equivalent to the claim the Quakers and Vikings shared the same morality, since both advanced considerations regarding the propriety of killing, though in the case of Quakers they were committed to pacifism and in the case of Vikings they recognized that, all else being equal, it was a good thing to go pillaging and murdering, as long as it took place in some other country.[68]

The four principles within principlism, he contends, are misguiding if they claim to bridge the gap between individuals who are moral strangers with real differences of moral vision. In fact, in the second edition of *The Foundations of Bioethics*, he labels adherents to the principles as moral fanatics.[69] He contends that there are competing accounts of how each principle should be worked out in particular situations and under different circumstances.

---

64. Ibid.
65. Engelhardt, "Four Principles," 144.
66. Engelhardt, *Foundations of Christian Bioethics*, 27–29.
67. Ibid., 35; Rorty, *Contingency, Irony, and Solidarity*, 59. As in principlism, Rorty reduces morality to a common morality that appeals to the interests of a community over its individuals through a common language.
68. Engelhardt, *Foundations of Christian Bioethics*, 31–32.
69. Engelhardt, *Foundations of Bioethics*, 2nd ed., 79.

For Engelhardt, autonomy can be reduced to the *principle of permission*; its basis becomes mutual permission to define morality and to act in certain ways that are deemed morally acceptable. Similarly, principles of beneficence and nonmaleficence are based on mutual agreement regarding what counts as good and what sequence those goods should assume. Among moral strangers, beneficence is dependent upon autonomy (or respect for other persons), and nonmaleficence is seen as necessary but not sufficient to show that an act is morally appropriate.

The principle of justice has no measure of acting rightly, and secular attempts to characterize restorative and retributive justice are reduced to concepts best understood in terms of autonomy. Similarly, distributive justice can encompass the good of giving persons what they are entitled instead of a larger concept of the good as human flourishing.[70] These issues, says Engelhardt, are actually reduced to concerns that fall under the beneficence principle. All of these principles are dependent in their meaning on the *principle of permission*, having little content or substance to them. Like Pellegrino, Engelhardt thinks the four principles can be recast, but unlike Pellegrino, he articulates his own vision in a theological rather than philosophical framework. He claims that the principles are evacuated of content when human beings seek a common fabric of secular morality.[71] It is the hope of the liberal state to overcome or transcend the particularities of specific smaller communities through sound rational arguments and to come to content-full moral agreement under the umbrella of a common morality. Those who do not agree can be dismissed as irrational. This moral catastrophe, as he calls it, is grounded in chains of permission and consent.

In *The Foundations of Christian Bioethics*, Engelhardt severely criticizes the faith/reason dualism in the Roman Catholic tradition for contributing significantly to the secular confidence in reason and a discursive rational universality.[72] He rejects both secular and Western Christian perspectives, while trying to articulate how his Orthodox faith puts bioethics in proper light. "Traditional Christianity" (his preferred term for

---

70. Engelhardt, "Four Principles," 137–38.

71. Ibid., 137.

72. Engelhardt, *Foundations of Bioethics*, 2nd ed., 79; Engelhardt, *Foundations of Christian Bioethics*, 45. Dennis Sullivan ("Defending Human Personhood," 292) suggests that Engelhardt's intense critique of secular bioethics was somewhat blunted by his conversion to Orthodoxy, though Meilander notes that his conversion occurred before his second edition of *Foundations of Bioethics* in which his condemnations of the secular moral project had not yet waned.

the Eastern Orthodox tradition) uses first-millennium theological texts as contemporary guides for understanding Christian morality generally and bioethics specifically within the metaphysics and axiology of a more substantive morality.[73] From this perspective, a Christian bioethics is more liturgical than scriptural. It is founded on the desire to become united with God. This is a noetic (i.e., intellectual apprehension) experience but one rooted in and identified with a mystical experience with God.[74] This view is consistent with other contemporary Orthodox ethicists such as John Breck, who sees Orthodox ethics in teleological terms of a goal-oriented vocation rather than as the deontological application of rules.[75]

Within this faith context, the four principles can be a means to the goal of union with God. Autonomy, for example, becomes redefined as the freedom to pursue union with God as one's ultimate goal and purpose in making bioethical decisions. Views of other members of the community of believers are solicited rather than considered coercive. Authority is not in the consent of individuals but in choices made within the communion of saints, who are directed by the Holy Spirit to turn the moral agent humbly and selflessly toward God the Father. If individuals are unable to keep themselves directed to God, they may be persuaded to do so, using deception if necessary, in pursuit of their salvation and the goods associate with it.[76] Paternalistic infringement on autonomous choice is considered justifiable as a means to achieve a salvific end. In support of this view, Engelhardt cites the work of early church father John Chrysostom, who teaches that physicians could act paternalistically to the point of deception if necessary for the good of the patient.[77]

---

73. Engelhardt, *Foundations of Christian Bioethics*, 159.

74. Ibid., xix n. 6, 167–68. For a more comprehensive explanation of Engelhardt's distinction between noesis or intellectual apprehension and discursive reasoning, which he condemns as a wayward consequence of the Western Christian tradition, see ibid., 216 n. 31.

75. Breck and Breck, *Stages of Life's Way*. Breck emphasizes the need to seek out the right relationship between the absolute and the situational, to critique and yet to be more accommodating with the secular sciences, and to benefit from their practical and empirical evidence.

76. Engelhardt, *Foundations of Christian Bioethics*, 356. Engelhardt points to Augustine's position on deception, which prohibited it as spiritually harmful, as a major dividing point between his Eastern and Western successors.

77. Ibid., 362–63. Chrysostom tells of a sick man who refuses appropriate medicine in favor of a long drink of wine. The physician steeps a freshly kilned pot with wine, replaces it with water, and darkens the room to deceive the patient (Chrysostom, *Six Books*, 49–50).

The other principles are seen in the same light. In short, the four principles are recast within an Eastern Orthodox view of life that focuses all moral intentions and actions on the salvation of the individual through noetic experience that brings the believer closer to union with God. Engelhardt's public health views are consistent with this, but the only fully normative health care system is one that just involves believers in the Orthodox faith. Thus, religious communities should be free to opt out of public systems in order to practice medicine as their moral system sees fit. Government should not be involved in health care.[78]

Engelhardt can be admired for his bold explication of biomedical ethics based firmly on his faith perspective. However, his intense, single-minded pursuit of a full relationship with God neglects engagement in kingdom-redemptive work within the bioethical sphere of the created order. A concept of God's kingdom on this earth is distinctly missing from his work. In his bioethical framework, biomedical ethics cannot open up in response to contemporary reality and changes in human needs. It is frozen in time and fails to account for other aspects of the created order that influence medical relationships. It is covenantal in its focus on the relationship with God but fails to work out the implications of that relationship in temporal relationships with fellow human beings.

Paul Ramsey: A Protestant Voice Not to be Silenced

Beginning in the mid-1960s, vigorous debate developed among Protestant ethicists regarding what moral framework and methods should prevail in bioethics. Joseph Fletcher, who joined the Episcopal Church as a platform for social reform, built his situationalist ethic on the idea of the "loving act" in real-life situations rather than on rules and principles.[79] One of the most vigorous opponents to situationalism is Paul Ramsey. His prominence and commitment to a scriptural basis for bioethics led to a renewed

---

78. Ibid., 380. The government-payer Canadian system, for example, should be opposed because it does not allow opting out in favor of private insurance!

79. Jonsen, *Birth of Bioethics*, 42–47. Fletcher (*Situation Ethics*, 49–50) believed that the scriptural concept of agape should be translated into a utilitarian beneficence. He made few allusions to doctrines such as sin and salvation and even suggested that such doctrines were constituted Christian mythology. Gustafson ("Context versus Principles") has suggested that the seeds of Fletcher's situationalism can be traced back to a movement in Roman Catholicism after the Second World War. Following it's condemnation by Pope Pius XII in 1952, situationalism was carried forward mainly by Protestant theologians including Gustafson himself.

examination of the religious and philosophical underpinnings of bioethics among Protestant bioethicists.[80] Ramsey sees redeeming features in moral principles and rules for guiding the work of love as a biblical notion in medical relationships.[81] Principles such as "respect for persons" are a deontological requirement expressed as a canon of loyalty between a physician and a research subject or patient. This loyalty is expressed as faithfulness, exemplified by a biblical notion of covenantal but "inprincipled" love, which he adapts to medical research and practice through the influence of Karl Barth.[82] Ramsey is an ardent critic of Fletcher's anthropocentric and utilitarian ethic, in which love seeks humankind's good. For Ramsey, love commands theocentric obedience from humankind, and principles and natural law guide the work of covenantal love. These constitute his basic but not-well-developed covenantal approach to biomedical ethics. However, it still provides groundwork upon which to build a more contemporary covenantal ethic than that developed by Ramsey.

Ramsey uses principles to stress means of right conduct, as well as the calculation of ends.[83] He sees himself as a Christian voice in a wilderness of growing moral uncertainty and conformity created by the secularization of ethics. Specifically, Ramsey feels called to counter atomistic individualism, which he believes is the root cause and motive for the breakdown of marriage and parent-child relationships in Western society.[84] Ramsey's expression of his Christian faith in his bioethical thinking is controversial.

---

80. The controversy over situationalism paralleled that between traditional moral teaching and the greater biblical emphasis of Vatican II among Roman Catholics. Perspectives expressed in this controversy are captured in Outka and Ramsey (*Norm and Context*). James Gustafson ("Context versus Principles," 186–90) also systematically explicates the debate of context vs. principles. He notes particularly Reinhold Niebuhr, J. C. Bennett, and Paul Ramsey as principle defenders of moral principles and norms in contradistinction to contextualists.

81. Jonsen, *Birth of Bioethics*, 48; Ramsey, *Basic Christian Ethics*.

82. Ramsey, *Basic Christian Ethics*; Ramsey, *Deeds and Rules*.

83. Gustafson, "Context versus Principles," 190–91. Gustafson distinguishes prescriptive and illuminative uses of principles: "In the illuminative use of principles the center of gravity is on the newness, the openness, the freedom that is present, in which the conscientious man seeks to achieve the good and do the right. In the prescriptive use of principles the center of gravity is on the reliability of traditional moral propositions and their reasonable application in a relatively open contemporary situation" (191). Gustafson points out that interpretations of Ramsey's use of principles can be prescriptive or illuminative by either contextual moralists or devotees of moral principles, showing that the diversity of views goes beyond a simple, dichotomous "context versus principles" distinction.

84. Ramsey, *Ethics at the Edge*, 139.

Perspectives on Principles from Diverse Faith Traditions

His method of combating this secularization is fundamentally theological. But Hauerwas challenges Ramsey for not matching his witness with his execution in his book *The Patient as Person*, accusing him of leaving his theology behind in the preface.[85] By contrast, Gustafson praises Ramsey for his overtly professed commitment to his Christian faith as an ethicist.[86]

Ramsey's central notion is obedient love: that which such love permits is lawful and permitted without exception.[87] Obedient love is learned from faith in Jesus Christ, transforms justice that goes beyond natural law, and protects the vulnerable and weak from societal injustice.[88] Obedient love is the unselfish seeking of the neighbor's good, a concept tied inseparably to a biblical notion of the covenant. However, a primary concern of Christian ethics is the *relationship* with the neighbor, not the neighbor's good itself. For Ramsey, neighbor love is deontologically directed toward a right relationship as a matter of obedience.[89]

Paul Camenisch rightly suggests that Ramsey's writings evolve from a notion of obedient love into a concept that makes greater use of covenant ideas and terminology. Already in his early work *Basic Christian Ethics*, Ramsey describes obedient love as the basic Christian norm for ethics because of its association with the idea of covenant and with the reign of God.[90] Camenisch further suggests that Ramsey's increased emphasis on covenantal love helps to ensure care and protection of patients from potential harm inherent in the power exercised by caregivers and by society.[91]

---

85. Hauerwas, "How Christian Ethics," 15–16; Ramsey, *Ethics at the Edge*, xiii. According to Hauerwas, in *Ethics at the Edges of Life*, Ramsey responded to the accusation that he lacked theological content in *The Patient as Person* as follows: "I do not hesitate to write as a Christian ethicist. No more did I hesitate in my first major book on medical ethics to invoke ultimate appeal to scripture or theology and to warrants such as righteousness, faithfulness, canons of loyalty . . . *hesed* (steadfast covenant love), agape."

86. Gustafson, "Theology Confronts Technology," 386–92; Ramsey, "The Indignity," 56.

87. Ramsey, *Basic Christian Ethics*, 89.

88. Hauerwas, "How Christian Ethics," 22.

89. Ramsey, *Basic Christian Ethics*, 148.

90. Ibid., 388.

91. Camenisch, "Paul Ramsey's Task," 73, 81; Ramsey, *Deeds and Rules*, 44. Camenisch suggests this in two contexts. Ramsey invokes covenantal relations that transcend human will in order to assure individuals that they will receive adequate care and protection from societal encroachment. But he also condemns atomistic individualism as a source of act-*agape*ism that "eats away at moral relations."

Part One: The Rise and Dominance of Principles-Based Biomedical Ethics

The covenant is also a concept generally attractive to both Christians and non-Christians when deliberating moral issues. Camenisch notes that over time, Ramsey makes greater use of covenant terminology to extract moral wisdom within the human community or among professionals, being less concerned with appealing to overtly Christian insights for transforming or correcting the moral solutions. Camenisch gives the example in which Ramsey claims that his negative attitude toward *in vitro* fertilization comes from "the received principles of medical ethics" with no need to appeal to religious or other ethical criteria.[92]

I agree that Ramsey hints at common moral principles that are religiously neutral within his covenant ideas.[93] Still, his increasing use of covenant language at times drifts into a more generic form of relationship, one that is more tied to natural law than to a biblically presented concept. This may show his vulnerability toward common-morality thinking in his effort to engage secular colleagues. His movement from love to covenant allows better focus on relationships and increased engagement with non-Christians but at the risk of losing the biblical meaning of covenant. Thus, Ramsey seems caught in the modern dilemma of keeping the biblical basis of covenant upfront but finding covenantal language that is less biblically obvious in order to foster dialogue with non-Christians. His struggle resonates with many Christian ethicists today.

Ramsey does not speak out directly against principles-based ethics *per se,* and stated appeals to principles in Ramsey's writings are rare. Instead, he speaks about principles individually rather than in the context of a principles-based ethical framework. Ramsey makes a rule/principle distinction to address questions as to whether or not there can be exceptions to morally relevant rules and/or principles.[94] He starts with love and the love of others and then discerns what rules would be helpful in developing those relationships.[95] Initially making the distinction between rules and principles based on expected exceptions to rules but not principles, he later admits that exceptions can provide help for defining a more mature form of a principle.[96] In later writings, he tries to focus on the importance

---

92. Ramsey, "Shall We 'Reproduce?" I., 1350; Ramsey, "Shall We 'Reproduce?" II.
93. Camenisch, "Paul Ramsey's Task," 75.
94. Ramsey, "The Case," 74.
95. Ramsey, *Deeds and Rules*, 111.
96. Ramsey, "The Case," 72; Camenisch, "Paul Ramsey's Task," 84. Camenisch quite rightly concludes that Ramsey never makes claims that general moral principles can be shown to be absolutely exceptionless. He seeks moral continuity in his arguments that exceptionless moral principles can exist but fails to demonstrate that such

of *agape* as the ultimate norm in Christian ethics while using rules in a generic sense as distinguished from single acts.[97] Unfortunately, despite inconsistencies in usage, he retains the term "rules" over time, probably because of his strong opposition to act-*agape*ism and to the anti-rule theory of situation ethics against which he so firmly reacts.

Ramsey defines principles as *directions of action*, subordinate to *agape* as the ultimate norm. Jesus Christ's death and resurrection changes the relationship between *agape* love and rules/principles, allowing for a "fresh determination" of what should be done in situations not clearly covered by law or even by love's "own former articulation in principle."[98] Through Christ's resurrection, God's love is poured out. It is the source of richer meaning for moral principles and of a "fresh determination" of what should be done in situations requiring ethical discernment.

Ramsey has a linear model for moral reasoning. From the ultimate norm (*agape*, self-realization, etc.) emerge general principles from which situation-related action principles spawn definite-action rules. Accordingly, the movement of moral reflection is in the direction toward increasing specificity. Like an umbrella over this model, the Christian outlook leads to canons of loyalty in the moral life.[99] His appeal is always to *agape*. It is the principle of principles that gives full meaning to further principles.[100] *Agape* enters into all the specifications of the moral life. It expresses itself through principles and works to unfold the meaning of the life of love.[101] At one point Ramsey considers principles to be products of the relationship

---

an ideal actually exists now *and* in the future.

97. Ramsey, "Case," 73.

98. Ramsey, *Deeds and Rules*, 195

99. Ramsey, *Patient as Person*, 5. For Ramsey, informed consent is the cardinal canon of loyalty in medical practice.

100. Ibid., 86; Ramsey, "Case," 73–74; O'Donovan, *Resurrection and Moral Order*, 232–41. This central role for agape sounds like the ordering-principle of love of which Oliver O'Donovan speaks. As already mentioned, Pellegrino sees love as informing and illuminating the four principles.

101. Ramsey distinguishes *summary–principles*, which are used by the situationalists as summaries of past experiences or empirical generalizations from *general principles*, which hold more normative force and "comprise the texture of the moral life." In general, however, principles are necessarily linked to relationships in Ramsey's ethics. Gene Outka seems to agree with this distinction, objecting to the lack of distinction by situationalists between rules or principles that merely sum up previous experiences and those that have more normative force (see Outke, "Character, Conduct," 57).

between the *agape* love-expressing Christians and their neighbors.[102] He contrasts this with rules as *particular* directives of a definite action.

Despite such confusing attempts to distinguish principles from rules, Ramsey's main thrust should not be forgotten. He appeals to Christian confidence that, in performing a fidelity obligation (i.e., an obligation based on a covenantal fidelity to act in some way), unforeseeable future consequences will not retrospectively condemn the act as wrong. Christians should love those with whom they have moral relationships and honestly attempt to act righteously.[103]

Ramsey makes a few direct comments regarding principles-based ethics as formulated by Beauchamp and Childress. He tends to organize his medical ethics along the bioethical themes and problems of his day rather than around an ethical theory or framework. He addresses the dominant issues of the day and works through his basic ethical framework by deliberating on each one. Moral principles are instruments that help to implement the ultimate norm of love toward others, particularly the weak and vulnerable. When there are conflicts between duties or obligations that reflect different moral principles, Ramsey does not appeal to a common morality or a process that drives divergent concepts toward consensus or reflective equilibrium. He appeals to the *agape principle* and its requirement for neighbor protection.[104] Principles that are recognized from this ultimate principle are only part of the moral path to right actions and solutions.

In Hauerwas's view, Ramsey does not think of the four principles in the form cast by Beauchamp and Childress and other biomedical ethicists. The principles are perceived to be reminders, as Clouser and Gert suggest, or as legitimating categories shaped by a liberal culture.[105] Ramsey's idea of covenant love and fidelity contrasts starkly with the individualism of his liberal culture. Autonomy and the role of consent in medical research and medical care are particularly important for him in his rejection of such individualism. His acknowledgment of sin, his need to advocate protection for the needy and vulnerable, and his commitment to favoring human relations over rules all lead to a strong stand on informed consent.[106]

---

102. Smith, "On Paul Ramsey," 12. Seemingly in agreement with Ramsey, David H. Smith calls principles the products of the relationship between the one who loves (in the agape sense) and the neighbor who is loved.

103. Evans, "Paul Ramsey," 44–45.

104. Smith, "On Paul Ramsey," 14.

105. Hauerwas, "How Christian Ethics," 14

106. Ibid., 14–15. From his own Christian perspective, Hauerwas questions why

Ramsey does not stress a principle of autonomy. Instead, he emphasizes consent as "free and informed participation in medical decisions," made necessary by our weakness as fallen human beings who need protection.[107]

In *The Patient as Person*, Ramsey calls the "principle" of informed consent "the cardinal *canon of loyalty*." Through consent, the faithfulness that is normative for all covenants is specifically applied to human relations encompassed within the practice of medicine.[108] In his rejection of child participation in nonbeneficial experimentation, he combines relational and vulnerability concerns. Ramsey argues that the child has no sense of offering herself or himself solely for the sake of possible benefit for future persons.[109]

Ramsey addresses principles of nonmaleficence and beneficence indirectly. Nonmaleficence is, at best, insufficient as a principle distinct from beneficence. For instance, Frankena distinguishes four obligations that are captured under the principle of beneficence. These include the passive, negative obligation not to inflict evil or harm as the default in cases where there is conflict among these obligations.[110] By contrast, Ramsey's concept of beneficence echoes Jonathan Edwards's concept of the primacy of neighbor-love—that ultimate principle from which beneficence derives its justification.[111] Edwards notes that, in pure and absolute benevolence,

---

consent has played such a dominant role in medical ethics. He questions, for example, why some citizens should not be drafted to give blood without consent for the sake of helping others, noting that Ramsey also raises such a suggestion.

107. Ramsey, *Ethics at the Edge*, 157. While he does not stress the patient's absolute right to refuse treatment, he considers such a decision morally wrong if it is expected to lead to deliberate injury to one's health.

108. Ramsey, *Patient as Person*, 5.

109. Ibid., 14.

110. Frankena, *Ethics*, 47; Beauchamp and Childress, *Principles of Biomedical Ethics*, 4–5. Beauchamp and Childress consider these obligations to be norms. The more passive "do no harm" obligation is the sole norm for the principle of nonmaleficence, while the other obligations fall under the principles of beneficence. Moral norms include principles, rules, rights, virtues, and moral ideals (12–13). In other places, they do not make clear distinctions between norms and obligations. In fact, in their attempts to justify the validity and normativity of a common morality, they state that appeals to a common morality are normative, and thus have normative force, if they establish "obligatory moral standards for everyone" (4). They go on, however, to argue that such norms have *prima facie* status; that is, the weight of value and importance that they assume are situation specific.

111. Ramsey, *Essential Paul Ramsey*, 25. Ramsey often uses the word "benevolence." Beauchamp and Childress (*Principles of Biomedical Ethics*, 5th ed.) make the following distinctions with regard to benefit to others: "*Beneficence* refers to an *action* done to benefit other; *benevolence* is the *character trait* or *virtue* of being disposed to

Part One: The Rise and Dominance of Principles-Based Biomedical Ethics

unity with someone else involves incorporating the good of another person as one's own good.[112] The template for such benevolence comes from God's righteousness through his faithfulness to the covenant he made with humankind. This righteousness is not corrective or distributive but is redemptive by way of God's grace in Christ, "with a special bias in favor of the helpless."[113]

For Ramsey, the *true* test of neighbor-love is not loving one's neighbor as one's self (as this can be self-destructive) but loving the neighbor as Christ showed his love for humanity. He calls this a *provisional* standard that is adopted by nearly all peoples.[114] Still, Ramsey sees the summary of the law as the *organizing principle* of all New Testament ethics. This summary is expressed in Jesus's exhortation to his disciples that they love one another as he loved them.[115] His love for them is the mark of their relationships to each other and to other human beings, even strangers and enemies. Ramsey notes that this link to Christ gives no rational explanation for how Christ's love for us shows more clearly our obligation to love our neighbor-other. "Reason alone teaches no such thing to be the meaning of virtuous benevolence."[116]

This is the crux of Ramsey's parting from a principlist interpretation of beneficence. Unlike the concept of beneficence of principlism, Ramsey does not distinguish between ordinary and extraordinary beneficence. To some, Christ's command is too idealistic to be practical.[117] To Ramsey, it is

---

act for the benefit of others; and *principle of beneficence* refers to a moral *obligation* to act for the benefit of others" (emphasis in original).

112. Ibid., 32.

113. Ramsey, *Basic Christian Ethics*, 14.

114. Ramsey, *Essential Paul Ramsey*, x–xi. However, Ramsey nowhere indicates that this is the foundation of an idea for common morality.

115. In John 13:34–35, Jesus lays down his new commandment as he explains that he will soon be leaving them: "A new commandment I give you: Love one another. As I have loved you, so you must love one another. By this all men will know that you are my disciples, if you love one another" (NIV). These verses summarizes Ramsey's Christian stamp on the Golden Rule, the one that binds covenant and love ideas at both the level of the God-humankind relationship as well as the Christian-neighbor relationship.

116. Ramsey, *Essential Paul Ramsey*, 38.

117. Beauchamp and Childress, *Principles of Biomedical Ethics*, 5th ed., 167. They recall Christ's parable of the Good Samaritan as an illustration of several problems in interpreting beneficence. They seem to empathize with "common interpretations" of the parable that treat the Samaritan's act as an ideal rather than an obligation of beneficence, since his actions have been interpreted as exceeding ordinary morality. This issue will be more fully discussed again in chapter 8.

Perspectives on Principles from Diverse Faith Traditions

the obligation of those joined in covenant with God. It is the faithfulness that comes with such a covenant. Yet, Ramsey states, paraphrasing Edwards, "the old creature passed away, yet not perfectly; all things are made new, yet none perfectly."[118] Ramsey's biblical view of beneficence goes well beyond the principlist requirement of nonmaleficence and the minimal, if any, requirement for self-sacrificing beneficence.[119]

As with the other three principles just mentioned, justice for Ramsey is always considered in a relational context. The biblical notion of justice involves meeting the needs of others, and this represents the measure of God's righteousness to others.[120] Ramsey suggests that love-transformed natural law is the legacy of Jesus's teachings and eschatology. According to Hauerwas, Ramsey believes that this idea has become ingrained in the laws and practices of Western civilization. As such, law should then be used to fulfill the commitment to neighborly love.[121] Similarly, natural self-preservation has been suspended in order that it does not become an obstacle to serving the needs of one's neighbor. The work of love should be free to confirm norms of justice and to create a redirecting and transforming influence on standards of natural justice.[122]

Distributive justice, however, is a difficult problem for Ramsey. If all human beings are equal in the eyes of God, then random selection and "first come, first served" are the only systems that would honor such equality. The ruling principle becomes the equal right of every human being to live, regardless of perceived differences in social or personal worth.[123] However, it is only in individual communities that have a singular purpose and *telos* that such random selection can be foregone in favor of other criteria for saving some lives preferentially to others.[124] As a result, Ramsey is hard pressed to make decisions about what is needed in the face of scarce resources. Once a loving relationship to one's neighbor is established, then love needs to be enlightened concerning what is the actual good for that

---

118. Ibid., 40.

119. I will argue in chapter 8 that this forced distinction between beneficence and nonmaleficence is necessitated by the minimal requirements for participation in the common morality.

120. Ramsey, *Basic Christian Ethics*, 14. For Ramsey, such justice is primarily redemptive rather than distributive or corrective in nature.

121. Hauerwas, "How Christian Ethics," 22.

122. Ramsey, *Essential Paul Ramsey*, xv.

123. Ramsey, *Patient as Person*, 256.

124. Ibid., 257.

neighbor.¹²⁵ In the end, Ramsey admits that he does not know how to determine priorities in medicine when resources are scarce, calling society "largely an unfocused meshing of human pursuits."¹²⁶

PRINCIPLISM FROM ISLAMIC AND JEWISH PERSPECTIVES

In recent years, Islamic views have become more widely expressed in bioethical literature. One recent Islamic view tries to fit the principles into a heavily legalistic interpretation of divine revelation. G. I. Serour, an Egyptian obstetrician-gynecologist, outlines the importance and use of the four principles in biomedical ethics from an Islamic perspective. He believes that distinctly different ethical theories emphasize one principle over the others.¹²⁷ To the four principles, however, he adds the principle of protecting human subjects from commercial exploitation. Serour also distinguishes between legal and ethical duties. Law is generally associated with negative duties aligned with nonmaleficence, while biomedical ethics focuses on beneficence as a positive duty. He supports a pluralistic social vision of secular legislation that protects minority faith communities in countries where the laws may be shaped by dominant religious beliefs.

Sharia law is the set of instructions that regulates daily activities for many Muslims.¹²⁸ Islam has no divine predeterminism, and thus Muslims have relative freedom to make moral decisions. According to Serour, Islam puts a strong emphasis on thinking, respect for persons, and learning, even about worship.¹²⁹ Contrary to some contemporary perceptions of Islamic intolerance, passages in the Qur'an forbid attempts to compel or coerce others to believe in a faith contrary to one's convictions. Thus, autonomy

---

125. Ramsey, *Basic Christian Ethics*, 116; Smith, "On Paul Ramsey," 10–11.

126. Ramsey, *Patient as Person*, 269, 275.

127. Serour, "Islam and the Four Principles," 77. He says libertarians always prefer autonomy, utilitarians prefer beneficence and nonmaleficence, and egalitarians favor justice. As mentioned earlier, Clouser and Gert ("A Critique of Principlism," 223) propose similar preferences for specific principles within specific ethical theories in their critique of principlism.

128. Ibid. Sharia law consists of 1) the Qur'an, 2) the Sunna and Hadith, which contain additional saying of the Prophet Mohammed, 3) the opinions of Islamic scholars, and 4) Kias, which compares and draws analogies of previous judgments with contemporary issues.

129. Ibid., 80. Serour quotes from the Hadith: "One hour of thinking is better than a night of worship."

Perspectives on Principles from Diverse Faith Traditions

is seen as the free will and desire of any individual to learn in accordance to one's own beliefs.

Under Sharia law, the believer is instructed to do good (beneficence) and to avoid harming one's neighbor (nonmaleficence) to the point of not offending or hurting feelings. Justice for individuals is expressed as rights and duties granted in Islam regardless of race or social status, while distributive justice is discussed in terms of food and care for Muslims and non-Muslims alike. Serour notes the long history of these principles in Islamic medicine as expressed in sources such as the Hippocratic Oath, the 500-year-old teachings of a famous Egyptian physician, and the content of a nineteenth century Egyptian medical oath. In the past few decades, numerous medical institutions across various Islamic countries have devised medical oaths that include three or four of these principles. Regrettably, however, Serour makes no mention of a morally distinctive Islamic bioethical framework within which the four principles can be recontextualized and grounded in the Islamic faith.

The ethical system that Serour describes is one in which God created the universe and allows humankind to responsibly enjoy the creation. Human beings exercise complete freedom to make moral choices but only according to the authoritative instructions within Sharia law. Both the emphasis on learning and knowledge (even over and above worship) and a rather distant relationship with God in decision-making suggest kinship with a common-morality motif. That is, thinking freely may find common ground among Islamic and secular bioethicists alike. Beneficence and nonmaleficence are linked to doing good and avoiding harm according to Sharia law, but the validity of these principles in contemporary Islamic medical codes has its earliest roots in the Hippocratic tradition rather than in a distinctly Islamic bioethical framework. Justice focuses considerably on the rights and duties of the individual believer, though distributive justice is also mentioned as applying to all persons. The tone and emphasis of moral decision-making is distinctly legalistic and individualistic, albeit grounded in Islamic law.

Avraham Steinberg outlines a Jewish perspective on the four principles in biomedical ethics.[130] Halakhah is the divinely revealed, written, and oral legal system of Judaism, including 613 commandments of Sinaitic origin, the Pentateuch, and interpretations of written law in the form of rabbinical decrees and customs. Authoritative sources include the Bible, the Talmud, and an extensive collection of codification and *respon-*

---

130. Steinberg, "Jewish Perspective," 67–72.

sa. Within Halakhah, a dispute-resolution mechanism resolves divergent views that impede otherwise decisive answers to ethical problems.

The relational model of decision-making in medical practice includes the physician, patient, and a qualified rabbi. The covenant between God and the Jewish patient is mediated by the physician, who is an instrument of God's goodness directed to the patient, forming the core of a temporal physician-patient covenant. The four principles are included but modified in medical practice by other Jewish moral and legal principles. In contrast to rights-based ethics that minimizes socially shared values, Jewish ethics sees moral fulfillment through obedience to God-given moral norms and requirements. It relies on a rich Halakhic interpretive literature to deal casuistically with specific cases. In a framework of Halakhic rules and regulations, the four principles are completely *prima facie*; that is, *prioritization of principles* for any given case is paramount for decision-making. The moral and legal weight of each ethical principle is derived from Halakhic law in the context of the particulars of a specific case. In addition, the preservation of life dominates Jewish medical practice, overriding any religious or ethical precept and forcing acceptance of treatment through a rabbi or other authoritative source. Not accepting potentially healing treatment makes the person, at best, "a pious fool."[131]

Steinberg agrees with Pellegrino and Thomasma that autonomy in Western culture has become inappropriately dominant. According to Jewish tradition, autonomy combines divine providence and human freedom of choice, interpreted within the proper moral context. For example, when Jewish rules or regulations are violated, a person's autonomous wishes may be abrogated and coercion sanctioned.[132] Also, it is generally agreed that human behavior and actions are both humanly free and divinely determined in a tension whereby neither predominates.

While beneficence and nonmaleficence are considered positive and negative sides of the same principle coin, all levels of beneficence are promoted over simply doing no harm. The moral essence of the Torah is the imperative to love one's neighbor as one's self. The Jewish person does right and good deeds because God acts beneficently and mercifully toward humankind.[133] According to Steinberg, the Jewish concept of justice

---

131. Ibid., 66–67.

132. Ibid., 69. This is reminiscent of the Eastern Orthodox position of Engelhardt, Jr. (*Foundations of Christian Bioethics*, 354–66), which sanctions deception above autonomous consent if its enactment leads to a better path toward salvation and its associated goods.

133. Ibid., 71.

in biomedical ethics asks what human life should be, which is contrasted with principlism's emphasis on distributive justice, which is preoccupied with issues of economic resources. Justice is established by divine commands and is implemented by imitating the divine quality of justice in the world.[134]

Jewish bioethics integrates faith into bioethical deliberations and decision-making. The communal nature of Jewish bioethics is nurtured by the long and complex traditions of laws and interpretation and by the direct role that rabbis and other faith authorities have in contributing to decision-making. Thus, the autonomy of individuals in Jewish law is tempered by the importance of relational interaction with each other in community as a reflection of their relationship with God. This and the considerable (sometimes coercive, in some Jewish traditions) moral sway of religious leaders regarding important moral decisions are important keys in a rich moral framework. However, for those who subscribe to the common morality, such religious beliefs are considered too particular and threatening to consensus building.

---

134. Ibid., 72. Here he refers to Ps 119:137–44, particularly verses 143b–44, "but your command give me delight. Your statues are always righteous; give me understanding that I may live" (Today's NIV).

4

Richness and Depth of Understanding within Faith Traditions

The elegance of the four-principles approach is that it need say nothing about the deep, and some claim untraversable, philosophical chasm separating these two types [i.e., utilitarian and Kantian] of philosophical theory.... Similarly, it is neutral between the various religious moral theories and indeed between different versions of the same religious theory.... Of course, this moral-theoretic neutrality is not to everyone's taste.[1]

—RAANAN GILLON (1994)

DIVERSITY AMONG ROMAN CATHOLIC AND ANGLICAN BIOETHICISTS

In *Principles of Health Care Ethics*, Raanan Gillon invites an international group of English-speaking health care professionals to consider the "common moral theme" of the four *prima facie* principles of Beauchamp and Childress and their scope of application. In his contribution, Gillon concedes that Beauchamp and Childress fail to provide a method for resolving conflicts between principles in particular situations, but he supports their promotion of principles as a common moral language dealing with moral issues in front of a backdrop of common moral commitments.[2] He

---

1. Gillon, "Four Principles," 325.
2. Gillon, "Preface," xxi.

feels that moral agents should focus on understanding the scope of shared commitments and the different beliefs on which they are often based.

This chapter deals with the diversity of views of principlism within religious traditions, focusing in this first section on different perspectives within Roman Catholic and Anglican traditions. Bioethicists in these traditions directly address the role of principlism in biomedical ethics and show the diversity of responses even within traditions. These theologians and bioethicists mainly accommodate principlism. They avoid any in-depth analysis of the secular basis for its core faith beliefs and for the worldviews that distinguish principlism from a biblical ethical framework. There is no appeal for a distinctively biblical bioethical framework, and thus none is proposed.

Anglican Views

Citing Hans Kung's exhortations for peace among religions through the pursuit of a world ethic, Anglican ethicist Ronald Preston suggests that the four principles may provide such a common level of agreement in bioethical decision-making.[3] He sees hope in MacIntyre's suggestions of learning a new first language of moral reflection in order to cope with the moral fragmentation of Western ethics. On another level, Preston distinguishes what he calls the "simple rationalism of the Enlightenment" from a rationality that acknowledges the conditionality of human experiences. He suggests that an element of "interest-free" thought that transcends ideological elements and crosses religious, philosophical, and cultural barriers could be possible. Thus, he falls back on the natural-law tradition in his appeal to common conceptions of human nature that rise above specific religious and cultural contexts.

Preston presses the notion of a basic morality reflected in the four principles, though agreement about such a morality may come about for very different reasons. However, his basic morality premise seems to trump his Christian faith when he contrasts a secular-humanist faith perspective with the Christian worldview—that of humanity as image-bearers of God in need of restoration through Jesus Christ. Christianity is lumped together with other faiths almost as an add-on to an underlying morality, with the former needing to conform to the latter as a matter of common necessity.[4] Preston tries to anchor a common morality that

3. Preston, "Four Principles," 23.
4. Ibid., 26–27.

Part One: The Rise and Dominance of Principles-Based Biomedical Ethics

transcends religious particulars in the context of necessary emotional and social dimensions. Benevolence and non-maleficence directed toward relationships and a common good within medicine need an empathic dimension that goes beyond the four principles. He finds grounding for moral judgments in "the power of reasoning discernment," the process of weighing conflicting claims based on different principles. Unfortunately, justification for choosing the right moral choices remains suspended in uncertainty, subject to the preferential whims of the kind of personal intuitions that MacIntyre is so concerned about.[5] For Preston, the four principles provide a way into dialogue with those of different fundamental beliefs. His acceptance of the common-morality premise of principlism brushes aside the enriching perspectives that religious commitments can bring into the dialogue. His Christian faith commitment seems secondary to a faith in the power of reasoning discernment; his faith must accommodate a common morality.

By contrast, John Habgood offers an Anglican perspective that draws heavily from eighteenth-century moralist Joseph Butler and his general principles of enlightened self-interest, benevolence, and conscience. Habgood interprets Butler's concept of benevolence as a "luminous self-evidence" naturally inherent to humans. Conscience dominates Butler's principles, it being the capacity for moral reflection through which internal moral values are brought to bear during moral deliberation. Its utility is particularly needed when other principles are in conflict, and appeal is made to one's conscience to make a moral judgment.[6] Habgood grounds human freedom and dignity in the individual's relationship with God. Preserving the respect of others assumes that such persons know what is best for themselves, even if the decisions and actions of such persons are perceived as unwise. This individualistic notion avoids confronting the dangers of conformity to societal norms in societal interactions involving biomedical decisions. In articulating a concept of autonomy as the dignity and rights of persons, Habgood avoids taking a position on the difficult task of working as a Christian in a public arena among non-Christians.[7]

Referring back to Butler, Habgood describes beneficence as a principle needing limits set by justice and veracity in the pursuit of well-being. Veracity, he claims, keeps beneficence reined in between sentimentality

---

5. Preston seems to secularize natural law to accommodate a common-morality idea, "topping up" a common morality with values of religious belief in a typically dualistic fashion.

6. Habgood, "Anglican View," 57.

7. Ibid., 60.

and an overprotectiveness that infringes on human dignity (autonomy), such as in the traditional paternalism wherein caregivers decide what is best for patients without considering their preferences. Habgood emphasizes the primary need to respect persons as children of God, as though the other principles will fall into line if we keep respect in mind. Among those principles, justice constrains beneficence against favoritism and inequality in health care decisions. Public-health decision-making should more often involve lower level decision-makers, allowing more people to become involved in decisions affecting them personally. In this way, greater equity may be accomplished through a developed consensus of fairness.[8]

Habgood approves of the use of the four principles as middle axioms, though like Pellegrino and others, he is rightly leery of the dominance of autonomy.[9] Exercising the life of faith extends to implications of individual choices as a reflection of understanding of persons in relationship with each other and, ultimately, with God. Unfortunately, he gives no specific examples showing that these principles can give moral substance to decision-making for Christians and their communities. His analysis is accommodating to principlism, his idea of autonomy is quite individualistic, and he provides a superficial view of the importance of relationality in biomedical ethics. The biblical concept of love seems to be replaced by human conscience as a principle that can help to address conflicting principles.

Roman Catholic Views

John Finnis presents a Roman Catholic position that puts much trust in the guidance of reason in recognizing the four principles. However, "reason's full implications and morality's practical implications" can only be fully discharged via moral principles that guide one's life through doctrine, faith, and theology.[10] Finnis states that the most foundational moral principle is *willing possibilities* that are in alignment with integral human fulfillment, including basic human goods of life and health. Total happiness results from fully attaining them all, but this is directed by the most fundamental moral principle of openness to human fulfillment: love of God

---

8. The communitarian model in the Oregon health care system solicits just such participation, though being attentive to the larger picture may have value in making wiser allocation decisions as their early experience showed.

9. Ibid., 63.

10. Finnis and Fisher, "Theology," 31.

Part One: The Rise and Dominance of Principles-Based Biomedical Ethics

and of one's neighbor as one's self.[11] He links moral principles (including the four principles) firmly with natural law in light of (and supplemented by) revealed divine law.

For Finnis, true beneficence is serving humankind and mediating God's healing power.[12] He distinguishes three forms of maleficent behavior in health care practice: lying, killing, and mutilation. Moral actions are chosen after reflection involving faith in reason and the authoritative wisdom of the church. In his moral judgments, reason provides the final guidance.[13] He calls the contemporary concept of autonomy "a false principle of autonomy that becomes a vehicle for the profound injustice of a beneficent maleficence" when it is used to justify mercy killing the infirmed and disabled.[14] *True* autonomy is seen in a communitarian sense; it follows the *principle of subsidiarity*, wherein larger communities or institutions help smaller ones to best care for their needy members. Finnis focuses on justice as fairness when emphasizing the Christian concern for the poor and needy. Mercy can go beyond justice and non-maleficence to heal evil except in the case of mercy killing, in which mercy breeds injustice and the negation of autonomy. For Finnis, the four principles are helpful tools for understanding bioethical problems, yet the principles must refer back to the authoritative elements of Scripture and the declarations of the magisterium, as well as strongly rely on reason.

Roman Catholic Bernard Hoose acknowledges the positive contributions of the four principles, as well as the complications that religious perspectives can bring to the application of principles. Hoose respects the right to self-determination, the need for information relevant to a decision, and rights to privacy, confidentiality, and promise-keeping. He identifies ontic evils (those actions not considered inherently morally evil or wrong) in discussing the principle of double effect and suggests that intention should be taken into greater account.[15] As well, Hoose discusses

---

11. His description of happiness has elements of eudaimonism, an ancient Greek idea of happiness or the well-lived life taught by ancient Stoics and Perpatetics. Wolterstorff (*Justice*, 149–79) and Annas (*Morality*) provide an in-depth examination of these influences.

12. Ibid., 34, 37.

13. Finnis and Fisher, "Theology," 38–40. Regarding the importance of reason in preserving basic human goods in making choices, he writes, "The good provides *a* reason against such a choice, and because that good cannot rationally be 'outweighed,' that choice will be not merely against *a* reason but against *reason*" (emphases in original).

14. Ibid., 41.

15. Hoose, "Theology," 45–48.

Richness and Depth of Understanding within Faith Traditions

distributive justice and the importance of human relationships. Fidelity to others is construed as a biblical concept exemplified in ancient Israel and characterized by kinship bonds, covenantal bonds, and relationships with aliens or strangers.[16] In addition, risking accusations of paternalism, he prioritizes fulfilling the principle of non-maleficence and respecting those caregivers whose conscience may require care decisions that are contrary to the patient or a surrogate.

ANALYSIS OF CHRISTIAN RESPONSES TO PRINCIPLISM

The Anglican perspectives of Preston and Habgood attempt to accommodate principlism but fail to demonstrate the clash of faith commitments between Christianity and principlism. Preston tries to fit Christianity into a common-morality mould along with other religious faiths, attempting to overcome religious differences rather than encouraging moral dialogue with rich religious content. Habgood shows better insight into the pitfalls of principlism, noting its dominance of autonomy. But in my view, his notion of autonomy is too anthropocentric and individualistic. Conscience is considered to be as important as love in terms of being an overarching principle. The four principles are subservient to conscience and other more general principles. Beneficence is constrained by justice and respect for individuals' right to make bad medical decisions for themselves. In general, he relies too heavily on the works of Butler and provides few novel Christian insights.

Variations within the Roman Catholic tradition usually revolve around differences between interpretations of the grace/nature dualism. Laurence Cunningham characterizes the Roman Catholic "worldview" using themes such as the world as a gift from God, the presence and influence of sin, a balance between the goodness of that creation and the sin that distorts it, and the cumulative experience of church traditions.[17] Albert Wolters analyzes these themes as variations of the nature/grace motif. He considers these distinctions to be *supra*-theological, in the sense that they are conceptually more fundamental than theological beliefs and are often unconsciously practiced. Wolters further categorizes variations of

---

16. Ibid., 51.
17. Naugle, *Worldview*, 34–38.

PART ONE: The Rise and Dominance of Principles-Based Biomedical Ethics

the grace/nature relationship within Christian traditions.[18] The Thomist tradition sees grace as supplementing nature (what Wolters refers to as *gratia supra naturam*, wherein grace is the *donum superadditum* to nature).

The critiques of Pellegrino, Finnis, and Hoose are derived from this religious motif. Finnis is committed to the power of reason and inadequately accounts for the need for Scripture to overcome the influence of sin. Loosened from its scriptural mooring, natural-law theory gropes for some common basis for law and morality within the created order.[19] Hoose acknowledges that the four principles serve as reminders of important moral elements rather than as content-rich concepts. He is minimalist in considering nonmaleficence to be the minimum requirement for bioethical actions.[20] However, he does see the importance of giving attention to medical relationships, including respect for caregivers as well as patients.

However, Pellegrino is less accommodating to principlism and provides the most in-depth critique among these perspectives. While giving credit to Beauchamp and Childress for their efforts to bring together participants with different basic beliefs into the bioethical dialogue, he cannot accept principles-based ethics *per se*. Such an ethical framework is detached from any grounding in the sources of authority accepted by the Roman Catholic Church. It privatizes religious beliefs for the sake of a common morality and inadequately accounts for virtues in ethical discourse. With boldly explicit references to his faith, Pellegrino moves forward with his own philosophy of medicine wherein virtues that guide the moral agent (usually the caregiver in medicine) to realize and apply principles are moved front and centre. His answer to principlism is the merging or synthesis of principles-based and Thomist virtue ethics. In this sense he follows faithfully his predecessor Thomas Aquinas, the master synthesizer of church teaching and Aristotelian ethics. However, he also recognizes the overarching principle of love that elevates the expression of

---

18. Wolters, "No Longer Queen," 65–68. Wolters considers the nature/grace dichotomy as a worldview in a narrow sense that may be considered part of a large Christian worldview. Other conceptual forms of the nature/grace dichotomy include *gratia contra naturam*, grace opposing nature; *gratia iuxta naturam*, a two-realm conception expressed in the Lutheran tradition; and *gratia intra naturam*, a Reformed Christian view wherein grace restores or renews nature. Wolters elaborates further on the implications of belief in these categories elsewhere (see Wolters, "On the Idea," 14–25; "Christianity and the Classics," 189–203).

19. Cochran, "Bible," 183. See also Finnis and Fisher, "Theology" and Hittinger, "Theology."

20. Hoose, "Theology."

Richness and Depth of Understanding within Faith Traditions

grace. By contrast, in principlism there is no single overarching principle that helps to resolve conflicting principles in specific situations.

Unlike principlism, the core of Pellegrino's philosophy of medicine is beneficence expressed as care within the physician-patient relationship. In this sense, beneficence dominates autonomy, though he puts substantial weight on respect for both caregiver and patient. Unfortunately, he writes little about other relationships within medical practice, and his emphasis on physician authority and virtue carries undercurrents of soft paternalism.[21] Despite these misgivings, his efforts to overcome the influence of principlism and secular bioethics in general are highly commendable. Using the neo-Calvinist language of structure and direction, he tries to reconceptualize the four principles and give them religious *direction* through the primary guiding virtue of love in each case or situation.[22] The central point of his critique of principlism is the perceived misalignment of the principles with virtue. This contributes to an imbalance of their relative importance and expression within the secular cultural context, wherein autonomy and individual rights are held disproportionately high in authority while beneficence is not given sufficient expression. The independent status of nonmaleficence is doubtful, except as a reminder that a lack of beneficence is unethical.

Like Pellegrino, Engelhardt boldly digs deep with his critique. He holds that principlism is groundless by its nature. Its principles are reducible to a principle of permission by which any interpretation is valid as long as parties agree. He perceives the religious depth of the problem: that the moral authority of God is replaced by that of rational dialogue and consensus agreement based on reason alone. He repeatedly castigates the Roman Catholic nature/grace dualism for its rationalistic approach to the study of God and the created order. While Engelhardt advocates for retention of distinct faith communities, his idea of societal pluralism envisions a public forum of moral appeasement for the sake of outward peace. He does not express the missional need to present religious reasons for moral positions in the public forum. For him, the separation between faith communities of religious (private) and secular (public) morality is an

---

21. Pellegrino, "Four Principles," 357. He condemns paternalism, however, as diametrically opposed to beneficence and in polar relationship with autonomy.

22. Wolters (*Creation Regained*, 87–88) uses these concepts as a "short hand" for the biblical themes of creation, fall, and redemption. Structure refers to the essence of a created thing by virtue of God's creational law, whereas direction refers to sinful deviation from the structural ordinance and its renewed conformity to that ordinance through Christ.

unfortunate fact of life. But this falls into the hands of principlism and its common-morality premise. Such a position stifles the mission of Christ's command to reveal the full impact of the gospel on our moral lives as members of the larger society around us.

His conversion to the Eastern Orthodox tradition strengthens this separation while promoting additional separation from other Christian traditions. In my view, in *The Foundations of Christian Bioethics*, his theology distorts his vision of medical practice and public health through a quest for union with God that at times runs roughshod over other normative expressions of the created order, such as honesty and full disclosure. Engelhardt's perspective is in line with other Eastern Orthodox perspectives wherein belief and worship are inseparable. Timothy Ware notes that Christianity to the Orthodox believer is a liturgical religion.[23] Alexander Schmemann calls the Orthodox view *the* Christian worldview; it is a sacramental way of the church seeing the world and cultivating the kingdom through its experiences.[24] In Orthodox anthropology, human beings are priests of creation.[25] Food is transformed into divine love meant to bring humans into communion with God.[26] Christ restores true life, making it a sacrament and communion with God. The creation is regained and humans again assume their role as priests serving creation.[27]

Between these two committed Christian bioethicists, one can see the impact of different variations of a Christian worldview on specific bioethical practices. For example, Pellegrino would consider lying and deception to be anathema to good, virtuous Christian medical practice. It would breach the virtue of honesty and the principles of respect for persons and beneficence even when viewed within his Thomist framework. Engelhardt, on the other hand, repudiates the dualistic Thomist view of life and is particularly troubled by its emphasis on rational discursive

---

23. Ware, *Orthodox Church*, 271. From his interesting Reformed Christian perspective, James K. A. Smith (*Desiring the Kingdom*, 25, 34, 46–47) calls for human persons to develop into embodied agents of love and desire, shaped by liturgies that aim our desires toward the kingdom of God or to false gods. Smith separates worship/liturgy from worldview in that human beings worship before they cognitively articulate a worldview. According to Smith, we worship in order to know.

24. Schmemann, *For the Life*, 7–8.

25. Naugle, *Worldview*, 46–47.

26. Schmemann, *For the Life*, 14. For the Orthodox, says Schmemann, human beings are to live eucharistically, in that they must acknowledge God as creator and gift-giver and must express their profound gratitude. Adam's sin is seen as making the world material, whereas before his sin, it was life in God (18).

27. Naugle, *Worldview*, 52; Schmemann, *For the Life*, 20–21.

processes in bioethical deliberative discourse. Interestingly, the central role of liturgical living resonates with James K. A. Smith's recent exhortation for Reformed Christians to capitalize on new opportunities for them to witness in postmodernity through a fresh appreciation of liturgy and worship.[28] Smith cautions against attempts to impose a rationalist substantiation of the truth of the Christian faith on a pluralistic culture, a process sometimes described as the Constantinian agenda.[29] However, I think Smith and Engelhardt part company in important areas. The former would not likely justify deception and lying to patients, nor would he condone overriding personal health care decisions of individuals by spiritual counselors or spiritual leaders, even with the intention of fostering spiritual unity with God. Such myopic fixation on a single, most important life goal disempowers patients and conflicts with the biblically inspired mandate to recognize and work with normative directions and structures of medical relationships. In other words, while church counsel is very important, final patient decisions should reflect patient conscience and personal accountability to God.

Paul Ramsey's ethic comes out of theological ideas amalgamated from several Protestant Christian traditions. He is not constrained by dualistic dogma; instead, covenantal love becomes a central theme rather than tangential addition. Ramsey puts more importance on working out principles in covenantal relationships than do either Pellegrino or Engelhardt. Though his principles/rules distinctions are often inconsistent or confusing, Ramsey's requirement of principles or rules to guide right living provides an ethical framework to combat the situationalism of his day, against which he consistently reacts. The biblical notion of covenant provides the grounding for his principles, which are given meaning through the God-humankind covenant.[30]

Ramsey addresses the principles of autonomy, beneficence, and justice as though they are concepts within moral themes. They neither stand alone nor form the main struts of a moral framework but rather

28. Lyotard, *Postmodern Condition*; Smith, "Little Story." Smith draws heavily from Jean-Francois Lyotard's account of postmodernism and his critique of meta-narratives and autonomous reason.

29. Smith, *Who's Afraid*, 73–74. Unlike Engelhardt, whose response to both secular and rationalistic Christian perspectives is to develop Eastern Orthodox health care organizations, Smith suggests a Christian apologetic of postmodernity that promotes laying everyone's presuppositional baggage on the bioethical discussion table and narrating the story of the Christian faith regarding how its message applies to bioethical issues.

30. Smith, "On Paul Ramsey," 12.

are perceived as actions or motives within relationships. He ties informed consent to his notion of fidelity and loyalty, which in turn are cornerstones of his covenantal relationship between caregiver and patient. Beneficence is at the core of covenantally sanctioned action toward one's fellow human being by way of the biblical command of love of God and one's neighbor. As a result, nonmaleficence has no real role as a negative reflection of positive benevolent action. Still, distributive justice is problematic for Ramsey in a health care context because he has no way of determining who should receive care when limited resources require the delivery of care to some but not others.

Insofar as his analysis of the four principles looks back to biblical covenant and the command of love for guidance and meaning, I think Ramsey provides the first Christian response that acknowledges covenantal relationships as the focus of biomedical ethical reflection. His crusade to counter situationalism and his deontological bias explain his preoccupation with informed consent, his emphasis on the protection of children and adolescents from human research, and his lack of a formal ethical framework that can serve as an alternative to principlism. Beneficence is the central and organizing principle of his covenantal and relational ethic, justice is inexorably linked to agape love, and autonomy is understood in covenantal rather than individualistic terms. In addition, he shows the total inadequacy of nonmaleficence within a Christian understanding of beneficence and love for one's fellow human being. This is all the more surprising given his persistent deontological preoccupation with rules and principles as generalizations of rules.

Ramsey lays important groundwork for a covenantal focus on human medical relationships founded on God's faithfulness through undeserving gracious love for humankind. He pays particular attention to the poorest and most vulnerable; as identified by Goheen and Bartholomew, the failure to do so is one of the dangers of a Christian worldview in our contemporary world.[31] His philosophy of medicine is more implicit than that of Pellegrino, but he creates a foundation both for William F. May's more comprehensive understanding of a covenantal ethic and for this current work. For instance, May envisions medicine as a covenanted profession and grounds this idea in the notion of covenant as the internal meaning of creation.[32] The character of this covenantal relating in medicine has

31. Goheen and Bartholomew, *Living at the Crossroads*, 23,

32. Gilbert Meilaender ("On William F. May," 107–8, 117–18) writes that May sees the task of ethics as creating possibilities to transform the way ethical issues are considered rather than focusing on specific quandaries. Those issues become mysteries to

elements not only of caregiver philanthropy but also of indebtedness to patients. This tension is only fully resolved through the reflective image of God's covenantal relationship with human beings and the undeserving grace he grants that holds it together, despite our infidelity.[33]

While these are important beginnings toward a covenantal ethic, such an ethic needs to be further developed in light of the increasing complexity of medicine today. Consequently, principlism needs more in-depth critique, and an alternative ethical covenantal framework needs to be more fully developed. In part two of this book, I will articulate how a biblical covenantal ethic can open up the normative structures and meaning of relationships within medicine and can recontextualize the four principles in their most meaningful and practical way. First, however, I will provide my own in-depth critique of principlism. Unlike previous critiques, I will explore the presuppositional foundations of principlism and the worldviews out of which its contents have developed. While I will touch on the relationship between worldviews and their philosophical expressions, I will engage in a more robust discussion of the relationship of worldview, philosophy, and theology in chapters 6 and 7.

THE PRESUPPOSITIONAL ROOTS OF PRINCIPLISM: A REFORMED CHRISTIAN CRITIQUE

The Notion of Worldview

In this section, I will offer my critique of principlism at a level that others have not comprehensively addressed. I will also show how principlism is a manifestation of secular worldviews of our age. Understanding the root of principlism at this level is necessary in order to set the stage for a Christian response to principlism that exposes the latter's lack of moral authority and justification. Only by understanding principlism's presuppositional roots and core beliefs can a Christian ethical framework be developed and the redemptive aspects of principlism be revisited and renewed in light of biblical teaching.

---

be explored more than puzzles to be solved. Moral responses should resemble ritual more than technique and are better approached through image, symbol, and story. His covenantal ethic is a corrective vision.

33. Ibid., 119.

PART ONE: The Rise and Dominance of Principles-Based Biomedical Ethics

David Naugle notes that the term *Weltanschauung* was first used by Immanuel Kant.[34] Kant conceived of *Weltanschauung* as a supersensible power of the mind that underlies what is otherwise mere appearance. By the end of the nineteenth century, the term *Weltanschauung* or "worldview" became commonly associated with an intellectual understanding of "the higher questions of religion and philosophy" regarding the cosmos.[35] Wilhelm Dilthey was one of the first philosophers to systematically address the concept of worldview, possibly driven by "reverential awe for the mystery of life and the sense of the sacred in human life."[36] He defines worldview as the incorporation of beliefs, emotional habits, and tendencies relating to the world and our life in it. Worldviews emerge from our mental structures as attitudes to, and knowledge of, life.[37] Worldviews are distinguished by means of principles, purposes, and preferences that govern human actions and give meaning and unity to life.[38] Kant suggests that it is possible to develop *one worldview, believed and lived out by all, by virtue of our common capacity to reason.*[39]

According to Dilthey, religious worldviews are rooted in "a relationship to the invisible" and give meaning to an order of life that includes an appraisal of life and an ideal of practical conduct.[40] All types of religious worldviews retain spiritual traits, particularly "an unshakable epistemic confidence and a fixity upon the transcendent world."[41] Jewish, Arabic, and Christian theologies represent *historical transitions* from a primal monotheism that fostered the philosophies of the Enlightenment thinkers

---

34. Naugle, *Worldview*, 57–58. Betz ("Zur Geschichte") and Meier ("De Geburt") provide further in-depth reading on the origins of worldview as *Weltanschauung*. Other books that explore the concept of worldview include Wolters (*Creation Regained*), Schaeffer (*Complete Works*), Walsh and Middleton (*Transforming Vision*), Holmes (*Contours*), Pearcey (*Total Truth*), and Goheen and Bartholomew (*Living at the Crossroads*).

35. Orr, *Christian View*, 365.

36. Kluback and Weinbaum, *Dilthey's Philosophy*, 8.

37. Dilthey, *Selected Writings*, 141.

38. Ibid.; Hodges, *Wilhelm Dilthey*.

39. Goheen and Bartholomew, *Living at the Crossroads*, 13. James Sire (*The Universe Next Door*, 16; *Naming the Elephant*, 12, 124) has identified prominent competing worldviews in our culture as Christian theism, deism, naturalism, nihilism, existentialism, pantheistic monism, and postmodernism. Each of these worldviews develops and finds its validity from a core religious orientation toward either the true God or toward one or more idols.

40. Dilthey, *Dilthey's Philosophy*, 34.

41. Naugle, *Worldview*, 89.

Richness and Depth of Understanding within Faith Traditions

through a "monotheistic idealism of freedom." Their transcendent orientation is a historical product of "sacerdotal techniques," while their *true spirit* is that of the *human spirit* that is freed from moral rigor and personal restrictions.[42] As Naugle notes, for Dilthey, there is no god's-eye point of view.[43] Rather, worldviews maintain an inescapable skepticism about truth and the nature of things.

Sander Griffioen rightly cautions that Dilthey maintains eschatological hope in a metaphilosophy that is elevated above the competition of worldviews. This hope embraces a new concept of reason that is critical of traditional standards of truth, including those of Christianity.[44] However, Dilthey's conflict of worldviews is not analogous to a biblical battle of the spirits. There is no Holy Spirit in this competition, just competitors vying for the right to redefine how faith in Reason should ultimately play out.

I prefer the definition of "worldview" presented by Goheen and Bartholomew; that is, it is a framework and expression of "basic beliefs embedded in a shared grand story that are rooted in a faith commitment and that give shape and direction to the whole of our individual and corporate lives."[45] As such, philosophy and systematic theology are theoretical reflections on those basic worldview beliefs. The claim of truth within a worldview can be neither proved nor disproved by science or philosophy.[46] Rather, religious faith gives direction to the worldview and its expressions. For worldviews such as modernism, truth resides in the power and authority of human reason. In the Christian worldview, truth is found in God's revelation to humankind in the created order and in his written Word. Metaphors such as "guide," "compass to life," or "roadmap" can characterize the central position of worldview in one's life.[47] In a pluralistic culture, Christian and non-Christian worldviews live side-by-side and sometimes clash.

Understanding Christian and non-Christian worldview distinctions is extremely important. Christians must keep one ear on Scripture and the other towards the surrounding culture in order to live out Christ's

---

42. Ibid. Dilthey (*Dilthey's Philosophy*, 35) writes, "A religious mind is always in the right when it comes to its experiences. But the progressing, rational mind recognized the faults of such an approach."
43. Ibid., 97.
44. Griffioen, "Worldview Approach," 104.
45. Goheen and Bartholomew, *Living at the Crossroads*, 23.
46. Griffioen, "Worldview Approach," 87.
47. Wolters, *Creation Regained*, 3–5.

command to be in, but not of, the world.[48] Wolters argues that such understanding helps Christians to keep constant watch for the influences of non-biblical thinking from our surrounding culture.[49] With this as background, in the next section, I will identify worldviews from which principlism is derived, analyzing their expression using various components of the framework and through the applications of its four principles.

Rationality and the Worldview of Modernity

The autonomy of human reason has formed the faith basis for non-Christian worldviews in Western thought. But reason is also deeply embedded in some Christian faith traditions. In the Roman Catholic tradition, Richard McCormick and others believe that reason is largely independent from Christian faith. Faith *motivates* obedience to, and *illuminates* our perception of, natural moral law. Reason is *informed* by faith.[50] As well, Goheen and Bartholomew suggest that scientism and confidence in reason has heavily influenced the thinking of evangelicals such as Carl Henry and Francis Schaeffer. For both, reason is a neutral entity that should support a Christian view of the world.[51]

By contrast, Roy Clouser has rightly countered that "reason is not autonomous nor is theorizing religiously neutral."[52] Contemporary Christian thinkers such as Alastair MacIntyre, Nicholas Wolterstorff, and Alvin Plantinga show that rationality has a profound influence, it being an

---

48. Goheen and Bartholomew (*Living at the Crossroads*, 108) credit John Stott with suggesting the need to engage in "double listening" to be properly equipped to live for Christ.

49. Wolters (*Creation Regained*, 29) speaks of the "intuitive attunement to creational normativity," which he equates with conscience. Through our conscience human beings witness the normative demands of creational law despite sin by virtue of their very constitution as creatures.

50. McCormick, *Critical Calling*, 204. Lisa Cahill ("On Richard McCormick") has critically appraised McCormick's understanding of the relationship between natural law and faith.

51. Goheen and Bartholomew, *Living at the Crossroads*, 15–16. Here, Goheen and Bartholomew give support to Hiebert's view (*Anthropological Reflections*, 38) that traditions of knowledge brought into a worldview strongly influence that worldview.

52. Clouser, *Myth of Religious Neutrality*, 97–98. According to Clouser, rational intuitions of self-evidence always include some intuition of divinity as well. Faith is an integral part of reasoning; reason is directed by some kind of faith commitment by all people.

integral presuppositional part of competing secular worldviews.[53] I agree with their premise that faith in rationality functions as *religious* faith, which spawned and grounds worldviews of the Enlightenment tradition. At the level of faith, rationality can become a synthetic intrusion into, and have a distorting influence on, a Christian worldview. Even when Beauchamp and Childress question whether "a heap of obligations and values unconnected by a first principle" have any hope of cohering under the power of reason, they quip, "Is our goal of reflective equilibrium more an article of faith than a demonstrable achievement?"[54] While this singular reference to faith should not be overinterpreted, I think it reflects genuine inner doubts about whether their common morality can overcome diverse core beliefs and be convincingly authoritative on ground as shaky as reason alone.

Christopher Norris argues that philosophical modernity searches for some grounding principle or assurance for knowledge that is objectively understood and mind-independent and that resists the challenge of skepticism and doubt.[55] However, modernism's faith in a better world through reason was shattered by wars and revolutions during the first half of the twentieth century. As a result, postmodernism abandons the modernist faith in the power of reason. Any distinctive set of values or belief system as expressed through pragmatic narratives can count as truthful.[56] Human lives make sense through the context of multiple, open-ended, ever-proliferating narratives and language games.[57] In addition, meaning systems are socially and linguistically constructed, each entirely tolerated and unprivileged.[58]

Modern and postmodern influences on the philosophy of ethics reflect fundamental changes in Western thought and culture.[59] As a Kantian idealist, Georg Hegel develops the first clear notion of modernity.

---

53. Ibid., 38, 157–58; MacIntyre, *After Virtue*; Hoitenga, *Faith and Reason*. Clouser contends that considering belief in God or a god to be non-religious is itself based on a religious belief, ascribing by default divine status to principles of reason. He cites the beliefs of Albert Einstein and Werner Heisenberg in the laws of logic and mathematics as religious in nature.

54. Beauchamp and Childress, *Principles of Biomedical Ethics*, 6th ed., 396.

55. Norris, *Deconstruction*, 7.

56. Bertens (*Idea of Postmodern*) and Rose (*Post-Modern and the Post-Industrial*) provide excellent analyses of postmodernism.

57. Norris, *Deconstruction*, 11.

58. Naugle, *Worldview*, 174.

59. Hare, "*In Vitro* Fertilization," 71–90.

Part One: The Rise and Dominance of Principles-Based Biomedical Ethics

His *freedom of subjectivity* principle embraces individualism, the right to criticism, and autonomy of action, marking the developmental culmination of the intellectual aspect of human beings. This means rejecting the reality of miraculous events and embracing the freedom to become acquainted with, and familiar with, nature and its laws.[60] Hegel traces the roots of this principle back to the rejection of church authority and personal interpretations of Scripture during the Protestant Reformation. From there, the foundation of morality changes from the command of God to the freedom of the human will.[61] This free, subjective will gains autonomy under universal laws.[62]

Postmodern Worldview and Truth by Consensus

Jurgen Habermas reveals the influence of postmodernism on Kantian idealists. As a committed Kantian himself, he believes that critical reason assumes the role of supreme judge and provides moral insights, but he emphasizes pragmatic, discursive, and linguistic aspects of understanding reality. Human thought and language become the foundation of structures of reality. Habermas is committed to achieving broad consensus on public policy matters through enlightened, democratic exchange among those with different, often conflicting, cultural views of what constitutes moral good.[63] In his model of communicative interaction, moral decisions are rooted in the "universality of an uncoerced consensus achieved through deliberation between free and equal individuals."[64] Thus, the moral standards created in distinguishing truth and falsity as well as right and wrong are immanent, embedded in languages, cultures, and practices. These standards possess a "transcendence" grounded not in a Hegelian transcendent Absolute but solely in their openness to critique and revision through the intersubjective recognition generated by the force of reasons.[65]

Postmodernists declare that all worldviews are products of human constructions and that human relations serve the interest of the stronger

---

60. Hegel, *Philosophy of History*, 440; Hegel, *Hegel's Lectures*, 549.
61. Ibid.
62. Habermas, *Philosophical Discourse of Modernity*, 17.
63. Norris, *Deconstruction*, 8.
64. Dallmayr, *Discourse of Modernity*, 65; Habermas, *Philosophische Diskurs Der Moderne*.
65. McCarthy, "Introduction," x.

party.⁶⁶ Objective truth is nowhere to be found. Alvin Plantinga criticizes this postmodern mentality of "creative anti-realism," wherein human thought and language are in some way *responsible for* the fundamental structures and entities of the world. This mentality clearly is in denial of created reality and the sovereignty of God over the cosmos.⁶⁷ Dallmayr suggests that Habermas promotes a contractual construct of individual cooperation and mutual agreement in the contractarian tradition of Hobbes and others. Its *telos* derives meaning from intersubjective understanding and consensus.⁶⁸ Eventually, formal structures emerge from experientially tested consensus-making over time and are reconfigured based on new experiences. Then, habitual, recurrent behavior leads to universal principles of ethics on the path toward the ideal of pure critical reason.

Very recently, Habermas's postmodern openness has shown an allowance for greater inclusion of religious perspectives at some levels of public discourse. Openly critical of Rawls's restrictive role of religion in political life,⁶⁹ Habermas has guarded empathy with Robert Audi's objection to Rawls's requirement for "adequate secular reasons" for any law or public-policy recommendations based on religious belief.⁷⁰ Religious traditions, Habermas argues, have "a special power to articulate moral intuitions." As such, in the *informal* public sphere, secular citizens should be open to possible truth content within expressed religious reasons.⁷¹ Yet, at the level of government policymaking and judicial rulings, only secular reasons count in order to maintain the neutrality among competing worldviews under the separation of church and state.⁷² Here, Habermas puts his liberal foot

---

66. Ibid., 186.
67. Plantinga, "Advice," 269.
68. Dallmayr, "Discourse of Modernity," 67–68.
69. Habermas, *Between Naturalism and Religion*, 123–24.
70. Audi and Wolterstorff, *Religion in the Public Square*, 25. Habermas (*Between Naturalism and Religion*, 105) notes Wolterstorff's contention that those who try to live out their religious faith strive for wholeness and integration in their lives and the truths inherent in that faith shape their whole existence, including its social and political aspects. Lisa Cahill (*Theological Bioethics*, 29–30) also speaks of the contest between missional agendas of Christianity, science, and business. Market capitalism is seen as a competing religion with its promise of salvation from unhappiness through commodities.
71. Habermas, *Between Naturalism and Religion*, 131–32. He also acknowledges that the pressure to critically appraise faith convictions may drive religious citizens to evade unreserved discursive scrutiny by "rationally justified reference to the dogmatic authority of an inviolable core of infallible revealed truths."
72. Ibid., 130. Habermas labels this position his *institutional translation proviso*.

Part One: The Rise and Dominance of Principles-Based Biomedical Ethics

down in resisting challenges by Nicholas Wolterstorff and Paul Weithman who want even this limited proviso of secular translation to be removed so that religious reasons should be allowed to stand on their own merits.[73]

Habermas hopes that welcoming openness, which he sees as a mentality of modernity, to all worldviews will lead to their replacement by a future community of unrestrained communication among equals, all accomplished through rational discourse. However, Griffioen cautions against this alluring openness.[74] I concur with Griffioen's cautionary note. In my view, principlism is the expression of this vision in biomedical ethics. The common morality is realized through the *sensus communis*, rational consensus that creates its own justification for both its grounding and for subsequent moral judgments and choices.

Despite disenchantment with modernism, its presence can still be strongly felt in formal cultural expressions. For example, biotechnology is alive and well with its promises of control over disease and human incapacity. Lambert Zuidervaart notes that residua of modernity, such as the modern construction of an epistemic subject, make possible the poststructualist notions of subject positions.[75] Smith adds that postmodernism does not cleanly break with modernism. Continuity is evident in the denial of grace by both modernism and postmodernism. They main-

---

73. Ibid., 133–35; Audi and Wolterstorff, *Religion in the Public Square*, 160. Habermas understands that Weithman (*Religion and the Obligations of Citizenship*, 3) wants citizens to base their judgments on their concept of justice grounded in their own substantive worldview. Habermas is concerned that religious claims could evolve into an authoritative governmental agent of a religious majority that imposes its will in violation of democratic procedures. Weithman (*Religion and the Obligations of Citizenship*, 142) rejects such concerns, arguing that such positions should not gain sufficient public support to put them in power if democracy is working properly! Habermas concludes that the empiricist understanding of a liberal democracy envisions all political parties striving for the largest possible shared basic goods such as money, security, and leisure time. By contrast, Wolterstorff represents a party that aspires to other competing goods, what Habermas calls goods of salvation.

74. Griffioen, "Worldview Approach," 96, 103–4.

75. Zuidervaart, "Good Cities," 149. Seeing this uneasy co-existence in a positive light, Zuidervaart claims that modern subjectivism awakens us to God-given creative potential: "In all these ways we who inhabit a postmodern culture are deeply indebted to modern thought, even as we seek ways to escape its destructive dilemmas. So the challenge that modernity sets before us is to be postmodern without becoming antimodern and to recover medieval humility and ancient wonder without embracing the narrow parochialism and rigid stratification of a premodern world." For Christians in the Reformed tradition, this means proclaiming the story of a good creation redeemed by Jesus Christ and of a God who loves mercy and justice with the promise of a new heaven and new earth.

tain a theme of self-sufficiency and naturalism while having a mutual disenchantment with the world.[76] Also, with modernity comes a loss of gratuity, while postmodernism disembodies. As a result, relationships are reduced to facts and algorithms.[77]

Principlism: A Postmodern Worldview and Vestigial Remnants of Modernity

According to historian Albert Jonsen, contemporary bioethics is inadequate for addressing the bioethical challenges of science and biotechnology. It lacks strategies for resolving complex issues such as the moral status of the human embryo, organ donation, and end-of-life issues.[78] The emotivism and expressivism of the early twentieth century, he believes, have contributed to this moral insufficiency. G. E. Moore, for example, writes that the notion of "good" is intuitively perceived, with no foundation as a natural property.[79] A. J. Ayer and Charles Stevenson claim that ethical statements only represent emotive feelings that attempt to persuade others to approve or disapprove of actions or events.[80] By the 1940s, the notion of ethical claims having a basis in rationally discernable natural facts was replaced by a preoccupation with the emotive and linguistic aspects of ethical expression.[81]

In the wake of these new notions of ethics, *metaethics*[82] arose in the early second half of the twentieth century out of frustration with the

---

76. Smith, *Who's Afraid*, 26; Hughes, *Worship as Meaning*. Smith gives Graham Hughes credit for the last point.

77. Cayley, *Rivers*, 220–29. Mary Hesse ("How to Be Postmodern," 457) notes that feminists such as Ann Seller conclude that the best way of reaching satisfactory interpretations of experience is through open conversation within some human community. She notes the similarity of this conclusion with those of Gadamer, Habermas, and Rorty.

78. Jonsen, *Birth of Bioethics*, 3. Attributing much of this inadequacy to principlism, Clouser and Gert ("A Critique of Principlism," 219) call the reliance on the four principles "a mantra . . . this ritual incantation in the face of biomedical dilemmas that beckons our inquiry."

79. Moore, *Principia Ethica*.

80. Ayer, *Language*.

81. For a full discussion of Stevenson's critique of the pseudo-concepts of ethical terminology, see Stevenson, *Covenant of Grace Renewed*.

82. Jonsen, *Birth of Bioethics*, 72–73. According to Jonsen, the term was coined by A. J. Ayer in 1949. At this time, moral philosophy distinguished first order discourse that concerned discourse over what actions and policies are right or wrong

PART ONE: The Rise and Dominance of Principles-Based Biomedical Ethics

modernist dream that a better life could be achieved through autonomous human capacity and industry, motivated by a myth of progress.[83] For a quarter century, moral philosophers analyzed the language of ethics, debating distinctions such as right and wrong, good and evil, and fact and value. But truth became relative and historically contingent.[84] Principlism arose as an expression of such a postmodern idea of moral truth.

However, even several years after the establishment of principlism,[85] opportunities arose for moral philosophers to find philosophical grounding regarding bioethical positions and policies. One example typifies the triumph of postmodern influence when the reflective method of principlism is applied. In 1982, a Royal Commission in the United Kingdom was charged with examining the social, ethical, and legal implications of developments in human-assisted reproduction.[86] However, after attempts at sound philosophical reasoning, commission chair Warnock rejected deontological and utilitarian arguments. She confessed that the commission had adopted a relativist position, despite her previously expressed strong contention that a metaethical focus on ethical language trivializes ethics at the expense of normative ethics. She stated categorically that, while on moral questions there could be better or worse judgments, there was no such thing as a correct judgment.[87] Colleague Richard Hare mused that the Commission simply found some conclusions that most of the

---

from second order discourse, which probes the meaning of terms such as "right" and "wrong."

83. Naugle, *Worldview*, 173; Goheen and Bartholomew, *Living at the Crossroads*, 107–09.

84. Goheen and Bartholomew, *Living at the Crossroads*, 110, 113. The philosopher Jacques Derrida is a formative champion of a focus on language as the basis of what can be known. He considers language to be the most fundamental aspect of reality itself. In this thinking, modernist optimism about facts is challenged by belief in a return to nominalist reality in which there is no objective ontological standing, just a framework for reality imposed by our minds on the particulars of the universe. O'Donovan (*Resurrection and Moral Order*, 49–51) points to Herman Dooyeweerd's claim that nominalism prevails when special sciences attempt to investigate a specific aspect of reality without considering its coherence with other aspects that philosophy helps to provide. Dooyeweerd (*New Critique*, vol. 1, 558–66; II, 564–67) also sees the perceived separation of faith and reason as a nominalist construct incompatible with a Christian worldview.

85. Beauchamp and Childress, *Principles of Biomedical Ethics*, 1st ed.

86. Jonsen, *Birth of Bioethics*, 309.

87. Warnock, *Question of Life*, x, 96.

Richness and Depth of Understanding within Faith Traditions

members could sign, arriving at consensus for its own sake rather than through hard philosophical work.[88]

It appeared that postmodernism had encroached on biomedical ethics.

Principlism clearly has elements of a postmodern worldview. Moral judgments derive from a consensus of moral friends or strangers who look to intuition and persistent debate in order to arrive, hopefully, at moral agreement.[89] On the other hand, it can be argued that the dominance of autonomy over other principles is a remnant of the individualism promoted by modernism. Despite the claim of Beauchamp and Childress that autonomy has only *prima facie* standing alongside other principles, others rightly point to the pervasive dominance of autonomy in biomedical ethics.[90] Seeking universal moral norms from a common morality also represents a remnant of modernity, yet its "objectivity" stems from a postmodern consensus of subjective expression and persuasion, denying privilege or primacy to any one set of beliefs as bearers of truth.[91]

Moral decision-making in principlism is rooted in historicism, in which history is a "categorical matrix of all meaning and value."[92] Over time, moral judgments change because of the contingencies of culture.[93] O'Donovan exposes the powerful influence of historicism on contemporary ethics. When creation is not recognized as a complete design, presupposed by any historical contingency, the goodness of created natural structures becomes confused with sin and disorder and the integrity of created structures as irreducible totalities is lost. The end of times becomes the historical end of temporal existence rather than does the coming of Christ on the clouds. Such is the teleological goal of reflective

---

88. Hare, "*In Vitro* Fertilization," 71–90; Lockwood, "Warnock Report."

89. Michael DePaul (*Balance and Refinement*, 2–4; 13–23) nicely summarizes the coherentist method of reflective equilibrium that undergirds much of consensus-determined morality.

90. Pellegrino and Thomasma, *Christian Virtues*, 117–24; Evans, *Playing God?*, 158–65. Pellegrino in particular has objected that the principle of autonomy has superseded beneficence as the first principle of biomedical ethics due in large part to its loss of a communal focus and the failure to define its moral limits.

91. Beauchamp and Childress, *Principles of Biomedical Ethics*, 5th ed., 3–5, 401–05.

92. O'Donovan, *Resurrection and Moral Order*, 60.

93. Rawls, *Theory of Justice*, 20f, 48–51, 120f.

equilibrium theory without an eschatological focus on Christ and final moral accountability.[94]

Thus, principlism can be seen as a by-product of persistent aspirations of modernity, despite the reactive skepticism of postmodernity. Its use of coherence theory reflects the premise that certain non-religious epistemic beliefs will be favored *a priori*, that resolution of morally conflicting views must be attempted on a case-by-case basis, and that the commitment of the moral agent to particular beliefs is repeatedly tested. To achieve this, the pursuit of reflective equilibrium seeks grounding only in postmodern subjectivist preferences.[95]

In the process of achieving reflective equilibrium, *initial moral judgments* become *considered moral judgments* by filtering out initial ones that run the risk of being moral mistakes. Judgments are retained if no explanations can be found to render these judgments false or in error, though they remain revisable over time.[96] *Moral principles* can be induced from such judgments but are also considered revisable. The reiterative complexity of testing moral judgments and principles governs the confidence with which one decides whether the judgment or the principle should be adjusted.[97] Then, when *background or broader philosophical beliefs* about the nature of persons and the role of morality in society are considered, such beliefs are compared with the *narrow equilibrium* previously achieved between considered judgments and moral principles. However, like judgments and principles, *background beliefs are not assigned a privileged status.*[98] Otherwise, the accusation could be made that background beliefs threaten to coerce judgments and principles into agreement.

---

94. O'Donovan, *Resurrection and Moral Order*, 58, 60, 63, 67–68. Historicism denies a universal order of meaning and value given in creation and fulfilled in the kingdom of God. O'Donovan sees an idealist strain in all forms of historicism in which, at the end of time, history becomes conscious of itself. In my view, such groundless optimism breeds an evolutionary self-fulfillment of human ethical reflection that is the "grounding" of principlism's reflective equilibrium of moral deliberation and decision-making.

95. Daniels, "Wide Reflective Equilibrium," 258.

96. Rawls, *Theory of Justice*, 47–48. For Rawls, considered judgments are "rendered under conditions favorable to the exercise of the sense of justice . . . as a mental capacity." Accounts of this sense of justice, in turn, involve intuitive appeals that embody "various reasonable and natural presumptions." Thus, a sense of justice is foremost for Rawls in making such considered judgments. Unfortunately, these presumptions are not further articulated for Rawls.

97. DePaul, *Balance and Refinement*, 18–20.

98. Ibid., 20.

Richness and Depth of Understanding within Faith Traditions

This relativistic and temporally contingent process framework is driven by a reactionary aversion to any semblance of foundationalism and its modernist roots. It tries to ignore the profound and overarching influences of presuppositional, pre-theoretical background beliefs that are embedded in the basic core beliefs of each human being.

Today, the societal sense of moral urgency that spawned the Belmont Report has eased. Universities and medical schools have bioethicists and bioethics committees closely aligned with research ethics boards to oversee the protection of human subjects in clinical research. In its place is an urgency to find new life-extending therapies through medical science for progressively debilitating diseases like Parkinson's disease and cancer. Such urgency often side-steps ethical reflection and concerns in areas like human stem-cell research. The destruction of human embryos to obtain stem cells is considered acceptable by some non-Christians and Christians if resultant therapies benefit an already born, fully or near-fully capacitated human sufferer of disease. However, reflections on such weighty issues by Christians whose consciences question the destruction of early human life are often bereft of depth and imagination. The inability or unwillingness of many Christians to confront these issues with boldness and with intense, faith-enriching reflection has regrettably contributed to a thriving common-morality community. In the meantime, bioethics has moved to find whatever common ground can be found. Unfortunately, the basis of such agreement is at best of secondary interest. The agreement itself is its own authority and justification.[99]

Beauchamp and Childress claim that the common morality consists of "ordinary, shared moral beliefs . . . they make no appeal to pure reason, rationality, natural law, a special moral sense, or the like."[100] They further claim that principles are derived from shared moral beliefs they call *pretheoretical common sense moral judgments*, the basis of which is the existence of the common morality.[101] From this common morality mysteriously flow the four principles.[102] The common morality comprises

---

99. Louthan, "On Religion," 180. In his engagement with Richard Rorty, Alvin Plantinga shows how such consensus based on only rational opinion leads to a vacuous nominalism that can drift far afield from reality.

100. Beauchamp and Childress, *Principles of Biomedical Ethics*, 5th ed., 403. Other common-morality theories are cited as Frankena (*Ethics*) and Ross (*Foundations of Ethics*).

101. Ibid.

102. Ibid., 12.

those norms that "all morally serious persons accept as authoritative."[103] Thus, the grounding of principlism is in the principles themselves as direct derivatives of the common morality. I have shown that the common morality and its manifestations in principlism are rooted in worldviews that are grounded in faith in human reason. In modernism lies faith in reason as the universal norm for finding truth in this world. In postmodernism, faith in reason gives hope while sifting through the historical and cultural factors that make up contingent truth, that which is always revisable and unstable.

In my view, Beauchamp and Childress fail to substantiate a common morality of faithlessness. They do not deny that moral communities exist whose basis is faith in a moral source outside of our temporal existence. But they claim that these communities aspire to moral ideals, communal norms, certain extraordinary virtues, "and the like" that could not be obligated to persons who have faith in a common morality.[104] They claim the common morality is the public ethic with its common language and principles.

It is my contention that principlism is another private morality anchored in faith in reason alone. Since the true status of reason is that of a human capacity, not as an authoritative moral source, it imparts no superior moral status to the common morality. Unfortunately, no alternative worldview has seriously challenged the combination of postmodern and modernist belief at the core of common, universal morality, due in large part to the moral fragmentation of Western society. As a default, principlism has remained a popular default ethic. Its "mid-level" principles are considered more malleable within a pluralistic context than are *foundational principles* such as Hare's universalizability principle.[105] Ana Smith Iltis rightly points out that, while specification is touted by some as the solution to the foundational and methodological deficiencies of principlism, both specification and principlism are *theories without theories*. They lack a universally agreed-upon background theory or an overriding principle that gives guidance concerning *how* to specify and *how* to choose among principles and between conflicting specifications within a principle.[106]

---

103. Ibid., 3, 403. Elsewhere, they state that the combination of the common morality and the coherence model of justification "allows us to rely on the authority of the principles in the common morality."

104. Ibid., 3, 4.

105. Hare, *Freedom and Reason*.

106. Iltis, "Bioethics," 273–74.

Richness and Depth of Understanding within Faith Traditions

I have provided a look into the varied Christian responses to principlism, most of which express some appreciation for the common language that the principles provide for bioethical dialogue. Some responses provide more substantive critiques that include demonstrating the lack of moral grounding and authority of the common morality from which the four principles are derived. Others show the lack of a unifying principle or guiding moral authority for dealing with conflicts of principles in specific situations. In my own analysis, I expose the belief system and worldviews from which principlism developed. That is, principlism is grounded in a presuppositional faith in rationality. It has developed distinct features of modernist and postmodern worldviews from which it claims to draw its moral authority and justification for a linguistic framework for moral dialogue.

From a Reformed Christian perspective, this ethical framework must be challenged as an inadequate ethical framework for addressing contemporary moral reflection, problem solving, and policymaking. In the second half of this book, I will meet this challenge by developing a covenantal ethical framework that springs from the earlier work of Ramsey and May, grounded in moral authority outside of human or other temporal authority. More so than my predecessors, however, I will refocus on medicine as a relational discipline, paying careful attention to the normative expression of those relationships. With this ethical framework, I will re-envision the four principles in light of a biblical understanding of their place in God's created order.

As the first step in developing this new ethical framework, in the next chapter, I will provide the transcendent, biblical grounds for a covenantal ethical framework. Furthermore, I will give evidence that the biblical covenant theme as developed in the Reformed Christian tradition provides the most insightful conceptual framework for envisioning a covenantal ethic for biomedical ethics.

Part Two

A Modest Proposal for a
Biblical Covenantal Biomedical Ethic

5

Conceptual Support for Covenantal Biomedical Ethics

A covenantal ethic, above all else, defines the moral life responsively. Moral action (such as selling, refraining, respecting, giving, and professing) ultimately derives from and responds to a primordial receiving.[1]

—WILLIAM F. MAY (1996)

RECLAIMING A RELATIONAL CORE FOR BIOMEDICAL ETHICS

IN CHAPTER 1, THE major premises and structure of the principles-based ethical framework promoted by Beauchamp and Childress, also known as principlism, were reviewed.[2] In light of substantial critiques of this ethical framework over the past three decades as articulated in chapters 2, 3, and 4, its authors have attempted to address its perceived shortcomings in subsequent editions of their book *Principles of Biomedical Ethics*.[3] I conclude in chapter 4 that principles-based biomedical ethics should be re-examined regarding its basic presuppositions and core beliefs, providing such a critique by exposing the rationalistic core of its faith commitment expressed through elements of both modernist and postmodern

---

1. May, *Testing the Medical Covenant*, 52.
2. Clouser and Gert, "Critique of Principlism."
3. Beauchamp and Childress, *Principles of Biomedical Ethics*, 5th ed.

worldviews. In short, principlism reflects lingering modernist hopes of achieving a universal common morality based on rational consensus of all morally serious persons. However, in the spirit of postmodernism, such consensus seems achievable only by the outward acceptance of all views of truth as valid, as long as a dominant faith in logical, iterative persuasion prevails through the suppression of the expression of deeper beliefs that may disrupt a rational conclusion.

The diversity of so-called private views of truth reflects the moral fragmentation exposed by MacIntyre in modern society. Such fragmentation coincides with the replacement of God with human reason as ultimate moral authority since the Enlightenment. Christian responses to the rise and dominance of principlism also have been fragmented. Pellegrino provides the most in-depth Christian critique to date, reestablishing the moral authority of God's Word through the principle of love and a refocus of biomedical ethics on the virtues of the moral agent. But his refocus of the moral agent fails to address the relational complexity of modern medicine where moral agents with diverse faith commitments deal with tensions that such differences may generate. Ramsey and, subsequently but more systematically by, May provide insight into this by advocating for an ethic that seeks primarily understanding of relational aspects of biomedical situations and practice.

Recently, medical practitioners and educators have begun to recognize the merits of developing a covenantal framework in order to find deeper meaning in relationships between those of diverse moral beliefs.[4] Some advocate for a secular covenantal model that appeals to the Greek medical tradition for moral authority. That tradition claims moral authority in the tradition itself as conceived by human beings in the myths of the Greek gods. There is no link between the transcendent God of Scripture and humankind.

In light of this growing interest in the relational core of medicine and biomedical ethics, it is worth building on the work of Ramsey, Pellegrino, and May. However, the nature/grace dualism of Pellegrino obstructs a more holistic vision of created reality as all sacred and under God's providential care. In addition, the role of all caregivers, their relationships with patients and fellow caregivers, and their interrelations in medicine must each be valued and understood to give full attention and meaning to the

---

4. Cassel, "Patient-Physician Covenant"; Li, "Patient-Physician Relationship"; Brothers, "Covenant"; Coffey, "Nurse-Patient Relationship"; Nisker, "Covenantal Model."

needs of patients. In order to move forward and to provide a more in-depth and complete Christian covenantal ethical model for biomedical ethics, it is my contention that a covenantal bioethical framework rooted in a Reformed Christian worldview can address the loss of moral authority inherent in principlism and can restore full meaning to the ethos of biomedical ethics. A biblically based covenantal ethic offers a normative and rich understanding of human personhood and medical relationships. Such an ethic can enrich our understanding of medicine through a Christian social philosophy that avoids the pitfalls of reductionist views of reality and can more normatively contextualize the four principles of principlism.

I will begin this first chapter of part two by examining concepts of covenant used to describe and prescribe medical relationships in contemporary medicine. Contemporary appeals to ancient Greek medical or Christian traditions will be reviewed as justification for promoting a covenant framework for biomedical ethics, beginning with a brief allusion to various concepts of covenant in ancient times. I will then describe the historical development of biblical concepts of covenant, particularly in the Augustinian/Reformed tradition, and articulate previous attempts to develop and apply a biblical covenantal ethic to Christian ethics and bioethics. I will argue for further development of such an ethic because it can provide a meaningful relational framework and grounding in the covenantal relationship between God and all of humankind. The elements of such a framework will be described in chapter 6. In chapter 7, justification for a Christian social philosophy for medicine will be presented in light of the relational nature of medicine and the necessary encounters with the needs of strangers. This will lay the ethical groundwork for reconceptualizing the four principles of principlism in chapter 8.

COVENANTAL RELATING: HIPPOCRATIC TRADITION AND CURRENT APPEALS

The Hippocratic Oath: Then and Now

Agreements or pacts among different parties have been called covenants since the beginning of recorded history.[5] Biblical scholars have found

---

5. McCarthy, *Treaty and Covenant*, 31, 93, 126. Dennis McCarthy has presented linguistic and conceptual evidence for covenant relationships in various parts of the ancient world, mentioned in ancient Sumerian, Hittite, and Egyptian texts.

PART TWO: A Modest Proposal for a Biblical Covenantal Biomedical Ethic

striking similarities in the components of treaties among ancient peoples. For example, Dennis McCarthy notes that ancient Hittite treaties of the fourteenth century BC and Assyrian suzerainty treaties of the eighth century BC show similarities to covenants established between God and Israel in the Old Testament, particularly with regard to ritual practices and the role of mediators.[6] Against the backdrop of these Middle Eastern traditions and Israel's post-exilic period, a Greek medical tradition developed with a covenant concept understood most commonly through the Hippocratic Oath[7] (see Appendix 1).

The original purpose of the Oath is not known. W. H. S. Jones gives evidence that it may have been used to test the commitment of outsiders seeking membership into a clan-based medical community.[8] The Oath describes in covenantal terms the relationship between the medical apprentice Oath taker and his mentor.[9] It begins with the Oath taker swearing to numerous gods that he will fulfill obligations of the Oath (referred to in the Oath as "this covenant").[10] In gratitude for the gift of the knowledge of medicine, the apprentice considers his mentor equal in honor and respect to his own parents and his mentor's sons equal to his own brothers. He pledges financial help and free instruction in the art of medicine. This familial metaphor resembles the kinship metaphor describing Old Testament covenants as well as others described in the ancient world.[11] The Oath taker offers dietetic beneficence to the sick while pledging to keep them from harm and injustice while maintaining confidentiality. Specific codal

---

6. Ibid., 285–98. McCarthy suggests that Israel may have adopted ritual practices common to their neighbors but that they infused new meaning into them in the service of Yahweh (294 n. 39, 295).

7. Referred to henceforth as "the Oath."

8. Jones, *Doctor's Oath*, 29–33, 44.

9. Edelstein, *Ancient Medicine*, 56. According to Edelstein, the terms *covenant* and *law* were used interchangeably in Athens at the reputed time of the origin of the Oath, about 421 BC.

10. W. H. S. Jones (*Doctor's Oath*, 31) notes that an Arabic version from the first half of the thirteenth century is entitled "The Text of the Covenant Laid Down by Hippocrates," supporting May's contention that the entire Oath could be seen as a covenant.

11. Hahn, "Kinship By Covenant"; Bruggemann, "Covenanted Family," 18–23; Segal, *Rebecca's Children*, 3. Hahn, Bruggemann, and Segal further elaborate on the role of family and kinship in ancient covenants. Note also the parallel with use of the adoption metaphor in characterizing the new covenant in Christ in Eph 1:5 and Rom 8:23. In early Greek medicine, the physician Galen (c.129 to 216 AD) spoke of a previous ancient clan of Asklepiads who taught their sons anatomy and orally passed on the ways and secrets of their profession.

Conceptual Support for Covenantal Biomedical Ethics

prohibitions against harm include refusal to assist in suicide or abortion and abstinence from sexual relations with patients. The Oath ends with a blessing/curse formula; that is, the Oath taker asks to be blessed with fame for keeping the Oath and to be cursed among men if he violates it.[12]

Thus, the Hippocratic Oath contains a *code of conduct* regarding the behavior of the Oath taker to his *patients* and describes a *covenantal bond* with his *mentor*, an important point of distinction not often noticed by those who claim that the Oath defines covenantal roots in the patient-physician relationship. In addition, the covenant has an air of professional exclusivity in suggesting that the knowledge of medical practice should be shared only among those who take the Oath and enter into its promises and obligations.[13]

David Albert Jones notes there are a variety of contemporary views regarding the origin and philosophical influence of the Oath. He suggests that these views and the resulting appropriation of the contents of the Oath attest to the plasticity of meaning that can be derived from its content.[14] Three Hippocratic elements are common to early pagan, Christian, and Muslim versions[15]: an appeal to a transcendent witness or sanction, recognition that the aim of medicine is to benefit the sick, and the prohibition of deliberate killing, including killing of the unborn.[16]

Many contemporary versions have characteristically deleted any reference to transcendent authority, altering the meaning of the covenantal arrangement that was initially conceived.[17] Edelstein feels that the Oath

---

12. Meredith Kline (*By Oath Consigned*, 16–17), Gerhardus Vos (*Biblical Theology*, 137), and Dennis McCarthy (*Treaty and Covenant*, 96) all point out the important role of an oath as a ratification or sanction-sealed commitment in divine–human covenants in Scripture and frequently in extra-biblical treaties or covenants.

13. Ludwig Edelstein provides evidence that prohibitions to abortions, suicide, and sexual relations may have been introduced by a small group of reform-minded physicians influenced by Pythagorean ideals (a hypothesis also entertained more recently by Nigel Cameron (*Life and Death*)). Edelstein (*Ancient Medicine*, 6–51), May ("Code, Covenant," 29), DeVogel (*Pythagorus*), and Carrick (*Medical Ethics*) provide further readings on this and possible Epicurean influences.

14. Jones, "Hippocratic Oath"; Rutten, "Receptions of the Hippocratic Oath." David Jones notes that groups as diverse as Nazi physicians and the British Medical Association have invoked the Oath as a source of authority for their practices.

15. Jones, *Doctor's Oath*, 22–27. The earliest Christian version was produced in the tenth or eleventh century. W. H. S. Jones also provides an Arabic version from the early thirteenth century.

16. Jones, "Hippocratic Oath." Jones provides a comprehensive analysis of these versions.

17. See, for example, the version adopted by the World Medical Association (World Medical Association *Declaration of Geneva* 1948, amended 1968, 1983).

Part Two: A Modest Proposal for a Biblical Covenantal Biomedical Ethic

was taken with free conscience in ancient times and that the pledge to transcendent authority to do good deeds was motivated by the desire for eternal fame and glory among succeeding generations.[18] Robert Orr and colleagues have undertaken a review of contemporary versions of the Oath and their use among medical schools and medical associations.[19] They note that by 1993 only 11 per cent of Oaths mentioned an invocation of a deity. Unlike Edelstein, William F. May believes that this omission changes its fundamental character and that swearing to one or more deities affirms its religious character and "the ontological root of his [the oath taker's] life."[20]

Orr and colleagues suggest that such omissions may reflect a secularized, pluralistic society within which it is too difficult to find agreement on such matters of content.[21] Other important omissions in current versions include the protection of human life and accountability. Unfortunately, these omissions deprive the Oath of ethical guidance and a transcendent reference point. Leon Kass believes that the spirit of the Oath reflects and embodies a deeper view about character and virtue requisite for medicine rather than simply a codal list of "dos and don'ts."[22] It is this spirit that is lost in minimalist adaptations of the Oath. Reformed theologian Allen Verhey writes that, in practicing sensitivity to the ethical perspectives of others in a pluralistic society, Christians "should have the integrity to set medicine in the context of the Christian story, to form, inform, and reform medicine."[23] What, then, is the basis of recent invocations for covenantal relationships for medicine not based on the covenantal theme of the Christian Scriptures?

---

18. Edelstein, *Ancient Medicine*, 51, 61; Bailey, "Asklepios." By the time of the early church, Asklepios had become revered as a half mortal/half god who helped the poor of Greece. Asklepios's reputation was sometimes compared to that of Christ as savior, healer, and advocate of the lowly and poor. According to Bailey, Tatian even pointed out that Christ's death was not foreign to the pagans in that the god Asklepios suffered a similar end. Justin Martyr wrote in the second century that proclaiming Christ as crucified, dead, risen from the dead, and ascended into heaven was nothing new to his pagan audience, since their god Asklepios "was a great physician, was struck by a thunderbolt, and so ascended into heaven."

19. Orr, "Use of the Hippocratic Oath."

20. May, *Physician's Covenant*, 111.

21. Orr, "Use of the Hippocratic Oath," 386.

22. Kass, "Is There a Medical Ethic," 240.

23. Verhey, "Hippocratic Oath," 116–17.

Calls for Covenantal Relating in Medicine

Some bioethicists have recently expressed concern with the contemporary status of medical relationships and have suggested better relational models. Edmund Pellegrino argues that Mark Siegler's understanding of medicine as negotiated agreements between patients and physicians focuses too much on the *process* of relationship formation. Pellegrino redirects the focus toward the healing relationship as the architectonic principle of a theory of medicine that merges the phenomena of medicine with personal relationships.[24] Emanuel and Emanuel favor a deliberative model that portrays the physician as teacher and/or friend, and that envisions patient autonomy as moral self-development.[25] This choice is consistent with their model of a liberal pluralistic state made up of communities defined by shared conceptions of the good.[26] Suchman and colleagues suggest improving the identification of *empathic and praise opportunities* and what others have called "windows of opportunity" to improve sensitivity to the plight of patients within medical relationships.[27]

Calls for a covenantal concept or metaphor for developing human relationships within the practice of medicine have come from various segments of medical care in recent years. In 1995, eight prominent medical practitioners from diverse backgrounds and beliefs published a "Patient-Physician Covenant." These authors were motivated by a growing anxiety over changes in the structure and practice of medicine that threaten its fundamental values and the responsibility of physicians to their patients. The statement is meant to rally the profession around a renewed commitment to medicine as a moral enterprise grounded in a *covenant of trust*, a

---

24. Siegler, "Doctor-Patient Encounter," 627–44; Pellegrino, "Healing Relationship," 153–72; Pellegrino and Thomasma, "Christian Virtues."

25. Emanuel and Emanuel, "Four Models," 2221–26.

26. Emanuel, *Ends of Human Life*; Engelhardt, *Foundations of Bioethics*. 1st ed.; Engelhardt, *Foundations of Christian Bioethics*. Here Ezekiel Emanuel gives a full account of his communitarian model. In review and critique of this model, Baruch Brody ("Liberalism," 404) notes that it assumes a very similar version to that presented by Engelhardt in *Foundations of Bioethics*. However, Brody feels that Emanuel's version is developed more fully in his vision of sub-communities that 1) practice deliberative democracy through public debate and persuasion based on reasoned appeals to a shared common good and 2) envision persons as autonomous, deliberative agents who shape and sustain their community. Engelhardt's vision of medical practice and public health in his own inclusive community within the pluralistic liberal reality as defined by an Orthodox Christian faith is found in *Foundations of Christian Bioethics*.

27. Suchman, "A Model," 678–82.

Part Two: A Modest Proposal for a Biblical Covenantal Biomedical Ethic

greater concern for the sick, and better maintenance of "the soul" of the profession.[28]

Christine Cassel, one of the co-signatories, argues that physicians have a fiduciary (trust-based) responsibility to patients, the history of which can be traced to the myth of the demi-god Asklepios of ancient Greek medical tradition. Cassel draws a parallel between Asklepios's greedy acceptance of gold for medical services, rendered in Pindar's version of the myth, and contemporary inducements to put self-interest and self-gain before the values of the profession. Then as now, this grounding in trust is necessary to keep the beneficent focus on meeting patient needs. Cassel says that the physician's role has spiritual dimensions in the lives of patients and that medicine has a "transcendent significance to the activities of healing." Yet, she makes no appeals to moral authority beyond human common agreement.[29]

Citing Eric Mount's description of a Jewish covenantal accommodation of the vulnerable persons around us, Kyle Brothers argues that dialogue between the vulnerable patient and the physician provides a foundation that can lead to meaningful value sharing and patient empowerment.[30] He sees the chasm posed by major cultural differences as fostering a type of "otherness" that threatens communication unless both parties seek to understand each other's beliefs in their cultural contexts. Using the example of a young Sudanese woman seeking help regarding female circumcision, he explores legal, professional, and personal aspects while maintaining a creative, empathetic, and committed response to her situation as she presents it. For Brothers, the "special covenant relationship" requires presenting therapeutic options that meet the patient's needs according to the patient's preferences and desires. His emphasis is on patient empowerment, leading to less vulnerability of the patient in the relationship.

Jeff Nisker looks at a covenantal model to inspire teaching commitments in the "demoralizing climate" that he and others see as a threat to health care and medical education. He criticizes medical educators for a diminishing commitment to medical education.[31] In the medical

---

28. Cassel, "Patient-Physician Covenant," 604.
29. Ibid., 605.
30. Brothers, "Covenant," 1133; Mount, *Covenant, Community*, 144–47.
31. Nisker, "Covenant." Nisker calls the process of this diminishing commitment "demoralization by example." He adds that the bidirectional generosity necessary for a physician-patient relationship developed by Arthur Frank (*Renewal of Generosity*) applies just as much to a medical educator-student relationship.

educator-student relationship, Nisker seeks to capture the moral nature of medicine through inherent qualities of trust, generosity, commitment, empathy, and creativity not usually expressed in a contractual model. He appeals to characteristics of a covenantal relationship that others have offered, though not based on a tradition or a higher moral authority.[32]

From a nursing perspective, Sue Coffey explores whether a covenant concept can work both prescriptively and descriptively to better characterize the reality of daily interactions in nurse-patient relationships.[33] After briefly alluding to covenant in the Greek medical tradition, she credits William F. May with leading the contemporary resurgence of covenant as a prescriptive model for medical relationships, though she fails to note the biblical basis of his covenant idea.[34] Interestingly, her analysis *presupposes* the covenantal nature of the nurse-patient relationship, which can then be transformed and molded by the expressed views of nurses and patients. Coffey's study tries to create a theoretical framework of covenant through the testimony of experiences. She takes a feminist and care ethics viewpoint that emphasizes relationship, centeredness, situational particulars, and caring benevolence. This study is unusual in its assumption that there exists a structure for medical relationships that must then be formed according to the norms of practice, an assumption that will be further explored in chapter 7 as a Reformed Christian understanding of such relationships.

Physician David Landis has reflected on the tensions experienced in his medical training between protecting himself against the risks of emotional and psychological stress of patient encounters and providing maximum openness to patient needs. Some have advised that caregivers exercise protective distancing from personal, intimate emotional involvement.[35] However, such models have been criticized for their explicit and

---

32. Nisker does not even appeal to the "covenantal" devotion of the student of medicine to his mentor in the Hippocratic Oath!

33. Coffey, "Nurse-Patient Relationship," 308–23.

34. Meilaender, "On William F. May," 108, 119. As Meilaender notes, at times May speaks of the transcendent origins of covenant in generic terms while at other times he is clearer about his reference point in the God of Scripture. He even uses Calvin's spectacles metaphor indirectly, referring to ethics and theology as offering a kind of corrective vision for life issues. As if excusing the lack of theological specificity, Meilaender notes that May writes "very self-consciously as a theologian, but as one who is present not chiefly in ecclesiastical institutions but in the modern university."

35. Landis, "Physician Distinguish Thyself," 629–30; Fox, *Sociology of Medicine*; Lief and Fox, "Training," 15. Landis cites René Fox (*Sociology of Medicine*), who sees this detachment as a psychic counterirritant that focuses on information gathering

Part Two: A Modest Proposal for a Biblical Covenantal Biomedical Ethic

purposeful exclusion of affective, value-laden aspects of communication with patients.[36] During this training period, Landis experienced what he calls "a medical self," a new and unique self that emerged side by side with his original self. Personal experiences and emotions, he argues, can blur the distinction between the medical self and the personal self during patient encounters.[37]

Landis speaks of covenant development between the student, fellow students, and teachers. But for Landis medicine draws from a tradition of ideals. The student becomes covenantally bound to "the great healers and their art . . . to a medicine that was practiced . . . 'in the days of the giants.'"[38] He calls this a *transcendent* concept of the healing art. Landis draws a parallel with the student-mentor-mentor's family relationships of the Hippocratic Oath, suggesting that the medical student is reborn into a new professional family as a new self, the medical self.[39]

From this, it can be seen that some have used a secular concept of covenant to correct intuitively appreciated distortions of relationships within medicine. Such a covenant concept is often at best only loosely connected with ancient covenantal ideas while contributions from Christians such as May are sometimes cited but may be stripped of their biblical moorings. The increased interest in covenantal models coincides with efforts to address the overemphasis on patient autonomy that has largely replaced traditional paternalism. This is exemplified by exhorting the caregiver to display patient-sensitive dispositions and virtues while resisting paternalism, all for the benefit of the more vulnerable partner in the relationship.

---

while distracting students from the affective aspects of their work. Talcott Parsons similarly cautions against the temptation to become assimilated into a personal role of intimate friend in favor of maintaining an Archimedean position outside of ordinary social roles.

36. Ibid., 631; Cassell, *Nature of Suffering*. Landis notes that Eric Cassell has characterized this tension as a paradox in which the desire to be open and attentive creates the risk of distress and emotional vulnerability that can limit that openness.

37. Landis, "Physician Distinguish Thyself," 633. Landis seems to make this distinction on vocational grounds, suggesting that plumbers develop "plumber selves" and mechanics develop "mechanic selves."

38. Ibid., 636. This is quite contrary to May's covenant idea for medicine grounded in the relationship between God and humankind, as will be discussed later in this chapter. Gilbert Meilaender ("On William F. May," 114–15) has intimated that May's covenantal ethic was heavily influenced by Ramsey (*Patient as Person*, xi–xiv) and that the latter was influenced by Karl Barth's idea of creation. For Barth, creation is the external basis of covenant, while covenant is the internal basis of creation.

39. Ibid.

However, secular bioethicists acknowledge no standard or ideal outside of temporal reality by which normative medical relationships can be modeled and their "rightness" tested. When perceived through covenantal relationships, medicine has the richest meaning of its goods and ends through biblical grounding that inspires moral character and imparts values that drive the content of relational involvement. Relationships within the practice of medicine should not be seen as a power struggle but as compassionate, skilled, and directed energy toward the needs of vulnerable human beings.

Christians need to respond to this surge of interest in developing covenantal relationships within various aspects of medicine. They should reflect on how the biblical covenant theme can be developed and be broadly appealing within a biomedical ethical framework in medicine. The creational origin of this theme links all human beings to God, providing a common moral grounding for such an ethic. Among the Christian traditions, the biblical covenantal theme has primary theological importance in the Reformed tradition of the Protestant Reformation. In the next section, I will present the covenant theme as developed in that tradition, providing evidence that a normative understanding of a biblical notion of covenant begins with the covenant between God and all of humanity at creation and ends in the new covenant in Christ.

COVENANTAL RELATIONSHIPS IN THE CHRISTIAN SCRIPTURES

Covenant with God: At Creation or Sometime Later?

In this section, various dimensions of the biblical covenant theme will be discussed, particularly those that distinguish a covenant of works (i.e., covenant of creation) and a covenant of grace.[40] The merits of a covenant theology and corresponding ethic for biomedical ethics that is relevant to all human beings will be articulated. Later, I will show the influence

---

40. The covenant idea is a central theme in the Reformed tradition, though it is in other Christian traditions as well. Preuss (*From Shadow to Promise*, 245ff.) and Hagen ("From Testament to Covenant," 7–15) articulate its role in the Lutheran tradition. Klassen (*Covenant and Community*) and Williams (*Radical Reformation*, 153–54, 161) present its place in the Anabaptist tradition. Trinterud ("Origins of Puritanism," 41–42, 49–55) gives Arminian and Deist perspectives. Very recently, prominent Roman Catholic scholars such as Pope John Paul II, Pope Benedict XVI, and Scott Hahn have shown the importance of the covenant theme and its link to creation. These views will be mentioned later in this section.

Part Two: A Modest Proposal for a Biblical Covenantal Biomedical Ethic

of natural law theory on covenant theology and its potential pitfalls if covenantal aspects are diminished or lost, including its replacement by a focus on human autonomy that pervades much of biomedical ethics. Finally, I will present different visions of the applicability of the covenant concept according to various formative Christian bioethicists, completing the groundwork toward the development of a covenantal ethic applicable to contemporary bioethics.

The covenant theme runs through the length of redemptive history, though its prominence varies among different Christian traditions. Within the Reformed tradition covenant became a central theme when biblical studies rediscovered the importance of covenant during and after the Protestant Reformation. E. Clinton Gardner points out that covenant thought within Puritanism in sixteenth and seventeenth century England and America was influenced by John Calvin's Genevan group and the Zwinglian group in Zurich.[41] In the Rhineland region, the void left by the rejection of Roman Catholicism was replaced by a moral authority based on divine law and the biblical covenant between God and humankind. These were civically expressed as natural law and social contract theory within a developing theological tradition among the Protestant exiles during the reign of Queen Mary I.[42]

Richard Greaves argues that Zwingli, Johann Oecolampadius, and Zwingli's successor Heindrich Bullinger all emphasized the contractual nature of the covenants between God and human beings.[43] As early as 1525, Oecolampadius surmised that a "natural law" was an inherent part of humanity since creation. Its basis is our innate reason and it forms the basis of ruler/subject civil relationships. However, difficulties in reconciling the notion of a pre-fall covenant of all human beings with the doctrines of predestination and election resulted in *covenant of grace* theologies wherein the concept of a divine-human covenant was limited to post-fall, redemptive relationships.[44]

Around 1580, however, a so-called *covenant of works* began to take root in Reformed theology. David Weir and Leonard Trinterud propose that the adoption of this covenant of works grew out of efforts to find a theological basis for moral, civil, and religious obligations binding *all*

---

41. Gardner, *Justice and Christian Ethics*, 55–56.
42. Trinterud, "Origins of Puritanism," 37–41ff.
43. Greaves, "Origins," 24.
44. Trinterud, "Origins of Puritanism," 42.

Conceptual Support for Covenantal Biomedical Ethics

human beings.[45] The idea of the natural law of the state contract was fused with the natural law of the covenant of works. Within a few decades, a distinction between a covenant of works and covenant of grace was recognized as the *double covenant idea*.[46]

David Weir argues that Calvin saw the divine covenant as an *instrument of salvation* offered after the Fall of humankind into sin rather than as a *relationship* between God and humankind made at the time of creation. By contrast, Peter Lillback counters that Calvin saw *all* humans accepted into a common covenant or adoption at creation, one that they could break through disobedience. While the covenant is not an organizing principle in Calvin's theology, it is an integral feature.[47] Calvin's notion of covenant permeates other key themes in his theology including the idea of adoption by God (by which he parallels common adoption with a common covenant), election, the church, the law, and the sacraments.[48] Within a given community are those who by special election will remain bound to God and those who are non-elect, destined to irrevocably break the common covenant. In the Old and New Testaments (called "covenants" rather than "Testaments"[49]), God's people are a mixed lot. That is, there are those who, like the Pharisees, seek justification in the letter of the law. But there are also those who seek justification in the faithful acceptance of the gracious offering of the Spirit that frees us from the law. This is the earthly reality of the church and human existence. It involves covenants with mixed membership of the faithful and hypocrites. Even those who are truly elect in the new covenant can stumble and thus necessarily and constantly need to be on guard against disobedience.[50]

---

45. Ibid., 48; Weir, *Origins*, 5–8.

46. Trinterud, "Origins of Puritanism," 48–49. Trinterud outlines the development of the common cause of both the Puritan religious movement and the parliamentary political movement, both having a common theoretical scheme of the double covenant: the covenant of works and the covenant of grace.

47. Lillback, *Binding of God*, 1, 27. Others formulate the covenant theme somewhat differently. Weir (*Origins*, 3) distinguishes the covenant idea from which emerges covenant theology from which, in turn, federal theology emerges. The latter consists of a prelapsarian covenant with Adam and a postlapsarian covenant with Christ as the second Adam. Vos ("Doctrine," 236) uses the covenant theme more as a means of organizing his theology whereas McCoy ("Johannes Cocceius," 359) delimits covenant theology according to the covenants of works and grace.

48. Lillback, *Binding of God*, 135–39.

49. Allen, *Love and Conflict*, 31–32.

50. Lillback, *Binding of God*, 224–25.

Part Two: A Modest Proposal for a Biblical Covenantal Biomedical Ethic

Calvin alludes to a conditionality of human obedience to God that suggests a covenant relationship. He links Adam prior to the Fall with membership in the kingdom of God and consequently implies a role for law and universal divine kindness in his doctrine of common grace concerning fallen humankind. The command not to eat of the tree of knowledge of good and evil was a test of that obedience. Adam needed to grow in wisdom toward perfection through obedience to God.[51] Lillback reminds us that at one point, Calvin actually calls Adam's relationship with God a covenant, sealed by the *sacrament* that was the tree of life.[52]

Following in the Calvinist tradition, Herman Bavinck clearly and convincingly teaches that God made a covenant with Adam and all succeeding human beings. As Spykman has noted, the Hebrew word for covenant (*berith*) does not appear in the creation account of Genesis 1 and 2, noting that it first appears in the text of the Noah account of Genesis 6–9. Mentioned first before the flood in Genesis 6:18 and laid out in detail afterward in 9:9–17, this covenant is made with Noah, his family, and all surviving living creatures on earth. It has elements of renewal of a creational covenant with the cosmos through his covenantal relationship with Adam. At the same time, it focuses on living creatures whose descendants will repopulate the earth and with whom he promises never again to destroy all life with a flood.[53] While the overt mention of a covenant here could be construed as the first covenant for all of humankind, the earlier absence of the term "covenant" by no means excludes its presence. Kline and Eichrodt rightly note that "the reality of a word may be found in biblical texts from which that word is absent."[54] Yet the basic elements are present: an introduction of God in his relationship with Adam, promises and obligations that define the community established by the covenant, and the blessing-and-curse formula that has a stated condition for fidelity and a penalty for infidelity.[55]

---

51. Ibid., 288; Calvin, *Institutes*, II. I, 241–45.

52. Calvin, *Institutes*, IV.XIV.18, 1294. In his exposition on sacraments, he writes, "One [sacrament] is when he gave Adam and Eve the tree of life as a guarantee of immortality. . . . Another, when he set the rainbow for Noah. . . . These Adam and Noah regarded as sacraments . . . proofs and seals of his covenants."

53. Kline, *By Oath Consigned*, 27. Kline considers the Noahic covenant as a reinstituting of the original creational arrangements under the Adamic covenant.

54. Ibid. Eichrodt, *Theology*, 17f. Hoeksema (*Reformed Dogmatics*, 221) cites additional Scriptural references to a covenant without using the word explicitly. Note as well the mainly inferential concept of a creation covenant in Calvin's writings presented in the previous section.

55. Spykman, *Reformational Theology*, 260. McCarthy (*Old Testament Covenant*,

Conceptual Support for Covenantal Biomedical Ethics

According to Bavinck, humanity was created in God's image as an organic whole, not as separate individuals. This organic whole is reflected in the parallel between Adam as the head of the covenant of works and Christ as the head of the covenant of grace. He notes that Augustine described Adam's relationship with God as a covenant. Bavinck defends a covenant of works idea based on the idea that Adam was created with the implicit task of seeking the highest state of humanity, albeit under a probationary command. He favors this term over "covenant of nature" since it connotes that eternal life could only be obtained through keeping God's commandments.[56] With Adam's sin, creation stalled in achieving its destiny. As head of the new covenant, Christ redeems and elevates creation toward its originally intended eschatological destiny while restoring the relationship of the elect with God the Father through the Holy Spirit.[57]

Others such as Charles Hodge, Geerhardus Vos, and Louis Berkhof support Bavinck's interpretation of the origins of such a covenant.[58] In distinguishing the Lutheran from the Reformed perspectives, Vos supports a covenant of works idea as the means for humankind to obtain the highest state of freedom and uprightness beyond an original state of uprightness. He defends the covenant of works and covenant of redemption on the basis of the principle that God is to be glorified in all things.[59] For Berkhof, the creational relationship was covenantally qualified, established after creation and belonging to the administration of God's created kingdom.[60] Meredith Kline and O. Palmer Robertson support the concept but favor the more fitting term "covenant of creation" rather than covenant of works.[61] I agree with this corrective change since the term "covenant of works" connotes too great a distinction from a "covenant of grace" and in so doing implies a lack of grace in God's establishment of the covenant with Adam and thus all of humankind at creation. Indeed, God established his covenant with humankind through grace. However, despite these terminological differences, conceptually Bavinck appropriately links

---

1–10) gives an extensive review of these elements of covenant.

56. Bavinck, *Reformed Dogmatics*, 564–79.

57. Hielema, "Herman," 4–6, 72, 88–92, 114, 120–99.

58. Hodge, *Systematic Theology*; Vos, *Biblical Theology*, 37–51; Berkhof, *Systematic Theology*, 211–18.

59. Vos, "Doctrine," 234–67.

60. Berkhof, *Systematic Theology*, 272–301. On this point he differs from Spykman (*Reformational Theology*, 259, 260), who sees God's dealings with creation more intimately connected with covenanting. God covenanted his world into existence.

61. Kline, *By Oath Consigned*, 27–37; Robertson, *Christ*, 67–87.

Part Two: A Modest Proposal for a Biblical Covenantal Biomedical Ethic

the covenants of works and grace as standing and falling together. The law of God applies to both.[62]

Some Reformed theologians such as John Murray, G. C. Berkouwer, and Herman Hoeksema have raised concerns about the concept of a covenant established between God and humankind at creation.[63] While agreeing that, after creating humankind in his image, God established the provision involving a condition, a promise, and a threat for a possible future of "indefectible holiness and blessedness," Murray still refuses to consider the relationship with Adam a covenantal one. He cites the lack of an oath confirming the promise and no redemptive provisions as the source of his reluctance to call the Adamic relationship covenantal, preferring the term "Adamic administration." He calls the first or old covenant the Sinaitic one.[64] Hoeksema admits that the pre-fall relationship of God and Adam was covenantal in nature. Yet he refuses to call it a covenant of works, denying that it was a means for Adam to "work himself up to the highest state of eternal life and heavenly glory."[65] Similarly, Berkouwer objects to the connotation that the creational covenant involved finding God's favor through works or achievement of fulfillment of his law rather than through his grace alone. For him, the works/grace distinction creates a false antithesis.[66]

In my view, the evidence is compelling for a covenantal relationship between God and humankind through Adam. Despite Murray's objections, the main elements of such a covenant (i.e., divine initiative to condescend into a relationship with humankind as a gracious gift out of love, the promise to keep that relationship, and a condition of obedience) are present in the Genesis account of God's relationship with Adam. Perhaps most importantly, such a covenant provides the foundation for redemptive covenantal history and administration that encompasses all of humankind. It does so through an initial relationship with God from the beginning of created time, a period of relational disarray resulting from human disobedience, and the ultimate redeeming of that relationship. That redemption could only come from the once-and-for-all sacrifice of God through the death and resurrection of Jesus Christ for those who are

---

62. Bavinck, *Reformed Dogmatics*, 579.

63. Murray, "Adamic Administration," 49; Berkouwer, *Sin*, 207, 208; Hoeksema, *Reformed Dogmatics*, 217–20.

64. Murray, "Adamic Administration," 50.

65. Hoeksema, *Reformed Dogmatics*, 217.

66. Berkouwer, *Sin*, 208.

obedient to him. As such, it brings into sharp focus the meaning of Christ as the second Adam in Romans 5 and 1 Corinthians 15.[67] Jeremiah also draws a parallel between creational and redemptive covenantal perspectives, a point made by Calvin and, later, by Spykman and others.[68] It also defines the true and genuine nature of religion which identifies God as the God of the covenant from the beginning to the end of time.[69]

Bavinck also necessarily links this creation covenant with the core of our ethical existence. A biblical covenantal ethic provides the ethical anchor for all of humankind and its activities, including biomedical ethics: "Only in this covenant does the ethical . . . unity of mankind come into its own. And this ethical unity is requisite for humanity as an organism."[70] Just as God covenants with humankind through Adam, God judges the whole human race. All human beings are privileged as rational and moral beings. They are created free to serve him willingly, guided by council, admonition, invitation, and warning.[71]

Natural Law, *Imago Dei*, and Moral Responsibility

The role of natural law is important in covenant thinking in both the Genevan and Rhinelander traditions. It points to a transcendent moral order by which all temporal moral and positive law is measured.[72] Jean Porter points out that natural law has shaped the scholastic interpretation of scriptural narratives in stages of progressive moral pedagogy. However, she also admits that the church's understanding of natural law has been influenced by classical Greek pagan authorities. As basic human inclinations, natural

---

67. Kline, *By Oath Consigned*, 28–29.

68. Jer 33:20–26; Spykman, *Reformational Theology*, 261–63. O. Palmer Robertson (*The Christ*, 19–21) also makes a compelling argument that this passage refers to a covenantal relationship that has existed since creation rather than to the covenant with Noah.

69. Bavinck, *Reformed Dogmatics*, 569–70.

70. Ibid., 578.

71. Ibid., 570–71.

72. Gardner, *Justice and Christian Ethics*, 62. Gardner summarizes this nicely: "Natural law presupposed the capacity to discern the basic precept of the moral law through reason. . . . Since the fall, only certain 'relics' of the law of nature remain in the hearts of all people. Such imprints are indispensable . . . for they provide an essential basis for human community."

law should be developed through communal deliberation into common moral practices.[73]

Russell Hittinger agrees that scholastics led by Thomas Aquinas closely associate the necessity of divine teaching through the covenantal relationship with God with a full understanding of the law of nature. However, Hans Urs von Balthasar insightfully cautions us that the scriptural idea of law directs normative action in the context of the covenantal relationship with God. If law loses its covenantal framework, it quickly transforms into "an ethic of autonomy—the very antipode of covenantal ethics."[74] He relates this to today's emphasis on autonomy in law and ethics: "In modern Western legal culture, however, natural law is typically invoked as a principle of autonomy. . . . Natural law has no history, but is rather the ahistorical lever that can be applied to all historical communities."[75] In my view, von Balthasar is correct. This loss of the covenantal roots of natural law, under the influence of Enlightenment thinking, distorts human autonomy in biomedical ethics. This loss is at least one of the sources of distortion in principlism wherein autonomy becomes the dominant principle.

The relationship that human beings have with God is in one sense a *double relationship*; that is, we are covenant partners with God as well as his image-bearers.[76] Human beings were created to reflect something of God's being. Our relationship with God should be a guiding template for our relationship with fellow humans. As God loves us, so also we should act lovingly toward those who depend on us. Furthermore, we should show grateful obedience toward those in authority over us as they in turn do to God. This interrelatedness in God's image includes a collective image of God for humankind.[77] All of humankind is included through the creation covenant with Adam. Since the Fall, humankind has been invited to engage in collective, renewed image-bearing through the new covenant in Jesus Christ, which concretely manifests as his church.

---

73. Porter, "Natural Law," 235–40. As discussed in chapter 1, principlism has adopted this method through its process of reflective equilibrium and its use of coherence theory.

74. Hittinger, "Theology," 406–7; von Balthazar, "Nine Propositions," 91–94.

75. Ibid., 408.

76. Konig, "Outline," 180–89.

77. Ibid., 184; Mouw, *God Who Commands*, 43–54. Richard Mouw deals with the tension often experienced between our personal relationship with God and our relationship with the church. He cautions against those such as Hauerwas, who would see individuals as subordinate to the community. Rather, Mouw advocates for a *normative individualism*, which acknowledges the need for involvement in human community but not at the expense of the relationship of each individual with God.

As recognized implicitly by Calvin and more systematically by his successors, God covenanted with humankind and with the cosmos during the act of creation. This covenant grants special status and responsibility to humankind over the rest of the creation order. As Bavinck argues, all of humankind is free to respond to God's offering of grace in an uncoerced way. However, with that response comes obligations of obedience and service as stewards of the created order and as witnesses to his wisdom and glory. Covenant-based responsibility includes moral responsibility for biomedical ethics that is applicable to all human beings by virtue of their common creational ancestry. True ethical unity of humankind cannot be achieved by consensus based on the faculty of reason alone but on a confessional unity with the true God through the covenant with him.

But sin distorts our relationship with God and with all other human beings, creating a global tension wherein humankind tends to move the focus of relationships and of knowledge away from God toward itself. Did the dualistic tension created by the scholastic synthesis of Scripture with classical Greek moral pedagogy foreshadow the secular moral methodology of principlism? If so, how can a biblical covenantal ethic persuasively renew the moral perspective for biomedical ethics? Should it and can it be purged from its pagan Greek moral tradition and become rooted in a creationally founded relationship inclusive of all human beings?

Divine-Human and Human-Human Covenants

Before addressing these questions, one needs to understand how Christian ethicists have tried to develop a covenantal framework for addressing biomedical ethical issues. In the following section, I will give representative examples of contemporary Christian ethicists who show how covenant as a dominant biblical theme can enrich our understanding of other major biblical themes. I will then show how some of these ethicists have used the covenant theme to capture the normative features of medicine and medical relationships.

Contemporary theologians and ethicists continue to expand our understanding of the divine-human covenant relationship. Gardner suggests that all Old Testament covenant relationships with God have three common elements: the establishment of an agreement between parties of unequal status, God initiating the relationship and dictating the terms, and the human party deciding whether to accept the terms of the covenant.[78]

---

78. Gardner, *Justice and Christian Ethics*, 30–34.

Part Two: A Modest Proposal for a Biblical Covenantal Biomedical Ethic

Meredith Kline argues that within a systematic formulation of a covenant theology, the divine-human covenant is defined generically in terms of law administration. While promise is a constituent of Old Testament covenants, divine law underlies every administration of such promise.[79] The *redemptive* covenant (i.e., that which was struck after the Fall) should not be reduced to its purpose of grace and the notion of election. For Kline, every covenant has a law component that unifies all biblical covenants.[80] He acknowledges such covenants as relational commitments, albeit *under sanction*, defined, secured, and expressed by the swearing of an oath.[81] Such an oath allows for an extension of covenantal relationships beyond those defined by bloodlines. Ridderbos shows that fulfillment of the covenant promise is not dependent on human fulfillment of the law for "Then God's covenant would no longer be a covenant."[82] Gordon Spykman advocates for a covenant theology whose normative structuring principle consists of God and responding human beings linked by the Word of God. This Word was given along with creation, forming both the bridge between God and humans and the boundary between God and the world. It "sets the horizon to all creaturely upreach" toward God, "touching on the very periphery of mystery."[83]

Joseph Allen identifies two types of covenant, distinguished by their participants and scope. The *inclusive covenant* is wholly creational, involving all living creatures in relationship with God the creator. The relationship does not always require active and conscious reciprocation; creatures need not be capable of covenanting with God. Rather, the covenant affirms their value as creatures, with human beings having a special responsibility for the care of God's good creation as obedient creatures. This inclusive covenant was established at creation: "The Christian proclamation is that God has created all people to live in covenant with God and with one another."[84] For Allen, by virtue of this covenantal arrangement, *all hu-*

---

79. Kline, *By Oath Consigned*, 33.

80. Ibid., 35.

81. Ibid., 16–17. McCarthy (*Treaty and Covenant*, 96, 175) agrees with the defining nature of the oath in ancient treaties and other covenantal relationships while Gerhardus Vos (*Biblical Theology*, 277) considers the ceremony of ratification or oath to be the very reason for calling the Sinai arrangement a covenant.

82. Ridderbos, *Epistle of Paul*, 135ff.

83. Spykman, *Reformational Theology*, 92–93. As we will see in chapter 7, such structuring principles constitute stable creational norms for relationships in the social philosophy of Reformed Christian philosopher Herman Dooyeweerd.

84. Allen, *Love and Conflict*, 39–40. Allen's idea of an inclusive covenant goes

man persons are God's children, whether they agree to it or not. Like the relationship of a child to its parents, we preconsciously entrust ourselves to God's care through the creational covenant. However, this covenant is never fully realized in this world but is maintained by an eschatological hope that "stands in judgment upon the brokenness of all human communities."[85] Allen's inclusive covenant has several aspects that are appealing for developing a covenantal ethic for biomedical ethics. The lack of a requirement for absolute reciprocation points to the inherent ontic value of human beings. Such inherent value has been bestowed with our status as God's special creatures created in his image. Such ontic value is inherent in the most vulnerable among us such as the unborn and those rendered less capable due to disease, even if they cannot reciprocate in the relationships. In addition, the inclusive covenant is available for each human being to lose if obligations of covenantal obedience are not met.

Allen also describes *special covenants* through which more specific moral responsibilities are shaped. They are distinguished from the inclusive covenant as strictly human relationships and by their special defining requirements, rights, and obligations. They also have common features such as the need for relational faithfulness, concern for the needs of others, and respect for the worth of other participants. Human beings are simultaneously involved with both covenantal relationships. Our participation in the inclusive covenant is *concretely expressed* through our participation in our special covenants.[86] Through the inclusive covenant, we are reminded that God is (or should be) the centre of our moral life. This covenant unifies the special loyalties of our special covenants. Sin can be expressed as the antithesis of the faith that binds us to God in that covenant. Allen believes that the most neglected characteristic of covenant love in human relationships in our time is the commitment to faithfulness to others. This is the commitment to responsibility for the effects of our actions on others and our commitment to care for others.[87]

---

beyond the concept of the creational or Noahic covenant between God and all of humankind. With almost pantheistic overtones, it captures the all-inclusive effects of sin on the created order by assuming covenantal relationships also between God and non-human creatures that is directly affected by sin.

85. Ibid., 41.

86. Ibid., 44–45.

87. Ibid., 74–80; O'Donovan, *Resurrection and the Moral Order*, 232–41. For Allen, covenantal love permeates both the inclusive and special covenant relationships by binding them as well as giving direction to their expression. Such love is like the ordering principle of which Oliver O'Donovan speaks and that I refer to later in this chapter.

PART TWO: A Modest Proposal for a Biblical Covenantal Biomedical Ethic

Covenant and Other Biblical Themes

Dennis McCarthy reminds us that the covenant spectacles should not be the only pair of glasses through which we understand the ethics of Scripture.[88] However, from a Reformed Christian perspective, in the tradition of Herman Bavinck and other neo-Calvinists, the covenant theme is "a golden thread weaving its way through the total fabric of biblical revelation."[89] Spykman reminds us that the covenant is inseparably linked with the concept of the kingdom of God. This dual idea "pulsates with the very heartbeat of all biblical revelation," providing the very matrix, enduring context, and directional orientation for living faithfully within the structural realities of creation. "By his royal/covenantal Word for creation the triune God makes us his covenant partners and citizens of his kingdom."[90] Through each aspect, we see the same redemptive history from a different directional perspective. Covenant can be seen as kingdom looking back to the covenant's creational origins. In turn, kingdom can be envisioned as covenant looking forward toward creational renewal and consummation. Seen in another way, covenant can be understood as a charter while kingdom is an ongoing program oriented toward an eschatological goal.[91]

In recent years, the importance of the link between the covenant and creation has also been emphasized by prominent Roman Catholic scholars. Joseph Ratzinger, currently Pope Benedict XVI, calls the covenant with God the goal of creation, "the love story of God and man." He calls the Sabbath the sign of that covenant.[92] Creation becomes complete

---

88. McCarthy, *Old Testament Covenant*, 87–88. In particular, he encourages us to remember the wisdom tradition with its attention to the mystery and majesty of God and creation. For some contemporary theologians including McCarthy, however, covenant was not such a continuous thread. For example, Nicholson (*God and His People*, 87) notes that some theologians like McCarthy and Wellhausen considered the covenant between God and Israel to be a late theological idea rather than a religio-sociological and cultic institution from the earlier time of their relationship.

89. Spykman, *Reformational Theology*, 11–12.

90. Ibid., 257.

91. Ibid., 258.

92. Ratzinger, *Spirit*, 26. Dumbrell (*Covenant and Creation*, 35) calls the Sabbath the particular covenantal sign of the notion of divine rest shared by humankind. Hahn ("Canon, Cult, and Covenant," 215, n. 26) notes that Pope John Paul II has referred to the Sabbath of creation as the first covenant. Just as the initial covenant of creation was signified by the Sabbath, says Ratzinger (*Many Religions*, 50–59), the new covenant in Christ was sealed in the Last Supper, in the blood of the new covenant offered by Christ in the cup (Luke 22:17–20). Roland de Vaux (*Ancient Israel*, 480–81) believes that the Sabbath is observed by humankind as the sign of the creation covenant and a

with God's establishment of the covenant. Ratzinger explains that creation provides the place and space for God and man to meet one another in covenant, a space for worship.[93] Furthermore, the "soul" of this relationship is worship, conceived as drawing all of reality into communion with God.[94] Spykman calls the covenant theme a comprehensive framework for understanding creation, the Fall, and the renewal of creation. It shares the same starting point with kingdom in that God covenanted his kingdom into existence at creation, and thus covenant with God existed from the time of humankind's creation.[95] The central and all-embracing nature of the covenantal concept "is the very foundation and framework for all biblical religion" and it "defines the fundamental structures undergirding all human relationships and every societal calling."[96]

It is this foundational nature of covenant that forms the basis of a covenantal ethic that can enrich biomedical ethics and provide the grounding that it otherwise lacks in principlism. According to Spykman, the comprehensiveness of the covenantal theme can be captured in six theses: 1) God's world exists in a pervasively covenantal context, 2) the covenant is creationally oriented, 3) the covenant was unidirectionally offered and bidirectionally implemented, 4) the biblical story is one kingdom plan of God's covenantal dealings moving toward perfect renewal, 5) the covenant promise encourages us forward as an eschatological hope, and 6) covenant

---

reminder of the first Sabbath at creation.

93. Ibid. Hahn ("Canon, Cult, and Covenant," 213), Wenham ("Sanctuary Symbolism"), Beale (*Temple*), and others identify the Garden of Eden as a special sanctuary in creation in terms of the divine–human relationship, noting a literary parallel between the Garden and the inner sanctum of the Temple. Hahn notes that the same Hebrew word is used to describe God's presence in the Garden in Gen 2–3 and in the tabernacle in Lev 26:12 and Deut 23:15.

94. Ibid., 27.

95. Spykman, *Reformational Theology*, 10, 257–59. Ridderbos (*Coming of the Kingdom*, 22– 23) sides with McCarthy in his caution against absolutizing one conceptual theme of redemptive history over others, but he favors the kingdom of God theme as being more universal in its scope than the covenant theme. It is my contention that a proper concept of covenant captures the breadth of God's promises of renewal to all of creation, giving proper attention to both pre-redemptive (creational) and redemptive (post-fall) covenants between responsive human beings and God. Bavinck (*Reformed Dogmatics*, 569) also acknowledges the creational origins of the covenant. For Bavinck, "If religion is called a covenant, it is thereby described as the true and genuine religion." Wright (*Climax of the Covenant*, 203) speaks of the Torah as "the covenant document" that desires to give life to believers while the renewed covenant in Christ is the badge of membership in the faith (156).

96. Spykman, *Reformational Theology*, 359.

Part Two: A Modest Proposal for a Biblical Covenantal Biomedical Ethic

guides our total way of life, calling us to live obediently as God's witnesses in his broken world.[97]

Craig Bartholomew agrees that Spykman argues for covenant and kingdom as the main themes of Scripture, with both being rooted in the creation covenant.[98] Bartholomew himself particularly favors the covenant theme but puts it in context with other themes through an analogy with a building with several entrances. Comparing the Bible to such an edifice, he considers covenant as one of its main entrances, giving one a unified picture of creation while doing justice to the historical outworking of redemption.[99]

The covenant theme also relates directly to the theme of the law of God as expressed in the created order and in the commands of God revealed in Scripture. Oliver O'Donovan stresses the importance of acknowledging the created order as the reality that God willed into existence, not as an order created by an Enlightenment-influenced human mind. This God-willed reality provides an objective reference for Christian ethics, which calls all human beings to lead lives in keeping with the order created for that reality.[100] But being tainted by sin, this order is clouded by a human inability to distinguish between what is naturally *right and normative* from what is simply deemed *right by human convention*. The certainty about the rightness of that order as an ethic of nature can only find ontological grounds in what God chooses to reveal.[101]

Without this, we find that "the very societies which impress us by their reverence for some important moral principle will appall us by their neglect of some other."[102] Advocates of principlism hope for moral consensus by rational convention while failing to see its lack of true moral

---

97. Ibid., 259–65. Robertson (*Christ*, 67–68) has noted that some in the church have forgotten this orientation, resulting in a deficiency in their worldview such that their vision is no longer kingdom-oriented but exclusively church-oriented.

98. Bartholomew, "Covenant and Creation," 11.

99. Ibid., 31–32.

100. O'Donovan, *Resurrection and Moral Order*, 16–17. "Christian moral judgments in principle address every man. They are not something which the Christian opted into and which he might as well, quite as sensibly, opt out of. They are founded on reality as God has given it."

101. Ibid., 18–19. Here O'Donovan criticizes Alasdair MacIntyre, whose solution to the voluntarism of modernity is a return to the teleological tradition set by Aristotelian ethics. However, O'Donovan notes that while the earliest Christian moral tradition was influenced heavily by Platonic and some Stoic influences, its realist substance came primarily from Scripture.

102. Ibid., 19.

Conceptual Support for Covenantal Biomedical Ethics

content without ontological grounds in God's revelation. Reconciliation of apparently conflicting moral principles also needs revealed knowledge of God's created order to distinguish between what is presented as sin-driven distortion of that order and what is renewed correction of that order by Christ's redeeming work. In this situation, one may feel forced to choose between a scripturally revealed ethic but without ontological grounding versus one based on creation but known "naturally," without the need for revelation.[103]

For a follower of Christ, Christian freedom involves Spirit-led interpretations of the character of created reality. O'Donovan terms this *creative discernment* of new situations under guidance of the Spirit, allowing for a deeper understanding of the situations that arise within the natural order around us.[104] Sharing in Christ's authority over the created order through his love, believers can perceive that order wisely by apprehending right relationships among living beings who are appreciated for their inherent value as creatures of God.[105] The covenant in Jesus Christ opens our eyes to the true and complete meaning of the created law of nature, first revealed to Adam, through the direction provided by the love of Christ through the Holy Spirit. Joseph Allen reminds us that the Old and New Testaments, coined by Irenaeus and his contemporaries, were once called the books of the Old and New Covenants. This unfortunate translational change from "covenant" to "testament" suffers a loss of the dynamic living reality of revelation and its association with the covenant idea.[106]

In a similar way, Scripture must be used to guide our thoughts toward a *comprehensive moral viewpoint*.[107] Quoting the commands in the Decalogue and the Sermon on the Mount, adding to these other commands and prohibitions, or deriving principles from parables and other biblical modes of moral teaching are all insufficient for making moral judgments. Moral deliberation and judgment should mirror how the New

---

103. Ibid., 19–20.

104. This creative discernment has important implications for Christians who wrestle with difficult bioethical issues

105. Ibid., 24–26; O'Donovan, *Begotten or Made?* Such an ontological basis for human value helps lay out a normative ethic for the value of the unborn, the disabled, and the vulnerable, which is lacking in many attempts to articulate the meaning of human personhood. However, such ontic value still requires a relationship to realize its full value; Peter Moore (*Enhancing Me*, 19) also notes, "in most religious philosophies, relationships are key to determining identity and value."

106. Allen, *Love and Conflict*, 31–32.

107. O'Donovan, *Resurrection and Moral Order*, 200.

Part Two: A Modest Proposal for a Biblical Covenantal Biomedical Ethic

Testament teaches us to understand the moral law of the Old Testament; that is, "attend to *principles of order* which are to be found within it."[108] O'Donovan distinguishes *pluriform codes,* which unsuccessfully try to cover the variety of moral relations, from *principles of order*. Whereas the former attempt to account for the diversity of moral situations that may arise in the future from those situations that have occurred in the past, the latter give insight into, and character to, the way in which moral rules are understood and obeyed. The *supreme ordering-principle* is the *love-command* or *summary of the law*.[109] This ordering principle transforms our obedient-love, which is our response to God's love to us through Christ, into neighbor-love, as taught and exemplified by Jesus's teachings.[110]

The covenant with God is not only a relationship but also a mission. Just as the kingdom of God can be considered a goal or end of covenant-related activity, covenant represents the mission toward the perfection of that kingdom. "To be in covenant is to engage in mission."[111] Christ overcame Israel's failure to be the light to its pagan neighbors and so the church, as a believing community, has become the new mission to the entire world. Through this community, God extends his gracious offer of covenant to all people and to all of creation. It is this mission that should motivate Christians in biomedical ethics to continually reassess and re-form a Christian perspective for bioethics. It also obligates Christians to witness to non-believers that the covenant with God embodies the full meaning for our understanding of all human relationships and for all pursuits of knowledge of the "natural" creation order. *In this way, Christian biomedical ethics seen through a biblical covenant theme and framework has global implications for all human beings.*

As mentioned earlier, Kline understands the covenant as the administration of God's kingdom and his lordship over the creation order through his people under the sanction of divine law.[112] Kline advocates for

---

108. Ibid.

109. Ibid., 203. This understanding of principles as guides for understanding the character of moral rules or commands rather than accounting for moral diversity based on past experiences seems applicable to a biblical critique of principlism and its conventional application in medical ethics.

110. Ibid., 232–34. Thus, this concept of ordering-principles binds covenant relationships and can envision normative actions and dispositions if conceived through the love of Christ. Such a concept of principles will be later explored as an alternative to those understood within a principles-based ethic such as that advocated by Beauchamp and Childress.

111. Van Gelder, "Covenant's Missiological Character," 196.

112. Kline, *By Oath Consigned*, 36.

Conceptual Support for Covenantal Biomedical Ethics

a covenantal terminology that theocentrically reflects the covenant theme. To represent the unity of covenant and kingdom themes, for example, he proposes the term "Covenant of the Kingdom." Within this continual covenant theme that cuts through all of redemptive history, he identifies a pre-redemptive component, or "Covenant of Creation." while the component graciously offered by God after the Fall is the "Covenant of Redemption." Such terminological correctives move away from the historical and more dualistically influenced covenant of works and covenant of grace.[113] The Covenant of Creation becomes the foundation for the administration of the Covenant of Redemption. Its omission would "deprive dogmatics of the conceptual apparatus required for a satisfactory synthesis of the work of Christ and the redemptive covenant."[114]

Like Lillback and others, William Dumbrell argues that the original covenant is implicitly evident in the creation account in Gen 1:1—2:4 and that the commitment created by that covenant was intended to achieve the purpose of creation. He points to Ps 8:5 with its reference to humankind's special created status, to God's invitation for Adam to join him in his Sabbath rest, and to the conditions imposed in the Garden of Eden as evidence of a special creational relationship with God.[115] Bartholomew takes special note that for Dumbrell, any covenant theology must begin with Genesis 1. Subsequent covenants are extensions of the creation covenant through which God pursues his creative purposes.[116] Bartholomew also links the creation covenant idea with *imago Dei* in Genesis 1. The image metaphor speaks strongly to the analogy between God's kingly reign over the cosmos and humankind's obligatory yet stewardly reign over creation. This analogy, he argues, points directly to all spheres of human activity.[117]

---

113. Ibid., 37.

114. Ibid., 29.

115. Dumbrell, *Covenant and Creation*, 33–35, 41, 44–45. Karl Barth writes that creation was the ground for the covenant; Dumbrell disagrees, arguing that the act of creation involved the inception of a relationship between his creation including human beings. This is most clearly shown in the devastating, cosmic proportions of the disorder brought on by the Fall. He later criticizes Charles Hodge for the same misconception, claiming that Hodge saw covenant as a means to an end rather than an end in itself.

116. Dumbrell (*Covenant and Creation*, 118, 120) and Bartholomew ("Covenant and Creation," 18–19) link this creation covenant with the Noahic covenant as the renewal of God's creative purposes and with the later Abrahamic and Sinaitic covenants through common themes relating to the land and to sanctuary.

117. Bartholomew, "Time for War," 106–7.

PART TWO: A Modest Proposal for a Biblical Covenantal Biomedical Ethic

Linking the covenant with God intimately with the act of creation, Spykman argues that at creation "God covenanted his world into existence. Covenant relationships are given in, with, and for all of created reality."[118] He considers the covenant with Noah as a covenant of new beginning with the human race as a whole, a renewal of God's relationship with Adam at creation. As mentioned earlier, the absence of the Hebrew for covenant (*berith*) notwithstanding, the elements of covenant are there before and after the flood.[119] The universal perspective inherent in the covenant with Adam and renewed with Noah reflects God's ultimate redemptive purpose. This perspective is further supported by the register of nations in Gen 10-11 and the steady list of outsiders who join God's people until the full re-emergence of all peoples at Pentecost.[120]

The Enlightenment moved away from the concept of a covenant relationship with God toward a post-creation God who was disinterested in human beings and the world. With the advent of social contract theory, human relationships were construed as negotiated relational deals in a society consisting of members who strive primarily to not harm one another. This anthropocentric focus further distances or rejects the idea of a relationship with a transcendent God or Other, the basis of which had previously formed the moral justification and grounding for behavior and actions within human relationships in Western culture. This explains the contemporary tendency to reduce covenant to more contractual models. Such models emphasize legal and formal protections meant to preserve the safety and autonomy of participants from intrusion by others, rather than cultivate relational growth and sacrificial dispositions.

As noted above, von Balthasar rightly expresses concern that loss of the divine-human covenant theme can lead to anthropocentric distortion of natural law theory with consequent derivation of law norms from human nature. An ethic of human autonomy that lacks a history and requires contractual relationships to protect moral identity is not far behind.[121] Kline's new terminology refreshingly captures the creational origin of covenant and reminds Christians that the root of human relationships

---

118. Spykman, *Reformational Theology*, 260.

119. Ibid. Spykman agrees with McCarthy (*Old Testament Covenant*, 1-10) on the basic elements of covenant in Scripture.

120. Ibid., 355-56. Spykman argues that it is not the "Hebrew particularism" of the Abrahamic covenant and its Old Testament successors but the original universal perspective that reflects God's redemptive goals.

121. von Balthasar, "Nine Propositions," 92-94; Hittinger, "Theology," 407-8.

Conceptual Support for Covenantal Biomedical Ethics

remains the divinely and graciously established covenant with God, not its human response.[122]

In summary, there is clear evidence in Scripture that the covenantal relationship between God and all of humankind began at creation, is maintained imperfectly for believers in God since Adam's disobedience and our redemption in Christ, and will be renewed and perfected along with humankind and creation when Christ returns at the end of time. Recent Roman Catholic magisterial works also support a universal creational covenant idea that speaks to its relevance for all human beings.[123] It is the relationship toward which all other relationships should be cross-referenced if the meaning of human life and of ethics is to be properly understood. Among the biblical themes, Spykman maintains that the covenant theme forms the foundation and framework for all biblical religion from which is derived the fundamental structures undergirding all human relationships and societal callings.[124] Bartholomew, Dumbrell, and others going back to Calvin argue that a creational covenant grounds the moral plight of all human beings from the beginning of time and provides the transcendent authority for moral living. A right understanding of that relationship between God and humanity is thus essential, not only for the Christian faith and for a biblical understanding of biomedical ethics but for all human beings.[125] Since the practice of medicine is carried out through a network of relationships, an ethical framework built around a biblical covenant framework can provide 1) transcendent grounding for bioethics where none exists in the current secular paradigm, and 2) a normative approach to understanding and actualizing normative relationships and structures in medicine as a discipline founded on human relationships.

BIOMEDICAL ETHICS THROUGH COVENANTAL SPECTACLES: A BRIEF HISTORY

Covenant Embedded in Contract: Veatch's Social Contract

Covenantal models for relationships in medicine differ among bioethicists of different Christian traditions. Robert Veatch's theory of medical

---

122. Kline, *By Oath Consigned*, 37. That is, the unity the covenant of creation with the covenant of redemption under the umbrella of the covenant of the kingdom.

123. Ratzinger, *Spirit*.

124. Spykman, *Reformational Theology*, 359.

125. Ibid., 93.

PART TWO: A Modest Proposal for a Biblical Covenantal Biomedical Ethic

ethics exemplifies an effort to retain some vestiges of a covenant idea in a theory that draws heavily from social contract theory.[126] Having once considered a calling as a medical missionary for the Methodist Church,[127] Veatch looks critically at Hippocratic, Judeo-Christian, and liberal traditions. Particularly harsh criticism is leveled at the Hippocratic tradition as too physician-empowering, too teleological at the expense of deontological obligations, and lacking any reference to social justice. He argues that the search for a universal basis for making moral decisions is less helpful than inventing a moral framework through a social contract by "rationally pursuing enlightened self-interest."[128] Gathering behind John Rawls's "veil of ignorance," human beings can create a community of moral rules that are mutually acceptable. He also believes in "the compatibility of theocentric perspectives with those of the founders of modern theories of social contract."[129]

Veatch proposes a social contract model that he assures can be acceptable to both those who profess to a pre-existing moral order (including those based on a transcendent God) and those who discover or invent their moral order. However, all participants would be bound by loyalty and trust in each other alone, not to God or other transcendent authority. Such binding is considered contractual but with a covenantal flavor and defined by specific binding communal qualities.[130] However, his apparent aversion to covenantal language suggests a preference for a more Hobbesian interpretation of binding relationships that emphasizes their legal and public aspects.[131] He therefore seems to relegate religious beliefs and practices to secondary importance behind an anthropocentric reliance on human relationships constructed by mutual agreement.

Very recently, in postmodern fashion but with a universalist twist, Veatch has acknowledged that religious belief should be considered valid

---

126. Jonsen, *Birth of Bioethics*, 329–30.
127. Ibid., 56.
128. Veatch, *Theory of Medical Ethics*, 120.
129. Ibid., 123.
130. Ibid., 125–26.

131. Ibid., 123–24. Acknowledging the central place of covenant in the Calvinist tradition, Veatch tries to tie this into Hobbes's affirmation of a law of nature initially created by God. But he admits that Hobbes (and Locke) was unable to reconcile natural law with contract theory. Veatch sees social contract theory as a way to overcome major differences based on religious beliefs and to work out an ethical framework by mutual agreement on basic moral principles. One can contrast this with Alasdair MacIntyre (*After Virtue*, 196, 250).

alongside secular belief in the collective development of contemporary bioethics. Ironically, his rejection of the Hippocratic tradition as groundless for contemporary purposes is replaced by a similarly groundless contemporary contract theory based on a rational consensus of contractual terms.[132] In his model, a covenant in medical practice would constitute a contractual agreement among responsible people, to be governed by one or more of his seven principles. He suggests ranking them, starting with *promise-keeping* as the greatest priority, followed by *honoring the autonomous status of each member of the community, honesty,* and so forth, ending with the moral necessity to produce good for each other as long as such activity is compatible with other principles.[133] One can see vestiges of a Christian covenant idea embedded almost unrecognizably in Enlightenment-rooted social contract theory.

Veatch's model is a form of principlism, reminiscent of the search for the common morality through iterative, reflective consensus building popularized by Beauchamp and Childress. While in recent years he seems increasingly willing to give increasing importance and validity to religious beliefs, his faith in the convergence of ideas based on common rational considerations still overrides any consideration for moral decisions based on transcendent moral grounding. Veatch proposes that principles mutually identified by both secular and religious bioethics provide common roots for a potential convergence of moral principles and beliefs into a fundamental common morality.[134]

Sturm's Covenantal Principle

Douglas Sturm envisions a covenantal principle for bioethics but within a social and theological context. In pursuing the scope and boundaries of bioethics, he believes that its focal point should be social theory, including social interpretation and social ethics but that its grounding should be theological. He proposes a "conjunction" of these dimensions

---

132. Jonsen, *Birth of Bioethics*, 329; Veatch, *Gifford Lecture*.

133. Veatch, *Theory of Medical Ethics*, 327–30. Veatch drafts a medical ethical covenant that incorporates his seven principles. These are beneficence, non-maleficence, autonomy, veracity, honesty, the avoidance of killing, and justice.

134. Veatch, *Gifford Lecture*. While insisting that his seven principles stand on their own, he notes in his Gifford Lecture that autonomy, veracity, honesty, and avoidance of killing can be subsumed under a principle of respect for persons. The latter adds an ontic and relational dimension lacking in the principlism of Beauchamp and Childress.

PART TWO: A Modest Proposal for a Biblical Covenantal Biomedical Ethic

in promoting a "relational principle" as more relevant in our time in light of "cosmological thought and social reality."[135] Sturm prefers the holistic, communal, and "full-bodied context" of a relational approach over more precise analytic ones. As a discipline developing through the input of those trained in other disciplines, bioethics remains open to creative change and reassessment.

In pursuit of a foundation for bioethics, Sturm agrees with William Glaser that each society develops a medical theory to deal with fundamental problems of the sick based on ideas about the universe, life, and humankind.[136] In light of a societal suspicion of "self-aggrandizing rationalization" but also of community ideologies that are often discounted as fringe perspectives, he sees a current tendency to return to critical morality through philosophical or theological reflection. In support of this trend, Sturm proposes adapting the process theology of Alfred Whitehead as the theological grounding for bioethics.

Sturm is drawn particularly to Whitehead's reformed subjectivist principle, which states that the experiences of subjects are intimately tied with all other subjective experiences. One's self contributes to the ongoing world while the world is the condition of the realization of that self. God acts through the world, and his valuation and intentions for the world move the world along in time toward future moments of "becoming." Communal relationships involve confrontations of "centers of dignity" (selves), which pursue their own ends and intentions through the drama of communal existence.[137] God is the dominant member of those relationships, and what matters is the quality of relationships. Self is confronted with demands of being in relationship with God, other humans, and one's self.[138] Sturm translates these three relational demands into principles of community, relationality, and autonomy, respectively. In traditional ethical language, says Sturm, these can be construed as the principles of the common good, equality, and liberty, which form the grounding for biomedical ethics. To these he adds a fourth *principle of covenant*, admitting to its origins in the Hebraic-Christian tradition that characterizes the relationships between God and his creation.

---

135. Sturm, "Contextual and Covenant," 135–36. Sturm was professor of religion and political science at Bucknell University and a member of the United Methodist Church.

136. Glaser, "Medical Care," 95.

137. Meland, *Realities of Faith*, 206.

138. Ibid., 207; Sturm, "Contextual and Covenant," 154–55. Sturm conceptually borrows from Meland here.

Borrowing from Bernard Meland, Sturm alludes to a pre-Fall covenant as a myth of identity between humankind and God. He also follows Meland's transformation of the notion of human sinfulness into one of dissonance. The initial covenant disobedience and the subsequent post-Fall dissonance is, for Sturm and Meland, "the strain implicit in the covenant relationship [rather] than in anything inherent in man himself."[139] This dissonance between the creation and God also creates tensions and conflicts when these principles are considered in bioethical contexts.[140] Sturm tries to support the validity of his four principles by arguing that other bioethicists have alluded to them in various ways.[141] He draws an analogy with Ramsey's confessional/personalistic concept of covenant-fidelity and the contractual model of Veatch.[142] However, Sturm finds that May's deeper relational emphasis of covenant more "closely approximates" his intention when he uses Whitehead's reformed subjectivist principle as the theological means for grounding bioethics.[143]

Sturm alludes to an anchoring "first principle," treating his covenant principle at times as such a principle.[144] Here he clearly differs from the principlism of Beauchamp and Childress, who have no unifying or priority principle that holds the common morality together.[145] Unfortunately,

139. Meland, *Fallible Forms*, 97–99.

140. Sturm, "Contextual and Covenant," 155–56.

141. Ibid., 156–59. For example, Sturm argues that Engelhardt focuses on the principle of the liberty of the individual, with autonomy as a regulative ideal for health care. Similarly, Leon Kass promotes his principle of equality through an Aristotelian anthropology of actualization of human potentialities involving an equalization of differences for the sake of providing an equality of treatment according to need. Sturm considers the "institutional ethic" of Jonsen and Hellegers as coinciding with his common good ethics by means of their theory of medicine as a provider of social justice for the human community at large.

142. Veatch's contractual model has already been discussed while Ramsey's covenant concept was touched on in chapter 3 and will be discussed later in this chapter as well.

143. Ibid., 158.

144. Sturm ("Contextual and Covenant," 135–36, 153–55). At one point he states that the relational principle is preferred over more analytical principles for understanding bioethics. At times, he seems to consider this first principle as the reformed subjectivist principle that provides a means to understanding the relation between God and the world. At other times he describes a relational or covenant principle as a myth of identity between the world and God that embraces his other three principles positively but is also a flashpoint for tensions and conflicts among these principles.

145. Beauchamp and Childress, *Principles of Biomedical Ethics*, 5th ed., 407. In fact, in their concluding chapter they even speculate whether their hope of cohering ideas toward consensus is based on faith!

Part Two: A Modest Proposal for a Biblical Covenantal Biomedical Ethic

Sturm's use of process theology as an interpretive framework for explaining our relationship with God fails to recognize the centrality of covenant as a root-metaphor in the historical-redemptive dimension of the biblical narrative. God is not just a dominant member of this network of relationships. The biblical concept of the divine-human relationship assumes a primacy that gives grounding and meaning to human relationships. His attempt to water down sin into a *relational dissonance* between God and human beings is particularly regrettable, since it is devoid of any Christian message of moral purpose and renewal by way of God's forgiving grace.

Christian Bioethicists in the Reformed Tradition

Ramsey's covenant idea in biomedical ethics was introduced in chapter 3 in the context of its close ties with the notion of obedient love.[146] He distinguishes between Christian neighborly love, which requires nothing in return versus a universal brotherhood or cosmopolitan spirit idea. Such Christian "enlightened unselfishness" requires thinking of one's self for the sake of others.[147] He also rejects the "ever more reducible notion of the 'dignity' of human life" as protection, "a sliver of a shield," against the abuse of any form of human life.[148] Specifically applying this to medical relationships, Ramsey focuses on the patient *and those who support the patient*.[149] His overriding concern for the autonomy of patient decision making results in an absolute belief in the sanctity of life and a rigorous insistence on informed consent as the cardinal canon of loyalty.[150] Unco-

---

146. Camenisch, "Paul Ramsey's Task," 73, 81. I refer in chapter 3 to Paul Camenisch's suggestion that Ramsey used covenant language more in his later writings to stress continuity in the moral life in terms that could be appreciated by both Christians and non-Christians. He also thinks Ramsey used the concept to give more substance to the argument to protect patients and research subjects from the power exercised by caregivers and society at large.

147. Ramsey, *Basic Christian Ethics*, 94, 157–61.

148. Ramsey, *Patient as Person*, xiii. I fundamentally agree with Ramsey here. Others such as Karen Lebacqz ("On the Elusive Nature") have tried to salvage the dehumanization of the embryo by claiming that it is owed respect while approving its destruction for research purposes.

149. I will highlight the importance of a biblical covenant ethic for understanding the patient/supporting other relationship in chapter 7.

150. Ibid., xii, 2–7, 124; Ramsey, *Ethics at the Edge*, 159–71. Informed consent is necessary because "Man's capacity to become joint adventurers in a common cause makes the consensual relation possible; man's propensity to over reach his joint adventurer even in a good cause makes consent necessary" (6). However, in later years, he

erced patient choice prevails, even when perceived by supporting others as not in the patient's best interest.

Ramsey stresses the importance of the divine-human covenant as the source for covenantal meaning. Obedient love is intimately associated with the covenant and with the reign of God in Christian ethics.[151] This covenant's link with interhuman relationships, however, is not always clear. Paul Camenisch notes rightly that Ramsey vacillates between attributing human relational obligations to human free will and appealing to God's performatives and mandates.[152] With regard to the latter, Ramsey also distinguishes the Christian faith commitment that motivates relational obligations from covenant responsibilities as an inner meaning of natural relations into which all human beings are born. Camenisch suggests that this vacillation may reflect Ramsey's overwhelming concern to forward the covenant idea for the sake of protecting patients and research subjects. Hauerwas agrees with this interpretation of Ramsey but in the wider context of creating a livable society that protects and respects its individual members.[153] However, Ramsey remains unclear as to whether covenantal relationships are initiated by an innate, "natural" human will or by intentionally modeling such relationships to a covenanting relationship with God. The problem with the former proposal is that covenant easily becomes contractual in spirit out of convenience and self-interest.

David H. Smith suggests that Ramsey's covenant with God must be a *conscious* relationship with God. This would run the peril of calling the unborn, or persons rendered unconscious, sub-human and not image-bearers of God. Smith argues further, however, that Ramsey's concept of creation avoids this conclusion by putting primary human value *in* the relationship with the creator. Such a relationship is not dependent on human capacity or even awareness of God by his created creatures but exists because of divine grace.[154] This juxtaposition of covenant and creational themes can be better conceptually envisioned through the concept of cov-

---

seems to favor a less absolute position on patients' rights to decide on their treatment of choice, accusing Robert Veatch of over-emphasizing patient rights and moving toward subjective voluntarism and "automated physicians."

151. Ramsey, *Basic Christian Ethics*, 388.
152. Camenisch, "Paul Ramsey's Task," 72–73; Ramsey, *Patient as Person*, xii.
153. Hauerwas, "How Christian Ethics," 27 n. 12.
154. Smith, "On Paul Ramsey," 13; Rusthoven, "Are Human Embryos." This is an important adaptation of a Reformed perspective on the relationship between creation and covenant themes to medical bioethics to give inherent ontic value to all human beings regardless of their capacities.

Part Two: A Modest Proposal for a Biblical Covenantal Biomedical Ethic

enant as a root-metaphor of Scripture. As mentioned earlier, Bartholomew contends that Old Testament covenant and creation-based literature tend to be antithetical, due in part to the static portrayal of the creation story.[155] If, however, the covenant notion becomes a root-metaphor that captures the dynamic, historical outworking of redemption through the successive covenant stories, then creation is transformed and renewed by redemption in Christ, rather than set against redemption.

Unfortunately, Ramsey's covenant-fidelity motif is not well developed.[156] Covenant and creation are cobbled together for the purpose of addressing a particular problem or situation. The creation theme helps to prevent the demotion of unconscious or unborn human beings to subhuman status. This perception of a utilitarian use of the creation theme to "save" the status of the unborn could have been avoided, however, by a more comprehensive presentation of the biblical notion of covenant and creation as they relate to the ontic value of human beings and the importance of the *imago Dei* motif. Therefore, try as he might to maintain a direct link between the biblical divine-human covenant and human relationships, Ramsey is caught in the contemporary preoccupation with protecting the autonomy of patients and research subjects as a primary objective of biomedical ethics. This preoccupation contributes to his reluctance to more explicitly and consistently use theological language when he expresses the meaning of covenantal relationships from his Christian perspective. Despite this reluctance, Ramsey's work provides some groundwork for other Christians to develop a biblical covenantal perspective more intentionally and more specifically to particular aspects of medicine. William F. May is the first to build more systematically on these covenantal foundations.

May proposes a covenantal model for medicine based on the new covenant in Christ. It is the starting point of a Christian perspective on covenant from which such a model of medicine can be developed. Unlike Allen, his inclusive covenant does not allude to the relationship between God and our first parents but between Christ and believers.[157] It is defined

---

155. Bartholomew, "Covenant and Creation," 32.

156. Thomist bioethicists Pellegrino and Thomasma (*Christian Virtues*, 80, 105) reject reductive contractual models of the physician/patient relationship as proposed by Veatch in favor of those based on a covenant of trust embodied in an ethic of virtue and trust. Within this covenant of trust, the patient's best interest comes before the physician's own interests. Seemingly aligned with Ramsey, they see this concept as the one most consistent with a Christian ethic in that the physician pledges fidelity to a binding promise to help.

157. May, *Testing the Medical Covenant*, 53. "For Christians, God's covenant with

Conceptual Support for Covenantal Biomedical Ethics

by the death and resurrection of Jesus Christ.[158] Its dynamic consists of giving and receiving. May sees the depth of this relationship in the created order. Meilaender observes that May looks to Karl Barth's characterization between "creation as the external basis of covenant" and "covenant as the internal basis of creation" wherein the created world acts as the backdrop that makes human relationships possible.[159] Humankind was given caretaker responsibility of creation but humankind's sin adversely has affected all of creation.

May notes that Ramsey considers covenant fidelity to be a governing principle that could be applied to particular bioethical issues. His faith in a covenanting God can become the basis for a canon of loyalty and for a principle of sanctity of life. May expands on this further. Our primary covenant with God measures all other covenantal relationships since loyalty to God requires loyalty to all of God's creatures.[160] May's main concern with Ramsey's covenant formulation is its translation of biblical moral commandments for living out covenant relationships into moral rules or principles, with a resultant loss of a theocentric focus. May acknowledges the attraction of rules- or principles-oriented approaches of bioethicists like Ramsey and James Childress for Christians. These approaches seem to address moral problems in a societal context "without divisive appeals to a particular religious commitment," and are thus particularly attractive to Christians in health care policy making positions.[161] Indeed, May states that their principles-oriented theories have philosophical and religious value in serving "a religiously pluralist and secular society." However, he expresses deep concern that Ramsey's covenantal emphasis falls short of a true ethic in that it deemphasizes the importance of the character and virtuous expression of the moral agent. Covenanted medical practitioners as moral agents not only follow a set of rules and principles. They also must

---

Israel structurally prefigures the inclusive covenant that will spread across the whole of humankind in God's Son."

158. Ibid.

159. Meilaender, "On William May," 114.

160. May, *Testing the Medical Covenant*, 54.

161. Ibid., 55. Elsewhere (*The Physician's Covenant*, 24–25, 31), May talks of closet Christian and Jewish moralists who suppress the resources of their religious convictions in their writings in medical ethics, considering society and the professions to be "confessionally indeterminate." May considers this a mistake because the images of shelter and rescue from suffering, sickness, and death through which caregivers are portrayed can only become clear in a religious milieu. And for May, religion is "whatever people attend to with their whole being. . . . The gods that enthrall modern men and women do not bless but threaten them."

Part Two: A Modest Proposal for a Biblical Covenantal Biomedical Ethic

develop character that affects more intimately their practice and thus relationships with patients and fellow caregivers.[162] May clearly sees the role of physicians as primarily moral agents rather than problem solvers.[163] Moral principles are procedural tools that are only helpful in the hands of properly dispositioned caregivers who practice a covenantal ethic.[164]

Covenant relationships involve a responsiveness and gratuitousness that may conflict without a transcendent origin and grounding.[165] Gratuitousness rises above a contractual agreement based on self-interest. It is more than the sum of gifts bestowed on us and more than the reciprocation of such gifts. The biblical notion of human covenant bonding presupposes a rootedness in God's gracious care as the source of human out-giving and receiving. Just as God cared for Israel as strangers in a foreign land, so they were expected to care for the stranger in their land.[166] May also realizes that covenant relationships need limits in order to avoid conflicting covenant obligations among various relationships. He considers covenantal relational involvement outside of appeals to God as *sentimentalization*. By contrast, covenantal involvement rooted in a transcendent Other reveals and teaches the normative limits of involvement.[167]

While May portrays the physician healer in Christian covenantal terms, he admits that there are appealing aspects to seeing physicians as contractors. For example, contractual associations provide legal enforcement of terms for both parties with stated protections and recourses, and presuppose honestly that self-interest primarily governs humans.[168] In

---

162. Ibid., 56; Mount, *Covenant*. Eric Mount agrees with May and promotes the open sharing of virtues of covenant communities of faith that may find resonance and relevance in fostering civic virtue. He emphasizes hospitality to the stranger as a pre-requisite for covenant.

163. Ibid., 141–42. Mount shows that the covenantal virtue of patience is manifest in medical relationships through listening attentively to patients.

164. May, *Testing the Medical Covenant*, 56; Pellegrino and Thomasma, *Christian Virtues*. May writes, "No ethic that adequately explores the medical covenant can focus simply upon the quandaries that emerge in medical practice and the bearing of moral principles upon those quandaries; it must also explore the identity and nature of those agents who profess medicine." His appeal to virtue ethics resonates with Pellegrino's critique of secular medicine today.

165. May, *Physician's Covenant*, 128.

166 The apostle John summarized the law of love: "In this is love, not that we loved God but that he loved us. . . . If God so loved us, we also ought to love one another," (1 John 4:10–11, NIV).

167. May, *Physician's Covenant*, 130.

168. May, *Testing the Medical Covenant*, 7.

Conceptual Support for Covenantal Biomedical Ethics

material terms, covenants are first cousins to contracts, given that they are agreements and exchanges between parties. But *in spirit*, contracts are external to the parties, while covenants are internal, preventing merely expedient discharge of obligations and promises. Covenants cut deeper into personal identity. They have *a gratuitous, growing edge* that comes from fundamental change in a person's being in a growing relationship.[169] In the context of the caregiver-patient relationship, May uses the term "transformational," going beyond expressed wants and responding to a patient's deeper needs. Teaching the patient by speaking the truth in love can avoid tendencies toward paternalism.[170]

A truly covenantal relationship with patients requires a virtue of fidelity that sets aside self-interest in favor of a *disinterestedness*. Such denial of self-interest is not meant to ignore patient needs in exchange for technical competence and precision but rather toward disinterested discernment, judgment, and action for the patient's well-being and best interest.[171]

May's preference for a covenant ethic in the healer-patient relationship seems motivated toward correcting the inherent power disparity in the relationship. In a biblical notion of covenant, the more powerful partner accepts some responsibility for the more vulnerable partner.[172] In all biblical covenants, God stresses care for the needy and requires that his covenant people attend to those who are widowed, sick, poor, and imprisoned. May emphasizes that the full meaning of a covenantal relationship comes from its grounding in the covenant between God and his people. In this light, suffering and death are no longer ultimate, feared, or necessarily overcome. Furthermore, through his death and resurrection, Jesus Christ "takes up death itself into the power of donative love" and allows others to participate in such power. One's beleaguered and fearful self is re-located

---

169. May, *Physician's Covenant*, 119–20.

170. May, *Testing the Medical Covenant*, 69–70. Others have also proposed that covenant has a transforming quality. Coffey ("Nurse-Patient Relationship," 317) sees the nurse–patient covenant as leading to internalization of values and beliefs inherent to the respective communities of the participants. Brown ("Character of the Covenant," 283–93) says that a covenant culminates in a shared identity and a new character.

171. Ibid., 68.

172 May, *Physician's Covenant*, 124; May, "Code Covenant," 29–38. May also acknowledges multiple ways in which the physician is indebted to patients and to society, a point conspicuously absent from past codes of medical ethics. May sees such reciprocity as a corrective to the otherwise philanthropic notion of the physician's commitment to fellow humans as a purely gratuitous act. Such an ideal, he insists, is a conceit of philanthropy.

Part Two: A Modest Proposal for a Biblical Covenantal Biomedical Ethic

in love within a dynamic of giving and receiving and is liberated from the terror of human suffering and death.[173] This enables caregivers to relate to the suffering of fellow human beings, freeing believers from the need to avoid ties with the suffering and dying. God is still there for the dying and for those who support the suffering and dying in their struggles.[174]

Kenneth Vaux explores covenant in the context of health care and medicine from a Reformed Christian perspective. Vaux speaks of Christ as the mediator of a new covenant but also as creator of the earth, through whom all things hold together.[175] He ties innovations in science and the moral decisions inherent in those discoveries to a cosmic understanding of the world, all of whose aspects and expressions belong to God.[176] Health is living out our existence as human persons in Christ, in whatever state we are. It is the command of God that gives wholeness of body, mind, and spirit, sustained by creational norms and God's grace.[177] We are partners with God who teaches us ways to heal and redeem this world. In line with Hauerwas and Ramsey, Vaux sees the worth of human beings and obligations to other persons as rooted in our belonging to God.[178] Vaux argues that within his tradition is an ethic of *koinonia* involving a called and covenanted community. The fellowship of believers happens only because God has joined individual members into one body and family.[179] As *ekklesia*, this community is set apart from the idolatry of the surrounding culture but called to serve as God's instrument to restore the created order of that culture through his grace. As such, this is a prophetic existence, forth-telling and fore-telling to the world what ought to be as well as what will eventually be.[180] In such a community, members are not autonomous as self-ruling creatures but are free and dignified moral agents who have their allegiance to God alone, existing primarily for each other rather than for themselves.[181] Each has a christocentric conscience and exercises it in the *koinonia* context that helped save the ethics of the early church from

173. May, *Physician's Covenant*, 124–27.

174. Rom 8:38, 39. "Neither death, nor life . . . nor anything else in all creation, will be able to separate us from the love of God."

175. Vaux, *Health and Medicine*, 14; Col 1:15–17. This christocentric view of creation and redemption hints at the inclusive covenant concept of Allen and May.

176. Ibid., 15.

177. Ibid., 34.

178. Ibid., 45.

179. Ibid., 106.

180. Ibid., 105.

181. Ibid., 106–7.

Conceptual Support for Covenantal Biomedical Ethics

antinomianism, a successor of which is the ethic of autonomy.[182] Vaux properly articulates a Christian view of individual believers that preserves human individuality and our individual relationship with God but promotes the importance of other church members who lend support and guidance along the path of Christian living.

Besides this allusion to autonomy, Vaux describes ancient moral structures that provided constraints on maleficence while implying encouragement to be beneficent. In pagan moral codes, the moral spirit was expressed primarily as negative sanctions. By contrast, for the ancient Israelites this spirit was one of positive beneficent action. For those in the new covenant, benevolence is a caring disposition leading to caring action in response to the life in Christ. This comes not as an inherent good but as a divine command to be righteous, do justice, and be concerned for others.[183] Like May, Vaux sees the new covenant as central to the Christian life for all who respond and believe. As such, it is inclusively offered to all but is exclusively defined by faith. Like Allen, he closely ties this covenantal relationship with God's love for us: we love because God loves us.[184] Vaux does not overtly appeal to a covenant ethic but acknowledges its central importance in more subtle ways. For example, he writes that an act cannot be right or wrong *in itself* in the context of faith. It is only compatible or incompatible *within the relationship with Christ*.[185] Such a link of moral right and wrong with relationality and Christ gets at the heart of a covenantal ethic grounded in God's Word.

Beyond the individual, Vaux also speaks of the church exercising a collective conscience through prophetic teaching and pastoral care. While decisions are ultimately personal, they need to be made "in the inner citadel of a person's (or a family's) relationship with God" and with support from within the faith community.[186] At one point, Vaux speaks of ethics as abandonment in the sense of giving way to God and others. He pictures

---

182. Ibid., 109. Vaux links the protective effect of the church community against heresy with the contemporary resistance to individualism. In this way he agrees with Pellegrino's critique of the dominance of autonomy within Western culture, worked out in biomedical ethics in principlism.

183. Ibid., 126. Vaux cites Lev 19:18 as one example of this refocused moral spirit: "You shall not seek revenge, or cherish anger. . . . You shall love your neighbor as a man like your self. I am the Lord."

184. Ibid., 127. He notes this link also in the earliest non-canonical text of moral instruction, the *Didache* (around 100 AD).

185. Ibid., 96–97.

186. Ibid., 98.

PART TWO: A Modest Proposal for a Biblical Covenantal Biomedical Ethic

ethics as coming from God, as a way of approaching bioethical issues using the guidance of specific commands that manifest as virtues, such as honesty, charity, and integrity.[187]

Vaux emphasizes Christ as the centre of Reformed ethics. Through Christ, a human covenantal community helps individuals exercise their moral conscience against moral individualism while promoting moral virtues that strengthen each community member as well as the moral fiber of the community as a whole. Vaux keeps us aware of the constant relational activity between each other as church members and between God and each individual. Both types of relationships are essential to living obediently under God's providential care. Out of the spirit of Vaux's Reformed approach to a covenantal ethic, I will develop a comprehensive and relational covenantal framework in chapters 6 and 7.

Hessel Bouma, III and his colleagues stress the importance of covenantal ethics from their neo-Calvinist Reformed tradition.[188] They agree with Allen on the distinction between inclusive and special covenants. However, whereas Allen's inclusive covenant includes all living things, including *all of humanity* in relationship with God *since creation*, these authors define the inclusive covenant as *Christians* being in covenant relationship with God *and with all of creation*.[189] Thus, the temporal side of this covenant is a post-Fall relationship between believers and God along with the rest of creation. While likely implied, their inclusive covenant does not explicitly acknowledge the redemptive potential for non-believers to rejoin a divine-human covenant established at creation.

The crux of their covenantal ethic is a loving response to those with whom one is in a caring relationship, acknowledging the more demanding and expectant nature of covenant relations compared with contractual ones.[190] They acknowledge that a minimalist moral view tends to prioritize the individual over the community. While they also speak of minimal rights and duties that are basic elements of their inclusive covenant concept, they are careful to note that negative rights such as not inflicting harm breed a one-sided individualism.[191] Bouma and colleagues

---

187. Ibid., 104. May (*Testing the Medical Covenant*) and Mount (*Covenant*) stress the importance of the virtue and character of those in covenantal relationships.

188. Bouma et al., *Christian Faith*.

189. Ibid., 88; Allen, *Love and Conflict*, 39–40. "Christians believe that they are in covenant with God and with all of creation. From this inclusive covenant flow the responsibilities of being a child of God."

190. Bouma et al., *Christian Faith*, 91.

191. Ibid. Much of their consideration of covenant focuses on individual rights

also see the root of all human covenant relationships in the covenant with God.[192] Importantly, they emphasize that this covenant is not just a theory or model. It is a reality that both motivates and conditions all other covenants. It also guards against the pitfalls of having an ultimate allegiance to finite creatures.

Ramsey, May, Vaux, and Bouma and colleagues give different insights into the value of covenantal thinking in reflecting on biomedical ethics. Ramsey's covenant idea is expressed as loyalty and fidelity in an effort to preserve patient autonomy and consent in medical practice and research settings. He does not delve systematically into a covenantal understanding of caregiver-patient relationships; his link of such relationships with the divine-human covenant seems weak and inconsistent. Smith argues that Ramsey implies the presence of inherent human value by putting such value in relationship with God the creator. However, in my view, this association with God as creator is too weak to support protection for the incapacitated and unborn. Vaux emphasizes partnership with God in living whole and healthy lives. He argues that the covenanted community is a gracious gift from God. It gives collective expression to serving God while providing community member support in resisting idolatry and cultural tendencies to lead self-ruled lives apart from God. Vaux does not develop a covenantal ethic, though he maintains the centrality of our relationship with Christ in discerning ethical action. He does not critique principlism but alludes to its principles briefly. Beneficence, for example, is conceived as a caring disposition in response to a life in Christ. Similarly, Bouma and colleagues emphasize covenantal ethics as a loving response to those with whom we have a caring relationship. They show the importance of the covenant with God on all human relationships. But they slip into a minimalist notion of rights and duties for all human beings, using Allen's covenantal language but restricting the inclusive covenant to believers in Christ. They also produce no in-depth critique of principlism.

Of these covenant-oriented ethicists, May provides the most systematic and in-depth study of the covenant theme in biomedical ethics. Recognizing that Ramsey's covenantal formulation loses theocentric focus with his deontological emphasis on moral rules and principles, May refocuses on covenant as relationships, particularly the patient-physician relationship. He stresses the more extended commitments and obligations of covenantal relationships compared to contractual ones. Only when

---

and duties.

192. Ibid., 94.

PART TWO: A Modest Proposal for a Biblical Covenantal Biomedical Ethic

grounded in the covenant relationship with God and focused on God's command to care for the widow, sick, and needy does the full meaning of covenantal relating develop and flourish. Unfortunately, May does not explicitly articulate a Christian worldview or philosophical basis for his covenantal ethic, nor does he satisfactorily account for the complex relational network of medical care. In addition, unlike Pellegrino he does not provide an in-depth critique or recontextualization of the four principles in light of his covenantal ethic.

The work of these Christian bioethicists has been a light in a discipline darkened by reliance on relative moral truth and faith in human reason to address bioethical issues. They each make incomplete contributions to the development of a covenantal ethic for biomedical ethics with their own distinct elements and emphases. An essential element of a covenantal ethic is a Christian concept of self or personhood that identifies the nature and character of the moral agents in medical relationships. In the next section, I will explore contemporary ideas of self in medical practice and lay the foundations of a biblical notion of self and personhood. This Christian anthropology will be linked to the development of a biblical covenantal ethic in the next two chapters.

BUILDING COVENANTAL RELATIONALITY ON BIBLICAL ANTHROPOLOGY

In this section, I will present a Christian view of human selfhood, a requirement for a robust concept of a biblical covenantal biomedical ethic. I will use the example of David Landis, presented earlier in this chapter, as a fractured self–identity, followed by a Christian concept of self, proposed by Christian philosopher Herman Dooyeweerd and further developed by Gerrit Glas and others.

Some appeals to covenantal relationships are corrective responses to the emphasis on protecting individual integrity and rights in our contemporary culture. However, applying this corrective may detract from a normative understanding of the role of the individual in covenantal relationships. Richard Mouw presents a concept of Christian individuality within, yet apart from, a culture founded on individual*ism*.[193] Scripture makes clear the direct accountability of individuals to God: we need to understand who we are in order to relate meaningfully to others. Allen's covenantal model stresses social aspects while pointing to God as the cen-

193. Mouw, *God Who Commands*, 43–54.

ter and ground of our individual being. In step with Mouw, he believes that a properly constituted covenant community fosters individuality rather than minimizes it in the communitarian sense.[194] In calling us each by name, God declares the worth along with the obligations of each human being in covenant relationship with him. We are accountable for our actions and for the intentions of our hearts.[195]

Applying a more secular perspective, David Landis postulates that physicians in our medical culture develop a "medical self" during medical training.[196] He contrasts what he calls the inner knowledge of one's pre-training personal self with a developing outside knowledge of the medical self. By means of a covenant with peers and the profession as a whole, the medical self grows in relationship with other medical selves and acquires the specific knowledge of the profession. Through fidelity promised under that covenant, medical selves promise to embrace their community and to maintain the distinction between the personal and the professional aspects of themselves. He suggests that creating a covenantal relationship with the profession of medicine offers the physician a corrective vision to see one's personal reaction to patients through "the generic glasses of my medical self."[197] That is, on entering the covenant with medicine, physicians should look at the reactions of their personal self to patient experiences through the spectacles of their medical self. In effect, they should depersonalize and universalize their personal experiences with patients in order to use that experience in the broadest possible way for the benefit of the largest number of future patients. He emphasizes that the medical self must be committed to remaining distinct from the personal self.[198]

Landis's covenantal model tries to describe what medical students experience emotionally and psychologically in their encounters with patients. Citing theologian James Gustafson, Landis believes that adopting a covenantal model for medical relationships enables medical students and physicians to *objectify their morality*. For Landis, such objectification contributes to the effectiveness of their actions.[199] Yet, Landis tries to inject

---

194. Ibid., 54. Mouw states, "[Human beings] are fitted for the service of a divine Ruler who calls each subject by name—but calls them nonetheless to participation in communities in which the shalom of God is exhibited."

195. Allen, *Love and Conflict*, 47–48. Members of a covenanting moral community are not interchangeable units in a utilitarian calculus balancing good over evil.

196. Landis, "Physician Distinguish Thyself," 632–33.

197. Ibid., 639–40.

198. Ibid., 639.

199. Ibid., 640.

Part Two: A Modest Proposal for a Biblical Covenantal Biomedical Ethic

a transcendent aspect to this model by appealing to *mythical associations* with past heroes and ideals of the profession, much in the spirit of the Greek mythologies. His notion of divided selves focuses on covenantal relationships with the profession and its co-members rather than with patients. The relationship with patients seems only to indirectly benefit from this professional covenant through its inherent obligations. These relational distinctions seem derived from the spirit and content of the Hippocratic Oath itself. In these relationships as envisioned by Landis, the medical student's selves seem detached in these relationships while at the same time interdependent on each other.[200]

In contrast to Landis's model, an overarching biblical covenantal ethic encompasses both professional and personal aspects of the physician.[201] It also involves covenantal relating between the caregiver and patient, not just among caregivers. Seen through this perspective, the "two selves" resolve into different, growing dimensions of personal expression and empathy. Both the personal and medical encounters are mutually enhanced if used in the spirit and expression of Christian covenantal love and its committed obligations. Landis's "dichotomy of selves" cannot be resolved because his "transcendent concept of the healing art" is merely a nostalgic reflection on "great healers and their art" from the ancient Greek past. These medical selves are united in their response to gifts such as patient donations of their bodies and time, mentor donations of time and instruction, and the ideals and traditions of ancient Greek medicine. Furthermore, Landis fails to consider the important conflicts between medical obligations to patients and personal obligations to family and friends that so often disrupt a physician's life. Both fall under obligations of covenant grounded in Scripture and need to be reconciled using Spirit-led scriptural guidance.

A Reformed Christian perspective provides a crucial and biblically normative understanding of self when seen in conjunction with covenantal relationships. In his insightful philosophical anthropology, the Christian philosopher Herman Dooyeweerd understands the human being as

---

200. This point recalls the two relationships in the Hippocratic Oath and the distinction made by Edelstein (*Ancient Medicine*) and May ("Code, Covenant") between the codal character of the patient-physician relationship and the covenantal character of the relationship between the mentor, oath taker, and the mentor's family.

201. In his analysis of the self psychology of Heinz Kohut, James Olthuis ("On Worldviews," 32ff.) shows how the Christian faith acknowledges God as "the ultimate empathic environment, the perfect, responsive love whose grace and mercy empowers us to seek forgiveness and obtain healing."

Conceptual Support for Covenantal Biomedical Ethics

an *enkaptic* structural whole. That is, a human being exists and functions as a whole but distinctly different "ways of being" can be identified; these include physical, biotic, psychic, social, linguistic, juridical, ethical, and other ways of being. Besides seeing these *structural* sides of human relating and functioning, Dooyeweerd also sees human selfhood in *directional* terms, as "the concentric directedness of the totality of a person's existence toward the Origin of meaning."[202] Self naturally looks toward a transcendent source of origin. True self cannot exist if this directedness is distorted or even absent. The intrinsic importance of religious belief is evident in the similarities between this definition of self and Dooyeweerd's definition of religion as "the innate impulse of human selfhood."[203]

Seen in this way, true selfhood is a religious unity specifying self-knowledge that is dependent on knowledge of God. Likewise, this selfhood should be interpreted through the understanding that human beings are image-bearers of God. Selfhood is dynamic in hearing and responding to the calling of God. Individual selves are also "rooted in" the spiritual community of humankind. In its fullest sense, our self is *both* individual and communal.[204] Peter Moore rightly emphasizes the importance of our relational identity in his comparison of the African concept of *ubuntu* with Western society's emphasis on self-reliant individualism.[205] *Ubuntu* connotes a principle of caring for one another to the extent that one is a person only because of, and through, other persons.[206] Addressing the value of *ubuntu* for overcoming the oppression of apartheid in South Africa, Archbishop Desmond Tutu argues that oppression deprives humans of fellowship or *koinonia*.[207] Such oppression can also come in the form of utilitarian disregard for basic human value. Our ability to relate may be limited, for example, by developmental immaturity or by loss of communicative capability through injury or illness and economic considerations may give cause to devalue the unborn and the incapacitated among us. However, given our created status as God's image-bearers, we possess an intrinsic value just a little less than that of angels according to the writer of

202. Glas, "Ego, Self, and the Body," 70.

203. Ibid., 78 n. 1. Glas quotes from *New Critique of Theoretical Thought* by Dooyeweerd (*New Critique*, 57): religion is "the innate impulse of human selfhood to direct itself toward the *true* or toward a *pretended* absolute Origin of all temporal diversity of meaning, which it finds focused concentrically in itself" (emphases in original).

204. Ibid., 73.

205. Moore, *Being Me*.

206. Ibid., 245–46.

207. Ibid., 254; Battle, *Reconciliation*.

Part Two: A Modest Proposal for a Biblical Covenantal Biomedical Ethic

the book of Hebrews. All human beings were created in relationship with God and by God's will, authority, and grace.[208]

Dooyeweerd's anthropology presents a biblical notion of the unity of human beings, refuting contemporary views of human beings that reflect a fragmented personhood and tension between the individual and society. Gerrit Glas notes that these views have led to insufficient attention to contemporary ethical and social contexts. Dooyeweerd's concepts of ego and selfhood emphasize interhuman relationships, the reality around us, and God as the origin of meaning.[209] However, for Glas, even Dooyeweerd's concept of self is still too anthropocentric. Glas favors a more dynamic view of relationships that mirrors the divine relationships within the Trinity of God. Still, Dooyeweerd's account of self or "the I" is fully relational since it relates the self to God, to others, and to itself.[210] Within this I-self relationship, an entity that Dooyeweerd calls the supra-temporal heart or spirit is related to the body as the totality of temporal self-structures. By extension, personhood is relational in nature and has its deepest meaning in the web of interpersonal relationships within a God-fearing community. This idea of personhood as interpersonal relationships begs the question of whether the unborn, particularly the human embryo, or the less-than-fully-capacitated are considered persons. Doubts would have to be cast if reciprocal relationality would be required. But relationality as caring is an image that better captures the biblical dimension of caring for the vulnerable as a divine requirement of true relationality with God and fellow humans.

Glas argues that virtue ethics is integral to Reformed ethics and "an important ally in the current moral debate."[211] However, he admits that virtue ethics needs to become more attuned to the specialization of medical care and the impact of new technological advances on normative,

---

208. Heb 2:6–7; Rusthoven, "Are Human Embryos."

209. Glas, "Ego, Self, and the Body," 74.

210. Ibid. Glas contrasts what Charles Taylor calls a punctual self with what Kierkegaard calls a self as a relation that relates to itself.

211. This emphasis on virtue in ethics is reminiscent of the ethical frameworks of William F. May ("Virtues"), Edmund Pellegrino and David Thomasma (*Christian Virtues*), and Celia Deane-Drummond (*Genetics*). Like MacIntyre (*After Virtue*), Pellegrino strongly advocates for a return to the Thomistic synthesis of Aristotelian ethics and Scripture as the solution to the fragmentation of morality. Deane-Drummond (*Genetics*, xxiii, 12–14, 143–52, 234–58) explores friendship as an integral dimension of Christian virtue ethics and extends its application to non-human creatures in the context of genetic interventions in the non-human world as possible expressions of love and wisdom.

creational structures.[212] He rightly expresses concern that the concept of evil is often neglected by ethicists, resulting in a *medicalization* of immoral behavior into a mental disorder. This can result in excusing evil actions and reducing the responsibility of the perpetrators.[213]

In my view, a Reformed anthropological approach does not envision a split self that evolves during medical training. Rather, the self of a medical trainee must develop mature and diversified conceptual understanding of patients as persons who petition help in time of need. In addition, the role of evil must be acknowledged in our presuppositional conceptions of the fallen creation order and its distorting influence. I agree with Glas, Dooyeweerd, and Mouw that selfhood should be perceived in dynamic terms, as a dynamic pilgrimage. Compared to traveling a life-path without Christ, a Christ-led pilgrimage results in directional diversion and change from that taken by unbelievers. Enjoyment is redirected from self-gratification to the enjoyment of glorifying God. The human relationship to God renews the relationship to other humans; it also renews one's perception of, and role in, the surrounding culture and in the rest of the creation order.

Allen uses the term *inclusive covenant* to characterize the initial relationship between God and all living things, affirming their inherent value in God's sight even if they are not capable of reciprocating God's act of covenanting. However, human beings are created in the image of God, setting them apart from other creatures and ensuring special inherent value even in the face of any incapacity to relationally reciprocate. The pre-Fall, creational character of Allen's inclusive covenant is analogous to the covenant of works presented systematically by Bavinck, Spykman, and others. The case is made for such a primordial covenant relationship largely because of the gracious and divine command nature of God's initiation of the relationship as an act of love and gift giving for the creature created in

---

212. Glas, "Persons and Their Lives," 50–51. Glas goes on to suggest that virtue ethics lacks the notion of a religious depth dimension and a vocabulary for evil, sin, and wrongness. David Novak (*Covenantal Rights*, 19, 20, 118) criticizes the lack of a concept of creation law in virtue ethics, resulting in its anthropocentric nature. He says its language has been easily translated into language that addresses competencies but not one that relates to commitment, benevolence, and malevolence. He does not mention Pellegrino directly but Pellegrino's critique of the dominance of autonomy in contemporary bioethics at the expense of beneficence addresses this concern.

213. Ibid., 52. Glas gives the example of Nazi physicians in concentration camps who suppressed their own shame and guilt through a splitting of behavior, showing emotionally touching gestures of affection one moment and murdering those same persons shortly after.

Part Two: A Modest Proposal for a Biblical Covenantal Biomedical Ethic

his image. Tragically, sin repeatedly broke the human commitment of that covenant until Christ unilaterally restored it through his death and resurrection, establishing a new covenant forever. Nonetheless, Paul makes it clear that the covenant with Adam defined his headship of humankind under the old covenantal relationship while Christ assumes headship of redeemed humanity through the new covenant. This new covenantal relationship is offered to all of humankind for those who repent and live out their covenant with Christ through their relationships with fellow human beings.[214]

May alludes to an inclusive covenant but seems to restrict the concept to the new covenant in Christ, although his reference to Barth's association of covenant with creation implies perhaps a belief in an original inclusive covenant as well. Thus, he does not present a full account of the role of covenant in redemptive history, starting from the covenant established by God at creation. In addition, while empathizing with the efforts of Christians to influence public policy through approaches such as principlism, May has genuine concern for a perceived diminution of the Christian appreciation for the importance of virtue and character of the moral agent. He makes no mention of the distortion of relational structures within the created order that plagues a principle-based ethic.

In my view, both Ramsey and May fail to sufficiently incorporate key elements into their covenantal frameworks. May is concerned about Ramsey's lack of attention to his Christian anthropology and about the direction of the moral agent. But he does not give sufficient credit to Ramsey's concerns about distortions of structural aspects of morality in the created order. Anthropology, faith direction, and creational structures all need to be addressed as a unity in order to develop a complete Christian covenantal ethical framework. Both Ramsey and May fail to present a systematic Christian philosophical framework for conceptualizing covenantal relationships. In chapter 7, I will show how Dooyeweerd's social philosophy helps to provide normative structure to medical practice while a covenantal ethical framework can keep a relational focus on both directional and structural aspects of practice.

Special covenants, according to Allen, are those established among human beings as living expressions of their created social nature. From the time when God realized that Adam was in need of companionship, this social aspect of humanity has played out through a multiplicity of relationships. However, what is the basis of these relationships? Ramsey

---

214. Rom 5:12–17; 1 Cor 15:20–26.

seems to be inconsistent as to whether these are social structures of the created order or human inventions. Why does this matter and how does the answer affect the understanding of a biblically derived covenantal ethic for biomedical ethics?

COVENANTAL ETHICS IN CONFESSIONALLY PLURALISTIC SOCIETIES

Rockne McCarthy and colleagues have outlined the three contemporary social philosophies of Western societies that influence the understanding relationships between different social structures.[215] In critiquing individualistic and communitarian social philosophies, they appeal to a pluralistic approach as that which is most normative from a biblical perspective. Specifically, they favor the pluralism espoused in the Calvinist tradition, which views an ordered reality of creation consisting of inherent structures that are realized by all human beings. There are distinct, independent spheres of social relationships with unique characteristics and focus. Seen through Dooyeweerd's Christian social philosophy, it is the sovereignty of each social sphere that inherently strives to withstand sinful distortion, such as when one or more social spheres tries to lord over others and usurp their authority, often with devastating consequences.[216] Biblical scrutiny of special covenants defined by such social spheres is a task requiring much-needed further reflection to develop a normative covenant ethic in biomedical ethics.

A Christian pluralist notion of social relationships should recognize the reality of a second dimension, that of confessional pluralism. This dimension envisions a world fragmented by contrasting faith communities. However, in contrast to the principlist belief in moral stability through a minimalist common morality exclusive of confessional beliefs, confessional pluralism strives to work with fundamental moral diversity. Each moral perspective is respected for its insights toward common concerns of all human beings.[217] Offering the example of Abraham Kuyper, McCarthy and colleagues show that common cause coalitions can be sought and struck among those of different faiths who have fundamental concerns about distortions in ethical actions regarding the environment and medicine. Such interfaith dialogue has begun to occur between Muslims

---

215. McCarthy et al., *Society, State, & Schools*, 15–19.
216. Ibid., 36–38.
217. Ibid., 39–40.

PART TWO: A Modest Proposal for a Biblical Covenantal Biomedical Ethic

and Christians with similar concepts of the created order and the human responsibility to that order.[218]

Eric Mount describes a general ethic of covenantal relationships that accommodates vulnerable "others." It is an ethic understood in Jewish and Christian traditions and has a potentially persuasive common good that can promote public responsibility.[219] Mount envisions a "global community of communities" where the rules of discourse guide the sharing of stories from different communities defined by covenanting around common goods. However, he presents the theme of covenant more as a metaphor for pointing to the interhuman and interdependent character of our existence as the ground for moral possibility and for reality that transcends our individual wants and needs.[220] Mount's approach differs substantially from principlism in its acceptance of views from different faith communities. Rather than stripping moral reasons of their faith-based justification and moral grounding for the sake of an empty consensus of permissive agreement, Mount welcomes diversity of moral justification while seeking moral unity through similar objectives of helping vulnerable persons.

Despite Veatch's encouraging invitation for greater input of religious views into bioethical reflections, he and others still fail to see, or accept, that foundational beliefs, religious or otherwise, *supersede* reason as the *justification* for moral positions. Belief in a common morality as a foundational belief has no grounding or authority other than mutual agreement. Faith in reason alone is insufficient for justifying moral positions. Any alternative to a reason-based framework must take into account a normative vision of the cosmos and its created order as well as an anthropology that properly accounts for human moral disposition, conduct, and responsibility. Sin is also a factor that is omitted from principlism. In a similar postmodern spirit, Sturm and Meland transform the biblical notion of sin into one of "normative dissonance" within all relationships. Sin becomes relational abnormality where the relational distortion is limited to human inadequacy. Sin as disobedience against God, expressed as wrongful

---

218. Ibid., 48. Egbert Schuurman ("Challenge") has recently suggested that such cooperative moral ventures targeting the environment may even be possible among reformist Muslims and Reformed Christians who have common elements in their cosmological view of creation despite differing foundationally in their idea of the nature of God, Christ, and salvation. Proceedings of such discussions were recently published (Jochemsen and van der Stoep, *Different Cultures*).

219. Mount, *Covenant*, 144–50. Wurzburger (*Ethics of Responsibility*) and Gellman ("On Immanuel Jakobvits") give examples of Jewish ethical positions.

220. Ibid., 157–58.

thought or action against other human beings, is stripped of its meaning and distorted into a normal tension in every relationship.[221]

THE CORE OF BIBLICAL COVENANTAL ETHICS: GOD'S FAITHFUL AND RECONCILING LOVE

In my view, both Sturm and Mount might have developed a more biblical principle of covenant had they pursued covenant as a root-metaphor as understood by Elaine Botha. Botha interprets the covenant as one of several central biblical themes that are woven within the biblical metanarrative. For Botha, the root-metaphor of covenant in Scripture sets the *direction* of interpretation and provides the relational context and meaning for themes like creation and redemption.[222] Scriptural metaphors, says Botha, are all qualified confessionally and fiduciarily. It is particularly *the fiduciary kernel of the scriptural root-metaphor of covenant* that makes a covenantal framework so well suited for biomedical ethics.[223] Covenant is the commitment of God's presence of engagement with us and world around us.[224] The biblical concept of covenant binds all human beings in a redemptive history from the beginning of created time to the complete renewing of the created order at the end of time. It also acknowledges that since Pentecost, the Holy Spirit has been at work giving evidence of the restorative work of Christ in a world not yet fully renewed and perfected. The Spirit's work is neither condemning nor exclusive. It is persuasive. The Spirit calls to all and accepts all who will hear and believe in language that speaks to the needs of the weak and the vulnerable.

A biblical covenantal ethic can help to give direction and meaning to the normative structures that constitute medical practice and research. This requires a philosophical framework that is inspired by biblical teaching regarding the creation order and that can discern the distorting influences of other unbiblical spirits of our culture. Such a philosophical framework has been developed by Christian philosophers in the Reformed Christian tradition and can be applied to enhance and renew our understanding of

---

221. Sturm, "Contextual and Covenant," 155–56; Meland, *Fallible Forms*, 97–99.

222. Botha, *Metaphor*, 220; Sturm "Contextual and Covenant," 155.

223. This terminology is reminiscent of Dooyeweerd's philosophy. While Dooyeweerd makes little reference to metaphor in his writings (and what he did say was usually not complimentary!), Botha (*Metaphor*, 113–16) makes the case that his concept of the religious groundmotive resembles the notion of root-metaphor.

224. Hunter, *To Change the World*, 241–43.

Part Two: A Modest Proposal for a Biblical Covenantal Biomedical Ethic

medical relationships and ethical principles. As mentioned earlier, Vaux sees the four principles of Beauchamp and Childress transformed from negative sanctions in ancient pagan moral codes to positive action commands for the Christian life that are fixed on Christ within the new covenant. However, a Christian social philosophy is needed to give normative force to medical relationships in terms of their internal structures and their relational interactions. A covenantal ethic is required to give biblical direction and proper relational context to the principles of principlism.

The spirit of openness inherent in a biblical covenantal ethic respects the diversity of faith communities in a world distorted by sin, yet also gives direction for human relationships through belief in Jesus Christ and the creation-renewing work inherent in that belief. This spirit of openness should be encouraging to bioethicists like Veatch and philosophers like Habermas who have begun to see the contribution to moral content that Christian perspectives can bring to biomedical ethics. As presented in the next chapter, Abraham Kuyper, Herman Dooyeweerd, and others have developed a Christian cosmology in which the created order is a diversity of distinct yet interwoven structures. Each individual thing or living creature is constituted by such a structure. Relational structures are also evident and need to be understood for the sake of normative relationships in professions such as medicine. The *confessional plurality* of foundational beliefs that is the reality of a sinful and not yet fully redeemed cosmos must be recognized and incorporated into the ethical aspects of our lives. A complete faith in purely rational persuasion in moral discourse reduces morality to legalistic and formal relations that resist depth of understanding out of fear of offense or coercion. Incorporation of faith commitments beyond reason alone bring forward the fullest meaning of moral positions that can lead to more fruitful dialogue as well as mutual respect for the profound differences that make up our pluralistic world.

As I have shown, contemporary appeals to covenantal relationships in medicine have been justified through both non-Christian and Christian traditions. As shown in this chapter, interpretations of biblical covenantal concepts differ according to the relation of covenant to other biblical themes in redemptive history, to the nature of the relationship to God and its effect on human relationships, and to its relationship to sin. From a Reformed Christian perspective, the covenant theme is central to our cosmology because human beings were created to be in relationship with God, other human beings, the rest of the creation, and themselves. A biblical covenantal ethic appeals to a common origin of our current human plight by virtue of a covenant established at creation by God. With human disobedience, that covenant was violated and the common recognizability of created structures, including relational structures within medicine, was distorted as a result of human beings repeatedly turning to false sources of authority and security.

Conceptual distortions within the current bioethical paradigm result in large part from the lack of an *ordering-principle*. As recognized and articulated by Allen, O'Donovan, Pellegrino, and others, for Christians that ordering-principle is the command to love God and our neighbor as ourselves. It gives full meaning and direction to guidelines, principles, and rules that guide our moral dispositions, actions, and judgments in our relationships with other human beings. Seen in this light, such an ethic for medicine can provide a helpful framework for open discussion not only among Christians but also with those with different faiths and basic beliefs. It provides hope that all morally concerned persons might see merit in biblically sound bioethical policies and decisions that, with the leading of the Holy Spirit, can benefit all human beings.[225]

Two characteristics that particularly distinguish the concept of biblical covenant from that of contract are the *steadfast* and *reconciling* nature of God's love. Pagan nations worshipped capricious gods that showed arbitrary behavior toward human beings, hardly a relationship of trust from which human relationships would be emulated. The ancient Israelites, and later the early Christians, needed assurance that their God was reliable and consistent in his promises and judgments.[226] This enduring responsibility goes beyond the legally stipulated, time-limited criteria of a contract. The reconciling characteristic is perhaps the most defining one. Unlike the legal release from responsibility that contract breaking allows, covenant with God entails a unilateral promise to keep that covenant *no matter what*. With this commitment comes a righteous stipulation to seek out repentance from the covenant breaker and to accept forgiveness when repentance is heartfelt so that covenantal integrity can be restored.

A biblical covenantal ethic welcomes engagement in moral reflection by those of any faith—secular or "religious"—who are willing to share insights derived from the persuasive force of their fundamental beliefs. Such moral sharing should occur in a spirit of mutual respect and openness. As noted by Bavinck, it is a covenantal obligation of Christians to articulate the ethical unity between God and humankind and strive to persuade

---

225. Mount, *Covenant*, 138–44, 151, 155–60.
226. Eichrodt, *Theology*, 38.

Part Two: A Modest Proposal for a Biblical Covenantal Biomedical Ethic

fellow human beings that true unity can only be achieved by common participation in the renewal of creation and its activities through obedience to the Word.[227]

I have shown the merits and promise of developing a covenantal bioethical model on the basis of the biblical covenant theme. It can fill the need for a well-grounded ethical framework that addresses the inadequacies of principlism. In the next two chapters, I will bring forward a vision of a biblical covenantal ethic for biomedical ethics that draws on covenant as a central theme in redemptive history as interpreted in the Reformed Christian tradition. I will show the importance of a Christian anthropology and social philosophy for understanding the network of relationships in medicine through a covenantal ethical framework. Then, in chapter 8, I will show how this covenantal ethic gives renewed normative meaning to the four principles in light of God's Word.

---

227. Bavinck, *Reformed Dogmatics*, 579.

6

Groundwork for a Contemporary Covenantal Ethic

I always write as the ethicist I am, namely a Christian ethicist, and not as some hypothetical common denominator.[1]

—Paul Ramsey (1974)

A BRIEF REVIEW

IN PART ONE, I trace the development of the principles-based ethical framework promoted by Beauchamp and Childress, present its core premises, and review critical appraisals of this framework by non-Christian and Christian bioethicists. While most critics give Beauchamp and Childress credit for their effort to create a common language and common moral denominator to promote bioethical dialogue, many are critical of the emphasis on process at the expense of moral content to which moral philosophy was committed in the past. Others are more accommodating to, than critical of, principlism. However, the depth of critique varies widely. Little attention is paid to the basic belief systems from which principlism draws its authority and justification and to the unbiblical nature of those systems. It is particularly disappointing that more in-depth critique has not been more forthcoming from Christian bioethicists whose input and influence has waned over the decades.

1. Ramsey, "Commentary," 56.

Part Two: A Modest Proposal for a Biblical Covenantal Biomedical Ethic

However, several bioethicists such as Paul Ramsey, Edmund Pellegrino, and H. Tristram Engelhardt stand out as Christian bioethicists who have provided bold witness in biomedical ethics by means of their distinct faith traditions. Of these three, Pellegrino probes most deeply into the nature of medicine. While praising Beauchamp and Childress for their promotion of moral dialogue through the mouthpiece of the four principles, he also exposes the lack of authoritative moral grounding behind principlism and the failure to develop a relational understanding of medicine. However, even Pellegrino fails to sufficiently expose the underlying worldviews from which principlism has developed and to consider the full network of relationships that constitutes contemporary medical practice. In chapter 4, I respond to these insufficiencies in a critical analysis of the elements of modernity and postmodernism that underlie principlism and of the faith in rationality in which both worldviews are grounded.

In chapter 5, I present the rationale and justification for developing a biblical covenantal ethical framework for biomedical ethics. In recent years there has been an increasing interest in covenantal ethics for medicine among caregivers, medical educators, and biomedical ethicists. A biblical covenantal ethic derives moral authority and grounding in a covenantal relationship established by God with humankind at the time of creation. Through this relationship, all human beings possess equal value and worth in the eyes of God. A covenantal ethic is proposed that is cosmic in scope; that is, it is relevant for, and can be at least partly and innately appreciated by, all human beings by virtue of our unique creational status as imagebearers of God. However, the fullest understanding and expression of this covenantal nature of human relationships can be achieved only through obedience to God as revealed in the Word of God. Thus, moral insight is found in its most meaningful expression through reflective understanding of human relationships with guidance from Scripture. The principles identified in principlism then take on new and deeper meaning within a biblical covenantal ethic, taking their place within a Christian worldview and theological context.

In this chapter, features of a biblical covenantal ethic for biomedical ethics will be presented and described. It will be argued that such an ethical framework provides a fresh perspective on biomedical ethics, giving substantially more grounding, depth, and moral content than principlism has provided. Key elements of any biblical ethical framework include 1) identifying a worldview, philosophy, and theology that give biblical authoritative grounding and guidance for moral character-building, reflection and decision-making, 2), articulating a biblical anthropology that properly envisions human authority and responsibility in our world in light of a normative relationship with God as creator and savior, and 3) focusing on the structural and directional normativity of those relationships that form the basis of medical practice. In light of the critical analysis of the worldview and philosophical basis of principlism provided at the end of chapter 4, I will now articulate an integrated covenantal ethic, Christian worldview, and social philosophical perspective for medicine. In the last chapter, I will take up the task of reconceptualizing the four principles of principlism in light of such a covenantal ethical framework.

INFORMING WORLDVIEW, PHILOSOPHY, AND THEOLOGY THROUGH THE COVENANT THEME

Christian Worldview and Biblical Theology of Covenant

Over the last thirty years, an increasing number of theologians have encouraged the study of Scripture as a narrative or story, partly in reaction to the historico-critical and moralistic approaches that have been taken in the past. In the early 1980s, Hauerwas claimed that narrative is epistemically fundamental for our understanding of God and of ourselves as contingent creatures.[2] Lesslie Newbigin encouraged an understanding of the meaning of human life as a story within the larger story of God's created reality.[3] Very recently, James K. A. Smith reminds us of the importance of narrative revelation, noting that its rich, multidimensional communication encourages the imagination to become fully involved in understanding God's creation through the unfolding of God's redemptive story.[4]

Understanding Scripture in this way also allows for an appreciation of biblical themes that are embedded in the redemptive narrative as

---

2. Hauerwas, *Peaceable Kingdom*, 17ff. Here, Hauerwas argues for the narrative character of Christian ethics.

3. Newbigin, *Gospel*, 15.

4. Smith, *Who's Afraid*, 75; Smith, *Desiring the Kingdom*, 45f., 68. In *Desiring the Kingdom*, Smith takes to task most conceptions of Christian worldview as too cognitive and propositional in nature, putting them perilously close to rationalist models. While praising Christian critiques of secular modernist worldviews, he believes that human beings are fundamentally oriented and identified by love and desire, both being affective expressions at a subconscious level. He argues that worldview as "knowledge" should be replaced by worldview as "social imaginary," an imaginative rather than intellectual understanding of the world that is more implicit in the practices of Christian worship and that is more authentically Augustinian.

Part Two: A Modest Proposal for a Biblical Covenantal Biomedical Ethic

presented in chapter 5. Goheen and Bartholomew link a biblical theology with a Christian worldview that identifies, articulates, and expresses its basic beliefs within the narrative story of the Bible.[5] Through inherent biblical themes such as creation, covenant, kingdom, law, sin, and mission, biblical theology helps us to identify fundamental and comprehensive signposts within the biblical story. These thematic signposts enable the believer to see the structure and orderliness of the creation and to map out the right direction throughout our dealings with that created order.[6] Among these themes, the covenant theme stands out as "a golden thread weaving its way through the total fabric of biblical revelation."[7] Its central position in redemptive history and its relational character make the covenant theme well suited as the basis for a normative understanding of relationships within creation, including those that form in the course of medical practice and research.

The biblical covenant theme expresses the relational essence of the biblical story and begins with the covenant established by the Trinitarian God. That covenant began as a divinely offered gift of relationship between God and humankind at creation. Over time, it has been violated repeatedly by human infidelity but repeatedly renewed by God's boundless grace through the prophets. That covenant was redeemed for all time through the suffering and resurrection of Jesus Christ. It is operative through the work of the Holy Spirit in all of created reality by way of Christians who strive to renew all aspects of the created order until its complete and perfect renewal by Christ at the end of time. Until then, our interpretation of Scripture remains under the often sinful influence of the cultures within which we must live.

Scripture is not used to articulate disconnected moral claims but to guide our thinking toward a comprehensive moral perspective.[8] As

---

5. Goheen and Bartholomew, *Living at the Crossroads*, 26–28. The entire biblical story could be considered a meta-narrative or overarching, a grand story that considers the true meaning of all events in history, within which are less comprehensive but nonetheless interrelated stories. However, the term *meta-narrative* has also been used to describe the grand story told within particular worldviews, so its meaning needs to be considered in light of the context within which it is used. For example, Goheen and Bartholomew (*Living at the Crossroads*, 109) distinguish between modernist and postmodern meta-narratives. They also distinguish biblical theology (not to be confused with biblical studies) from systematic theology, the latter of which is a theoretical endeavor on the same plane as philosophy.

6. Ibid., 29–30.

7. Spykman, *Reformational Theology*, 11–12.

8. Bartholomew, "Time for War," 26.

O'Donovan writes, Christians should look to Scripture for indications of moral structures and order in the world around us, not just for individual moral rules that match moral situations.[9] He suggests looking for principles of order such as the teaching of Jesus to the Pharisees: "For I desire mercy, and not sacrifice."[10] God's love-command is supreme among principles of order and has universal inclusiveness.[11] In grounding a covenantal ethic, it provides relevance for all human beings and their relationships.

Any theoretical accounting of the world and its cultures through theological and philosophical reflection must be informed through the confessional and creedal framework that constitutes the church as the body of Christ. As a holy, catholic communion of saints, this church constitutes an important aspect of biblical theology on which a Christian worldview is based. Every sphere of human engagement is given by God as part of the creation that unfolds in the face of human activity. Christian theorizing regarding distinct aspects of creation must emanate from a distinctly Christian standpoint.[12] In pursuit of such theoretical activity, the covenant theme can most comprehensively and most insightfully guide biblical insights toward normative expressions of ethical expression, including character and judgments, in biomedical ethics. Engaging in medical relationships is an ethically qualified activity.[13] It is thus important to grasp the full normativity of those relationships using a conceptual framework grounded in Scripture.

Normative expression of a biblical covenantal biomedical ethic requires the conceptual context of a Christian worldview. From such a worldview, biblical norms can be determined regarding professional competence and the relationships that constitute medicine. A Christian worldview also relates medical relationships to other aspects of our lives, including relationships outside of medicine. I will now present an exploration of variations of a Christian worldview, giving justified preference to a Reformed Christian worldview within which a biblical covenantal ethic for biomedical ethics can find expression.

9. O'Donovan, *Resurrection and Moral Order*, 200–4.
10. Hos 6:6.
11. O'Donovan, *Resurrection and Moral Order*, 200–4; Matt 9:13; Matt 22:37–40.
12. Smith, "Introduction," 18.
13. Jochemsen, "Normative Practices," 105. Henk Jochemsen and others have drawn insights from Dooyeweerd's social philosophy to advance a Normative Reflective Practitioner model for medical practice. In this model, they consider the principle of care as the normative principle of the ethical aspect and the *telos* of all caring practices. I will discuss this in more detail later in this chapter.

Part Two: A Modest Proposal for a Biblical Covenantal Biomedical Ethic

There is *one* Christian worldview held by the church at large in which Scripture is the central focus for giving direction to our perceptions of, and activities in, the world. But the church also has a long history of internal variations of that worldview, with different creeds and confessions reflecting different interpretations of Scripture.[14] David Naugle has identified four key elements or dimensions that gives a framework to a distinctly Christian worldview: 1) the existence of God, his nature, and his created order, including the moral order, 2) the human heart as core of our created likeness of God, embracing our selfhood and consciousness functions, 3) the appreciation of sin as blindness to the truth about God and his creation resulting in idolatrous perceptions of God and creation, and 4) the belief that our only hope of overcoming such perceptions is through the grace and redemption found in Jesus Christ.[15] Similar to the basic elements of a Christian worldview put forward by Albert Wolters, Naugle adds a Christian anthropological dimension based on our relationship with God, which was established at creation. This dimension is the essential spiritual orientation of the human heart, either toward God or away from him.[16]

A biblical covenant theme encompasses these elements, from which a covenantal framework can be developed for biomedical ethics. But fallible interpretations of scriptural texts reflect variations of the Christian worldview that represent an inner church plurality in a still-fallen world. Arthur Holmes has suggested that the Christian worldview is an "open-ended exploration"[17] and "an endless undertaking that is still but the vision of a possibility."[18] However, such openness requires vigilance in order to reap the fruits of fresh biblically based insights while resisting relativistic uncertainty that can erode biblical Truth.

James Olthuis envisions worldview as an ethical starting point regarding notions about how the world ought to function. It is also an integrator between faith commitment and a way of life that expresses such a commitment in concrete activities.[19] However, much like the fragmented

---

14. Smith, *Who's Afraid*, 57.

15. Naugle, *Worldview*, 290.

16. Ibid. Wolters, *Creation Regained*, 11–12. Wolters more specifically advocates for a Reformational worldview. Its basis is a Trinitarian confession that God the Father reconciled this sinfully fallen and distorted world through his Son and renewing it by way of the Holy Spirit.

17. Holmes, *Idea*, 4.

18. Ibid., 58.

19. Olthuis, "On Worldviews," 38.

morality that plagues our postmodern culture,[20] fragmented, concurrent worldviews can threaten faith communities.[21] Jacob Klapwijk argues that the Christian worldview has transformative power in challenging the ideologies of other worldviews. Human experience seeks validation in faith. In entering the praxis of callings and vocations in our largely secular culture, we must learn to integrate our experiences into the Christian vision of life.[22] Christian mission in society is transformative in nature, both rejecting and sanctifying the broken world around us.[23] This is the mission of Christian professionals, including those in medicine. Olthuis and Klapwijk agree that different expressions of the Christian worldview can legitimately exist when justified by inspired transforming forces. Such distinctive expressions result from interpretations of Scripture that reflect distinctly different perceptions of our relationship with the culture around us.[24] Differences in Roman Catholic and Protestant traditions might be perceived as quarrels within the same family. However, they can run deep and long, diluting the impact of the Christian mission to this world even though these traditions may still be considered within the same worldview.

I will next explore expressions of the Christian worldview from Roman Catholic, Eastern Orthodox, and Reformed traditions that have contributed significantly to a Christian understanding of biomedical ethics. I present the Reformed tradition as that which provides the richest source of Scriptural teaching for developing the biblical basis for a covenantal ethical framework.

---

20. MacIntyre, *After Virtue*.

21. Klapwijk ("On Worldviews and Philosophy," 43) argues that regaining a worldview is an urgent issue in contemporary culture, making the development of a Christian worldview essential to the health of Christian communities.

22. Ibid., 45–47.

23. Ibid., 47. Klapwijk refers to the apostle Paul's exhortation to "take every thought captive to obey Christ" (2 Cor 10:5).

24. Niebuhr, *Christ and Culture*. H. Richard Niebuhr's typology of the relation between our obedience to Christ and our response to the world around us captures these distinctions. Different Christian or heretical traditions can be seen as a basis for each relational type. These are: Christ against culture: Anabaptist; Christ in agreement with culture: Gnostics, Schleiermacher; synthesis of Christ and culture: Thomists; coexistence of Christ and culture: Marcion, two kingdoms of Luther; and Christ the Transformer of culture: Reformed traditions.

PART TWO: A Modest Proposal for a Biblical Covenantal Biomedical Ethic

Distinct Expressions of Christian Worldview

Non-Christian thought can influence or even distort the beliefs of different traditions within the Christian worldview. For example, the biblical themes of creation, sin, and redemption can be expressed and related to each other in very different ways. Roman Catholics often express the reality of the created order and interpretations of Scripture in dualistic nature/grace terms, believed by some to represent pagan influences in early Christian history.[25] Romano Guardini critiques the moral fragmentation of Western culture through such nature/grace spectacles.[26] In searching for the Christian corrective to the God-less, autonomy-oriented view of the created order of our secular culture, he rightly shows the necessity of knowing our relationship to God in order to normatively understand our relationship with ourselves and the cosmos. However, in Guardini's dualistic appreciation of reality, the priest is given superior status and privilege as the immediate purveyor of written revelation while the layperson is only qualified to pursue revelation in the so-called natural order.

In critique of the rationalism that pervades Western culture, Alvin Plantinga rejects reliance on rationality outside of belief in God in favor of a *properly basic* and entirely rational belief in God.[27] From a Reformed perspective, the problem of rationality in our culture is not one of reason versus faith but rather one of faithful versus unfaithful reason. Responding to MacIntyre's suggestion that reason has little or no place in Calvin's theology, Richard Mouw insists that Calvin sees reason as a means of understanding, not the source of, moral truth. Reason can only function effectively in proper relationship with God. Such proper reasoning must flow from trust in God.[28]

Recently, some Roman Catholic scholars have embraced a less dualistic and more relational perspective for biomedical ethics. Although a professing Roman Catholic, Lisa Cahill does not promote a secular/sacred synthesis. She expresses a more holistic appreciation of the context and historicity of moral knowledge, the reality of sin, and the social structures realized by the globalization of communications, finance, and science in our time. Cahill argues that Christian bioethicists must assume a prophetic role to promote human solidarity, compassion, and justice. They must be

---

25. Jaeger, *Early Christianity*.
26. Guardini, *World*, 9–12, 25–26, 54–60.
27. Plantinga, "Reason and Belief," 72.
28. Mouw, *God Who Commands*, 68.

Groundwork for a Contemporary Covenantal Ethic

inspired by the love of God and neighbor while combating "overly pragmatic and individualistic" approaches to biomedical decision-making. She believes that theological language and images do not hinder public discourse on bioethical issues. Rather, they can be effective in public settings, "not to dominate, alienate, or condemn, but to stimulate the emotions and imaginations of discussion partners."[29]

Moving further still from a dualistic perspective, Roman Catholic Patrick McArdle writes of the value of envisioning health care relationships through a covenantal perspective. He is attracted to the notion of covenant as a metaphorical basis for human interactions in health care based on mutual trust, care, and interdependence. For McArdle, covenant assumes that those in a position of power and privilege have responsibilities to assist the less well off. The term "covenant" most aptly describes the mutual recognition and enhancement of the status of involved parties in his vision of a relational model for health care.[30]

Eastern Orthodox bioethicists claim to see the created order in a non-rationalistic, non-dualistic way. However, in my view, their preoccupation with sacramental and liturgical aspects of faith impedes their development of a broader biblical perspective that captures nuances of the full historico-redemptive narrative, a narrative that may shed light on bioethical issues. This can lead to a myopic view of the creation order that insufficiently recognizes those spirits that subtly direct our attention away from service to God toward secular liturgies of consumerism and self-interest. On the other hand, their intense attention to the spiritual and relational aspects of their faith gives those of other Christian traditions reason to pause and reflect on whether such affective aspects of human nature are adequately captured in their own traditions.

For example, Alexander Schmemann believes human beings should relate to each other and the world as priests who strive to praise God in thanksgiving and worship in their daily lives in order to transform life into communion with God. Engelhardt's entire bioethical framework is based on such a priestly perception of human beings. Union with God is the focus of all activities and almost any means can justify this end, including lying and deception.[31] However, this tradition is inadequate for guiding believers to work out a deep understanding of structures of creation and

---

29. Cahill, *Theological Bioethics*, 36–38.

30. McArdle, *Relational Health Care*, 182–84.

31. Goheen and Bartholomew, *Living at the Crossroads*, 19; Schmemann, *For the Life*; Engelhardt, *Foundations of Christian Bioethics*, 186–90.

Part Two: A Modest Proposal for a Biblical Covenantal Biomedical Ethic

to engage others with an articulated vision of that created reality. Both Roman Catholic dualistic perceptions of creation and Eastern Orthodox inattentiveness to the human responsibility of redeeming the created order on earth leave both variations of Christian worldview wanting.

We turn now to a Reformed Christian worldview, particularly one that captures redemptive history through the spectacles of the covenant theme. In my view, this understanding of Christian worldview is most helpful for developing a Christian biomedical ethic.

In his review of the concept of worldview from a Reformed perspective, Wolters considers the concept of worldview to be "eminently suitable for Christian appropriation" if conceived as a comprehensive religious confession about the total scheme of things.[32] He shows that Abraham Kuyper first correlated the idea of worldview with that of Christianity as a culture-shaping force. As presented in chapter 5, the theological theme of covenant is a dominant theme within this tradition for understanding redemptive history. There is convincing evidence that God established a covenant with humankind at the beginning of the world, creating Adam in his image with the condition to love him, obey him, and care for his creation. Despite covenant-breaking, human disobedience, God established a covenant with a chosen people through Abraham. Israel was meant to be a light to all surrounding nations, to guide the remainder of humankind back to covenant-keeping with God.

After Adam's sin, God left each human being with a conscience, an inner sense of what the law requires of human beings in this fallen world. Human beings who do not recognize God or do so but refuse to acknowledge and worship him can still "do by nature things required by the law," even though in doing so "they are a law for themselves, even though they do not have the law, since they show that the requirements of the law are written on their hearts."[33] Wolters calls this natural disposition to do what is lawful "intuitive attunement to creational normativity."[34] I will return

---

32. Wolters, "On the Idea," 23.
33. Rom 2:14–15.
34. Wolters, *Creation Regained*, 29. He notes further, "Creational law speaks so loudly, impresses itself so forcefully on human beings, even in the delusions of paganism, that its normative demands are driven home in to their inmost being. . . . This does not refer to some innate virtue of 'natural man,' unaffected by sin, but to the finger of the sovereign Creator engraving reminders of his norms upon human sensibilities even in the midst of apostasy. God does not leave himself unattested; he refuses to be ignored."

Groundwork for a Contemporary Covenantal Ethic

to this idea in a later discussion about a revisited concept of "common morality" in light of Scripture.

Recently, John Witvliet has shown that the biblical theme of covenant is multidimensional and complex, with the new covenant in Christ culminating a covenantal historico-redemptive continuum.[35] The covenant theme is a primary theological matrix, permeating large portions of Scripture, the proper conceptualization and reading of which can draw together divergent traditions and interpretations.[36] Witvliet argues that celebrating the Lord's Supper, for example, could be understood as covenant renewal, while the liturgy can be seen as the actualization of the new covenant. Such conceptualization of covenant in association with these and other biblical themes shows the presence of covenant in communal communication with God. In this way, the covenant theme can help to bring about better interdenominational understanding and agreement.[37]

I have argued that the covenant theme provides sound biblical justification for a Christian ethic grounded in that covenant, a relationship from which covenantal relationships among human beings can be derived. From such an ethical framework, the normative aspects of human relationships that make up medical practice and research can be identified and normatively understood. However, we must also find or develop a Christian philosophical framework that provides an understanding of creational norms for social relationships. In my judgment, the social philosophy of Christian philosopher Herman Dooyeweerd provides such a framework that can be applied to medicine. I will begin by discussing the relationship between worldview and philosophy. I will then show the importance of developing a Christian philosophy that can give expression to the Reformed Christian worldview.

Relationship of Worldview and Philosophy

As shown previously in chapter 4, for Wilhelm Dilthey, philosophy is dependent on worldview. The latter encompasses a cohesive view of life and

---

35. Witvliet, *Worship Seeking Understanding*, 76–78; 2 Cor 3.

36. Ibid., 78.

37. Ibid., 79–86. Witvliet nicely weaves the themes of covenant, Eucharist, and liturgy, tying in the ethical obligations of Eucharist and liturgy in the language of covenant. Baltzer (*Covenant Formulary*, 171ff.), Vorgrimler (*Sacramental Theology*), and Stevenson (*Covenant of Grace Renewed*) give a more complete understanding of the potential for better transdenominational understanding by way of such thematic linkages.

search for ultimate unity that emerge from one's attitude and knowledge of life as a whole. Philosophy, on the other hand, deals more narrowly with products of our thoughts and the comprehension of reality.[38] Historically, the pursuit of metaphysical systems, says Dilthey, has failed, metaphysical systems are false, and therefore there is no place for metaphysics in philosophy.[39] In place of metaphysical systems, Dilthey puts forward a metaphilosophy of worldview.[40] A worldview, he says, is "an intuition which springs from our involvement in life."[41] He cites the influence of Hegel's religio-metaphysical experiences (reputedly resulting from his interpretation of early Christian documents) on his early thought as one example of such intuitions. The life involvements from which these intuitions are derived come about by means of our attitudes and personal relationships.

Emmanuel Levinas challenges the traditional emphasis on epistemology in philosophical reflections.[42] Rocking philosophy at its historical and conceptual foundations, he proposes that the top priority of philosophy should be the understanding of the demands of other persons with whom we are in contact. Consequently, ethics should be the starting point for such philosophical reflection. The very essence of philosophy, he argues, is relational. He promotes the idea of treating the other person as *absolutely* other, disposing of our own baggage of self-interests and priorities in order to selflessly understand others on their own terms. No commonality of beliefs or interests should be assumed between parties. This conscious attempt to shed personal bias and prejudice is reminiscent of John Rawls's veil of ignorance, although in his case Rawls hopes in doing so to gain rational ethical consensus with others within his theory of justice.[43]

In response to Levinas, philosopher Jacques Derrida fears that stripping relationship formation from interpersonal feelings and beliefs risks

38. Dilthey (*Selected Writings*, 141) goes on to say that, unlike philosophy, the development of views of life is slow, heavy work that involves the elevation of life to consciousness through knowledge of reality, an evaluation of life, and the achievement of will.

39. Naugle, *Worldview*, 83.

40. Ibid., 84.

41. Dilthey, *Selected Writings*, 146; Kluback and Weinbaum, *Dilthey's Philosophy*, 35. Dilthey understands the religious mind to have a fixation on a transcendent world that preserves idealism.

42. Levinas, *Totality and Infinity*; Levinas, *Otherwise*.

43. Rawls, *Political Liberalism*, 304–10. Rawls differs from Levinas, however, in that the communicating parties negotiate the terms of their social cooperation. Such detachment is out of step with Levinas's terms of association that evoke spontaneity.

reducing relationship formation to a process resembling the empiricist acquisition of knowledge through external sensory data. According to Christopher Norris, Derrida insists that some degree of mutual and shared understanding concerning common humanity is necessary for understanding others.[44] Rather than considered just a demand on us,[45] the other has a unique first person perspective on the world that we can enter by means of shared understanding. Edmund Husserl calls such commonality a shared cognitive-conceptual framework within a shared lifeworld of time and space.[46] This sharing of structural aspects of reality does not necessarily distort our appreciation of the perspective of others nor reduce their perspectives to passive projections of our own person. For Husserl, it is in our own experience that we can put ourselves in the place of others and comprehend how we differ from them.[47]

As one of the first philosophers to define a Christian worldview or lifeview, Søren Kierkegaard contrasts worldview with academic philosophy that is more narrowly concerned with cognitive pursuits.[48] He considers philosophy to be an objective, impersonal "comedy of abstract thought," while lifeview is at the heart of true philosophy, being the genuine love of wisdom and representing a set of fundamental beliefs that gives direction to the expression of one's everyday life.[49] Wolters introduces the concept of biblical *belief* as a biblical *worldview* that encompasses 1) central notions of creation as a given order of reality, 2) the Fall as an uprising against that order, and 3) redemption as the unearned restoration of that order through Christ. These notions are cosmic and transformational in nature. They unite all Christians in a fundamental worldview that provides the interpretive framework to work with our experience in all of its created richness.[50] The biblical theme of covenant encompasses each of these elements, making it attractive as the core of a framework for theoretical reflection on many aspects of our relationship to God and to the world around us.

Kuyper, Herman Bavinck, and their neo-Calvinist successors agree with Dilthey's idea that philosophy gives expression to worldview. In his

---

44. Norris, *Deconstruction*, 30.
45. Levinas calls the demand of others on us *radical otherness* or *alterity*.
46. Husserl, *Formal*.
47. Husserl, *Cartesian Meditation*.
48. McCarthy, *Phenomenology of Moods*, 136–37.
49. Goheen and Bartholomew, *Living at the Crossroads*, 12–13.
50. Wolters, "No Longer Queen," 2–3, 72–73.

Part Two: A Modest Proposal for a Biblical Covenantal Biomedical Ethic

typology of philosophy/worldview relationships, Wolters calls this the *worldview-yields-philosophy* model.[51] This neo-Calvinist model sees philosophy not as natural reason, as the Thomist model does, but as a discipline with a religious pre-theoretical commitment that gives direction and meaning to scientific pursuits. Most critical to a distinct Christian worldview is the judgment concerning whether to reject or to redefine the terms used in secular worldview and philosophical perspectives. The decision depends on whether the terms can be conceptually redeemed without accommodating unbiblical connotations when in dialogue with those professing non-Christian worldviews. Wolters feels comfortable with *terminological redemption* at this time in history.[52] Christians must work carefully when engaging postmodern peers who fear religious views may subvert the rationality of bioethical discourse and reflection. In expressing reasons for their views, Christians must communicate sincerity of conviction in ways that imaginatively express genuinely religious reasons that enrich moral understanding.

Herman Dooyeweerd relates both worldview and philosophy to religious ground-motive in his later writings. Ground-motive is a central driving force that governs temporal expressions of human religion and points towards the real or supposed origin of existence. It is the spiritual mainspring of a society, determining its entire lifeview and worldview.[53] Jacob Klapwijk coins the term *transcendental hermeneutical idea of philosophy* in an effort to keep philosophy's task distinctive and universally accessible regardless of worldview beliefs. It is transcendental in that it is accountable to presuppositions of theoretical thought that emanate from ground-motives and worldviews.[54] As philosophy, it requires a linguistic hermeneutic that governs textual interpretation and a philosophical hermeneutic to govern the interpretation of terms, propositions, theses, etc. All such interpretive modes flow from a context of pre-understanding that includes worldview beliefs. In this framework, Christians can work with the terminology of secular philosophies in the course of such dialogue but re-imagine such philosophies in light of normative structures recognized within the creation order through biblical insights.

---

51. Wolters, "On the Idea," 21–24; Bavinck, *Philosophy of Revelation*.

52. Ibid., 24.

53. Wolters, "On the Idea," 22–23; Dooyeweerd, *Roots of Western Culture*, 3–9. This description of ground-motive encompasses the idea of spiritual antitheses in modern society, a linkage which Zuidervaart ("Good Cities," 138) summarizes elsewhere.

54. Klapwijk, "On Worldviews and Philosophy," 53.

Goheen and Bartholomew argue that philosophical concepts arise from the basic beliefs of one's worldview, beliefs that answer questions like "who are we," "what's wrong with the world," and "how should/can it be fixed."[55] In his review of worldview in the area of social theory, Griffioen considers pretheoretical worldview orientation to be crucial to getting at the root of the theoretical issues in philosophy and the sciences.[56] Worldviews are guides to our understanding of the world, providing direction toward philosophical comprehension of the unfolding of structures of creation through human action.

By contrast, Paul Marshall questions the central role that philosophy has played in some Christian scholarship, particularly within the Reformed tradition. Philosophy, he says, is no more religious than any other human activity. Rather than making philosophy the starting point of all Christian scholarship, Marshall proposes that an "inner reformation of science" can begin anywhere in our Christian walk.[57] He makes the pursuit of scientific research (social research in his case) the first step, followed by the scrutinizing of such research by Christian scholars, including those in philosophy and other fields. He criticizes what he sees as an overly rationalistic approach to an inner reformation of science in Reformed scholarship. Marshall expresses concern over the perceived intimidation of Christian scientists by Christian philosophers who question the philosophical roots of the theoretical claims that stem from scientists' research.[58]

In my view, Marshall's concerns are not without merit but they also run the risk of being dangerously shortsighted. He rightly appeals for empathy and understanding by Christian philosophers for those who do research or engage in specific disciplines such as interpersonal clinical care in the various sciences. But he underestimates the necessity of training Christian scientists in Christian worldview and philosophy in order to engage non-Christian colleagues who will challenge the basic beliefs behind the interpretation of their research. While not all Christian scientists need

---

55. Goheen and Bartholomew, *Living at the Crossroads*, 24–25. Walsh and Middleton (*Transforming Vision*) and Wright (*Jesus*) also explore the importance of these and other fundamental questions that encompass a Christian worldview. In the tradition of Calvin, Kuyper, and Bavinck, Plantinga ("Reason and Belief," 72–73) considers belief in God to be properly basic and rational, in response to accusations that such a belief is irrational and thus not grounds for the justification of other beliefs.

56. Griffioen, "Worldview Approach," 106–9.

57. Marshall, "Epilogue," 187.

58. Ibid., 186.

PART TWO: A Modest Proposal for a Biblical Covenantal Biomedical Ethic

to be (indeed, should not be!) philosophers, they need to learn the tools of spiritual and academic discernment at the worldview and philosophical levels. With such tools, they can develop grounds and justification for the interpretation of their work in the public arena within which many of them engage peers. True discernment of the apostate spirits of our times requires knowledge of those spirits and their distorting influence on our scientific work.

As I have shown, while there are differences among Reformed scholars regarding the relationship between philosophy and worldview, there is general agreement that a Christian worldview encompasses a set of basic beliefs about our relationship to God and the created order derived from the biblical narrative. While all Christians can be guided in their daily lives by such beliefs, different callings and vocational pursuits can be further guided by Christian philosophy. Such a philosophy can provide a framework on which relational experiences in a particular science or vocation can be better analyzed and understood both for that discipline or vocation as well as in the larger context of relationships in other human endeavors. The biblical covenant theme permeates the understanding of the Christian life at both levels, giving ultimate meaning to the relationships that different callings entail.

Relationship of Reformed Christian Philosophy, Theology, and Covenant

Developing a covenantal ethic for biomedical ethics requires a Christian philosophical framework through which that ethic can be understood and expressed in medicine. The relationship of philosophy to theology is particularly critical in this regard. Wolters sees their relationship in terms of a direction versus structure analogy.[59] That is, Christian philosophy is a scientific discipline that focuses on understanding creational structures as both created unity and diversity. Theology (as systematic theology), on the other hand, is a scientific discipline that focuses on the direction of things as driven either by the evil that infects the world or by the cure that can save it through belief in Jesus Christ. Whereas Christian philosophy studies creation in light of categories in the Word of God, theology studies the Word of God in light of the structural categories of creation. Worldview, however, is prescientific. That is, it not only incorporates the teaching of Scripture through biblical interpretation but also incorporates everyday

59. Wolters, *Creation Regained*, 10–11.

Groundwork for a Contemporary Covenantal Ethic

experience acquired without formal scientific scrutiny, including elements from the surrounding culture.[60]

Goheen and Bartholomew distinguish biblical theology from systematic theology as two levels of reflection on the basic beliefs inherent in the biblical story.[61] The former seeks to understand and articulate the unity of Scripture through themes such as covenant and kingdom while the latter reflects on Christian beliefs at a more theoretical level. In this schema, Christian philosophy and systematic theology involve theoretical reflection concerning Christian belief and as such are on the same level relative to biblical theology and worldview. On the one hand, Goheen and Bartholomew contend, like Wolters and Spykman, that systematic theology requires Christian philosophical insight which in a sense precedes systematic theological work. On the other hand, systematic theology reflects upon core doctrines of Scripture that are foundational for the development of a Christian philosophy.[62] In this way they can be understood as co-dependent on each other as theoretical undertakings and as individually dependent on a biblically inspired view of humanity and the cosmos.

Spykman emphasizes the importance of explicitly delineating Christian philosophical foundations in the course of renewing Reformed systematic theology.[63] He notes particularly the positive influence of Dooyeweerd's Christian philosophy in repudiating the modern dogma of "the pretended autonomy of reason." This unifying view on our calling in God's world, including our task in theology, lends to Reformed dogmatics a deeper sense of life-relatedness, a more firmly structured place among the scholarly disciplines, and a more responsible directedness. As such, this view can open new doors to the possibility of ongoing theological reformation.[64] One of the fundamental tenets of this Christian philosophy is the belief in communion and communication between God and humankind. Through his Word, God discloses his sovereign will and elicits human responses to his will. This disclosure is a covenantal call to obedient living. I fully agree with Spykman that a right understanding of the

---

60. Ibid., 10; Goheen and Bartholomew, *Living at the Crossroads*, 27. Danie Strauss (*Philosophy*, 640) shows that the heart, as the core of human beings, can take an apostate direction that drives the thoughts and actions of human beings while salvation drives the heart in the opposite direction.

61. Goheen and Bartholomew, *Living at the Crossroads*, 26–27.

62. Bartholomew and Goheen, "Faith and Philosophy."

63. Spykman, *Reformational Theology*, 100.

64. Ibid., 101.

covenantal bond between God and humankind is essential to a biblical worldview, to Christian faith, and to Reformed dogmatic theology.[65]

The Christian theologian D. H. T. Vollenhoven considers covenant to be the essence of a definition of religion and religious belief. At the heart of our religious beliefs as Christians is the relationship of humankind to the God of the covenant and living in obedience to his law of love.[66] That covenant was established at creation and, as such, is an overarching theme for the cosmos. It signals the special position of humankind relative to other creatures in the cosmos. It represents the essence of the proper and normative direction of human thinking and activity toward other human beings and the world itself.

As mentioned above, this covenant theme also permeates theoretical reflection because a Christian worldview develops by means of seeing the world and its structures through the covenant theme. Compared to the kingdom theme, it provides a stronger and more direct expression of faith when relating to individuals and to aspects of the created order around us.[67] In the Reformed tradition, the covenant theme captures more of the essence of who we are and of our relationship to God and the world around us than any other biblical theme. It helps to understand the importance of obedient direction in our actions toward others and of obedient reverence to our duties and responsibilities to creational structures. Christian theology and Christian philosophy help in different ways to maintain that direction and to discover the duties and responsibilities of being stewards of the created order.

Need to Revisit the Four Principles

As explained in chapter 4, principlism springs from a culture wherein modernist and postmodernist worldviews have historically dominated the philosophical and ethical landscape. In failing to acknowledge God as transcendent authority, these worldviews and philosophies within secular culture fail to acknowledge the existence and influence of sin on efforts to understand the nature of moral truth. A biblical covenantal ethic developed in response to principlism is grounded in a unifying biblical theme

---

65. Ibid., 92–95.

66. Ibid., 100; Vollenhoven, *Introduction*, 77–93.

67. Spykman (*Reformational Theology*, 11, 257–59) calls these two themes together a bi-unitary index to the meaning of creation; while the covenant can be considered as an abiding charter, the kingdom is like an ongoing program.

that draws its moral authority and justification from the covenantal relationship with God. Its pervasive presence intersects with all other themes of the biblical narrative. Such an ethical framework is an overarching guide to normative activity within a Christian social philosophy and theology. Humankind has had a special relationship with God from the beginning of time, a relationship that gives guidance for direction to all interhuman relationships. Without such directional guidance, these relationships lose their true meaning.

Such an ethic can explore the normativity of the principles of principlism, the full meaning and nature of which can best be understood through the spectacles of a Christian philosophy of social relations. I agree with Pellegrino that those principles should not be discarded out of hand. They arose in response to social ethical needs and should be analyzed for what normative importance that they may retain. They need to be reconceptualized, guided by a biblical understanding of our covenantal relationships, duties, and obligations to God and to fellow human beings.

In my view, the normativity of the four principles should be revisited through a biblical covenantal ethic. Such an ethic engages them with the ethical core of medicine that focuses attention on the needs of other human beings. This engagement will be addressed in the next chapter. However, this effort also requires a biblical anthropology in order to gain a proper understanding of the meaning of autonomy, beneficence, nonmaleficence, and justice in light of what it is to be human and in relationship with God and others. A Christian anthropology of personhood uncovers the true meaning to what it means for human beings to be special creatures of God and have a special relationship with God. It is such an anthropology that I will explore in the next section.

IMPORTANCE OF PERSONHOOD FOR A BIBLICAL COVENANTAL ETHIC

Personhood and Principlism

Religiously rooted perspectives on personhood, linked to the biblical theme of divine-human covenant, contrast sharply with a principlist understanding of personhood. In a recent edition of their book *Principles of Biomedical Ethics*, Beauchamp and Childress devote a chapter to human moral status, methodically laying out perceived strengths and weaknesses

Part Two: A Modest Proposal for a Biblical Covenantal Biomedical Ethic

of different theories moral status.[68] For none of these theories do they appeal to some higher or non-temporal moral authority. Of the five theories that they claim deal with moral status, the relational theory is considered the weakest of those presented, concluding that "it leaves a nagging worry that social bonds and attitudes alone determine moral status."[69] Yet they offer no grounding to give moral justification for the moral legitimacy for any of these theories. Rather, they create admittedly abstract guidelines through the process of specification in an attempt to match compatible demands gleaned from several of these five theories.

Some of these guidelines compete with one another and are developed for illustrative purposes, *not as recommendations*.[70] Addressing the question of developing policy for the use of human fetuses in research, Beauchamp and Childress seem to grope for internal coherence and compatibility between and within guidelines. They claim that there is "nearly universal agreement" that very late-term fetuses are meaningfully different from a newborn. Nevertheless, they conclude that determinants of moral status are reduced to capacities such as sentience and cognitive ability. They seem seriously concerned as to whether moral justification can be given for downgrading the moral status of early human fetuses by such criteria, leading them to admit that this remains "one of the most difficult questions in biomedical ethics."[71]

Beauchamp and Childress then suggest that research on both vulnerable humans and animals "often has a compelling justification because of its potential benefits" to ailing human beings. They conclude that the real moral challenge is making the chosen answers *coherent* so that levels of risk of harm to different classes of human beings or animals should be allowed "only when a criterion of moral status permits unequal treatment."[72] They earlier define a criterion of moral status as a moral norm or standard that has the authority to judge or direct human belief, reasoning, or behavior.[73] It remains a mystery to their readers, however, what this moral norm or its authoritative standard should be. They rely on the views of others and find no consensus.

---

68. Beauchamp and Childress, *Principles of Biomedical Ethics*, 6th ed., 64–97. These include theories based on 1) human properties, 2) cognitive properties, 3) moral agency, 4) sentience, and 5) relationships.

69. Ibid., 80; Beauchamp, "Failure."

70. Ibid., 87.

71. Ibid., 91.

72. Ibid.

73. Ibid., 85.

Elsewhere, Beauchamp considers the term "person" to be too vague to resolve the problem of moral status and suggests replacing it altogether.[74] He admits that using capacities to distinguished human persons from animals and from human non-persons is virtually impossible. At the same time, he confuses moral status based on the capacity to make moral judgments with moral status based on affective experiences such as pain, suffering, and emotional deprivation. In the end he argues that, given such vagary of consensus about the meaning of personhood, the concept should be replaced. Unfortunately, he offers equally vague suggestions regarding the path to take for discussing substantive moral issues that involve specific nonmoral and moral properties, such as reason and moral motivations.[75] By offering no grounds for considering humans ontically distinct from animals and for considering all humans equally valuable at all stages of life, he can only be frustrated in trying to grasp the concept of human personhood, by whatever name they call it.

Christian Notions of Covenant

Philosopher Charles Taylor has argued that selfhood is linked to one's idea of "the good."[76] This traditional link has been lost in much of contemporary moral philosophy which focuses on what is right to do rather than what is good to be. As ethicist Margaret Somerville recently mused, the result is that we have become human "doings" rather than human "beings."[77] Taylor argues further that humans have some moral intuitions that are deep, powerful, and universal such that they are often considered to be rooted in human instinct. These intuitions include the concepts of respect for other human beings and of human dignity.

Taylor flatly rejects the naturalist tendency to adopt a reductionistic utilitarianism that ignores distinct moral frameworks that reflect analogous worldviews. Such frameworks give human beings qualified horizons that are constitutive to human agency and personhood. He makes the distinction between seeking to solve moral questions in universal terms and selecting a framework that makes the most sense of our moral responses within an optimally orienting moral space defined by a particular worldview. The latter framework provides our best vision of universally valid

---

74. Beauchamp, "Failure," 68.
75. Ibid., 59–68.
76. Taylor, *Sources of the Self*.
77. Somerville, *Ethical Imagination*.

moral commitments.[78] Such space is oriented toward "the good" as a core function of our selfhood, necessarily and only fully expressed in relationship to other selves.

Our very selfhood, he argues, is partly defined by this pursuit of moral questions that are motivated by a search for orientation toward "the good," and this pursuit is only complete when seen in relationship to other selves. Each of us is part of a web of interlocution or a communicative network.[79] Communication is mediated through a language of moral and spiritual discernment within a particular language community. A covenantal ethic gives moral content to the moral thinking and action within that network of communication while a Christian worldview provides moral space, orientation, and direction toward the most persuasive among choices of a higher life.

In conceptualizing the human being, a Christian covenantal anthropology also acknowledges the distinction between direction and structure. Human beings exist in ways both similar and distinct from other created beings. Speaking from a Dooyeweerdian philosophical perspective, Strauss proposes that the structural principle of being human includes normative psychical and behavioral aspects that distinguish humans from animals. The unique psychical, emotional, and ethical expressions as well as bodily structures are concentrated in the human heart or selfhood. This in turn belongs to a central relational dimension of creation that is grounded in our covenant relationship with God the creator. This relationship is subject to the love commandment; that is, that we love God and our neighbors.[80]

The structures that make up humanness and human expression fall under the influence of sin brought about by a purposeful covenantal rebellion. Human beings violated the obedience condition of the creation covenant, with devastating consequences for human beings and for creation as a whole. Despite this, God graciously chose to call human beings back into covenant through a special people who were again called to obedience. Israel was called to be a "priestly royalty" for extending God's presence throughout the nations.[81] God's people were to display to the world how a people can change when in covenant with God.[82] After Israel repeatedly broke covenantal promises, God sent his Son to once and for all over-

---

78. Taylor, *Sources of the Self*, 16–24.
79. Ibid., 36.
80. Strauss, *Philosophy*, 134–40.
81. Bartholomew, "Time for War," 2.
82. Ibid. Durham, *Exodus*, 263.

Groundwork for a Contemporary Covenantal Ethic

come sin and death and to redeem both Israel and the rest of humanity through his death and resurrection. In this way, all of humanity is directly beckoned to respond to the sanctifying Holy Spirit and thus back into full relationship with God.[83]

From a covenantal perspective, as mentioned in chapter 5, human beings are in a double relationship with God. From creation, human beings are at the same time image-bearers of and covenantal partners with God. The Genesis account states that at creation Adam was created in the image of God.[84] As creatures of God, human beings are not autonomous but are in relationship with God. Human beings are thus both creatures and persons. These concepts are in tension; to be a creature of God means absolute dependence on God, while to be a person implies a relative volitional independence from God.[85] When humankind's creatureliness is de-emphasized or the inherent relationship with God is ignored, human beings are sometimes seen as fully autonomous in purpose and will. Such distortion of the normative view of human beings is evident in secular anthropologies including that inherent in principlism. However, it is also important to understand differences in the biblical understanding of human beings as image-bearers of God.

A Christian community bound by covenant requires the maintenance of individual distinctiveness because each is accountable to God for dispositions of the heart and moral actions. Through this common image-bearing feature and the creation covenant that binds humankind to God, all human beings deserve mutual respect. God does not give discriminatory treatment to human beings based on individual characteristics. The early Reformers considered the original, pre-Fall righteousness of Adam to be natural rather than supernatural as suggested by the Roman Catholic Church. Human righteousness is the way human beings were intended to be as created creatures of God. With the Fall, human beings did not become less human. They lost direction and became unable to seek God on their own.[86] Each person has an old self under sin and a new self under Christ. That new self is renewed through knowledge of the image of its creator and is gifted to all human beings who believe.[87] In Lutheran

---

83. 2 Cor 7:1; Phil 2:12–13. While only the Holy Spirit can sanctify, human beings as persons must take responsibility when carrying out the fruits of that sanctification.

84. Gen 1:1, 26–28; 5:1–3; 9:6.

85. Hoekema, *Created*, 5–7.

86. Bavinck, *Reformed Dogmatics*, 551–53.

87. Gal 3:26–28; Col 3:9–11.

theology, the loss of original righteousness includes loss of the image of God. This results in a persisting dualism wherein the image of God stands beside and is detached from nature. Human good deeds are done but are considered earthly without God's grace, the acquisition of which bestows the ability to do spiritual good.[88]

As image-bearers of God, human beings reflect God in various ways. Just as God is relational with respect to the Father, Son, and Holy Spirit, human beings are necessarily social. This was recognized by God's gift of a human companion for the first human being. Despite authoritative views to the contrary,[89] there is good scriptural support for the retention of the image of God in fallen human beings.[90] Bavinck holds that *imago Dei* is not just a quality or aspect of a human being. It has ontic status. He cites various scripture passages alluding to post-Fall human beings as sons, likenesses, or offspring of God.[91] Christ, he argues, was born into this world fully and truly human. In conforming to the image of Christ, we are again becoming closer to God.[92]

Personhood and Covenant within Reformed Christian and Jewish Theology

Following Augustine's lead, Bavinck draws an analogy between the triune being of God as one and indivisible and the whole human person constituting dimensions of heart, mind, and will. Similarly, the body, soul, and mind of the whole human person are components of the image of God. Immortality appeared to be initially contingent on the ethical precondition of obedience to God. Adam's pre-Fall righteousness was a gift of

---

88. Bavinck, *Reformed Dogmatics*, 553–54.

89. Berkouwer, *Man*, 43–48, 56–59. Berkouwer acknowledges the difficulty of understanding whether human beings lost their image-bearing status with Adam's disobedience. He shows how Bavinck's distinction between image of God in the narrower and broader sense can be understood in light of certain scriptural texts (e.g., Gen 9:6; Ja 3:9; 1 Cor 11:7) and that the problem is prevalent in the Lutheran tradition. However, Hoekema (*Created*, 17) notes that Berkouwer, like Klaas Schilder, remains unconvinced that the image of God can be considered retained after the fall.

90. Hoekema (*Created*, 18–19) notes that Psalm 8 echoes Genesis 1:27–28 regarding humankind's status as bearing God's image. The lofty status given to humankind at creation relative to other creatures is clearly confirmed.

91. Bavinck (*Reformed Dogmatics*, 554) refers to Gen 1:26; Gen 9:6; Luke 3:38; Acts 17:28; 1 Cor 11:7; Jas 3:9 in support of his contention.

92. Ibid., 555. Again, Bavinck cites multiple passages to support his case (1 Cor 15:49; 2 Cor 3:18; Phil 3:21; Eph 4:24; Col 3:10; 1 John 3:2).

God but inconceivable without communion with God.[93] God's covenant with Adam required obedience, with the reward of eternal life. Extremes of Christian theological perceptions of the image of God vary from naturalistic views that attach the image to aptitude, potential, and free will to supernaturalistic views. The latter often perceive many human functions to be unnecessary or even debasing for a perfect Adam to have exhibited before the Fall.[94]

Such a Reformed perspective on personhood is also supported by some contemporary Jewish scholars. David Novak in particular has elaborated a Jewish perspective on personhood based on a Jewish interpretation of *imago Dei*. Attempts to create or realize an ontological or philosophical anthropology "out of its own operations" reduce humans to "the level of the immanent action of the world" and obscure or ignore any transcendent dimension. He argues that a normative ontological and theological anthropology germinates from the biblical creation story of human creation in God's image.

Novak rejects the earliest identification of the image of God with reason, as had been taught by the Jewish scholar Philo and his predecessors in ancient pagan philosophy, such as Plato and the Stoics. He further argues that a rational requirement for essential humanness is inconsistent with Jewish tradition since it would deny such human status to the unborn and severely disabled who cannot rationally perceive their surroundings. Such anthropology must be rejected because it has been used to justify killing those on the edge of the human community.[95] The image of God is a substantive, inherently meaningful internal quality rather than a capacity requiring participation in a relation to find any meaning.[96] Image-bearing makes possible a relational link or "covenant possibility'" with God that is grounded in revelation.[97] In a fallen world, the realization of this relational link requires special revelation.

Novak also acknowledges the need to include non-believers in ethical discourse. In doing so, he appeals to the tradition of *via negativa*. Non-believers can be considered humans as *shadows* of God that vaguely hint at something behind them.[98] This minimal but universal notion of the im-

---

93. Ibid., 558.
94. Ibid., 566.
95. Novak, *Law and Theology*, 108ff.
96. Novak, *Jewish-Christian Dialogue*, 129.
97. Novak, "Human Person," 48.
98. Ibid. Novak goes back to the etymology of *tselem elohim*, the Hebrew phrase

PART TWO: A Modest Proposal for a Biblical Covenantal Biomedical Ethic

age of God embraces a post-Fall, residual quality that still maintains both human distinctiveness from other creatures and the hint of a relational connection with God the creator.[99] Novak then turns attention to one common factor that binds all human beings, whether they are believers in God or not. That one factor that bestows true worth on each human being is God's concern for each of us. Novak argues that human apprehension of this is the core of human personhood and the normative response is to seek God. This represents our most basic right possible. Seeking God in response to God's concern for us develops the covenantal possibility that transforms human beings from shadows of God to images of God who live life in obedience to him.[100]

Interhuman relationships are grounded in this covenant because we respond to one another as equal concerns of God. Novak appeals to Levinas's philosophy wherein others make claims on us to help them by revealing their needs directly to us. In this sense, all of humankind have covenantal responsibility to each other because God is concerned about each human being as his image-bearing creature. We respond as fellow image-bearers of the true God. In hearing their voices we hear the voice of God. This allows for a vestige of the *imago Dei* as shadow that enables unbelievers to appreciate a law order in creation and full *imago Dei* status through a right relationship with God.

In my view, both Novak and Bavinck articulate very well both the core of a biblical anthropology and its relation to the covenant theme as being essential features of a biblical covenantal ethic. Both traditions directly relate the image of God and the covenant, seeing them as two intertwined biblical motifs through which *all* human beings are relationally linked to God. Our common conscience, says Bavinck, testifies to the reward of keeping God's commands. *In its relationship with God, the ethical unity of humankind comes into its own.*[101] But the fulfillment of that moral law written from creation on human hearts can be realized only by covenantally relating to God. Only through this relationship with God

---

for "image of God," and speculates that the noun *tsel*, meaning "shadow," is linked to "image" but in a more primitive and negative sense. He supports this with Psalm 39:6, where man is described as *be-tselem*, which can be translated as "mere shadow."

99. Ibid., 49–50.

100. Ibid. Novak visualizes the human reflection of God as a shadow prior to appreciation of God's revelation. He sees this as a conceptual protection against reducing human beings merely to worldly entities without a directing, distinguishing association with God.

101. Bavinck, *Reformed Dogmatics*, 578–79.

can human beings understand and appreciate their true personhood.[102] Covenant is also the essence of true religion. If all human relationships find their model and fulfillment in religion, then religion has the character of a covenant.[103] Sin spoiled or distorted created structures but did not alter the essence or substance of creation. The sinning human being is still a human being.

Human dignity is a term that has been increasingly used in contemporary biomedical ethics to capture the essence of human value, but its meaning is often divorced from any biblical grounding. However, a biblical understanding of the term has been explored. Novak argues that the biblical story of human creation in God's image is sufficient justification for claiming human dignity because of who we are, not because of what we can do or can make of ourselves.[104] In its most meaningful relational sense, human dignity ultimately stems from seeking God in response to his concern for us.[105] However, according to Daniel Sulmasy, the conceptual roots of a contemporary notion of human dignity are probably more Stoic than they are Christian. In the Old Testament, the Hebrew word for dignity refers to rank or position while in the New Testament the Greek word that is often translated as dignity connotes seriousness and discipline. Aquinas associates dignity with rank; kings are more dignified than their subjects. For Hobbes, dignity is bestowed by the authority of the community, while for Kant dignity is rooted in the capacity of moral choice.[106] For Sulmasy, every human being has intrinsic dignity by virtue of being a person. Meilaender explores the concept of human dignity as an inherent essence of human persons. The equality of all human beings is grounded in our relationship with God; we are equal in our vulnerability and covenantal relatedness to God.[107]

In my view, dignity has "common morality" connotations that ignore the connection of human worth with a relationship with God. I agree with Sulmasy that human dignity is ontically or intrinsically a property of all human beings, regardless of capacity. However, I think Meilaender better captures the essence of human dignity by linking it with our covenantal

102. Ibid., 571.

103. Ibid., 569.

104. Novak, "Human Person," 46–47. Novak's comment is reminiscent of Margaret Somerville's Massey Lecture in 2006, in which she bemoans the contemporary reconception of humans as *human doings* instead of human beings (emphasis added).

105. Ibid., 50.

106. Sulmasy, *Rebirth of the Clinic*, 24–33.

107. Meilaender, *Neither Beast nor God*, 92–104.

PART TWO: A Modest Proposal for a Biblical Covenantal Biomedical Ethic

relationship with God, our relatedness to other human beings, and our equal and universal vulnerability before God. This comes close to Novak's idea of human worth by means of God's concern for every human being. Given this, care must be taken to understand how others use the term in bioethical dialogue while in the same way being bold in using the term inclusive of its relational connections. Unlike David Landis's divided self, acquired during medical training,[108] human personhood and selfhood as the image of God maintains normative wholeness through the covenant with God. God's concern for all human beings, including the most vulnerable, should be the basis of human relating to each other in the same caring way.

Merging Christian Philosophy and Covenantal Ethics

Working from a Christian philosophical framework developed by Christian philosopher Dooyeweerd, Strauss stresses the value of a philosophical anthropology of human personhood through which we relate to the creation around us. According to this Christian anthropology, each human being exists in fifteen modal aspects found in the created order and understood as irreducible ways of being human.[109] In their temporal existence, each human being has a richly varied normative structure that must be seen as an enkaptic whole. Each irreducible way of functioning retains its distinctive wholeness while functioning within the whole human being. This is important because without this in mind, there is a tendency to reduce human beings to one or a few aspects at the expense of others, thus reducing the appreciation for the complexity of human existence and activity. For example, like Egbert Schuurman, Strauss cautions against the *technicism* of our age that reduces human health and illness to scientific abstractions.[110] This is a specific manifestation of contemporary technological society, as described by Jacques Ellul. Technicism permeates all spheres and activities of human life. Its characteristics are rationality and an artificiality that opposes and gradually replaces our natural

---

108. Landis, "Physician Distinguish Thyself," 44–49 and chapter 5 of the current work.

109. Dooyeweerd, *New Critique*, vol. 1, 24; Chaplin, *Herman Dooyeweerd*, 55–59, 63–67. Chaplin calls all living and non-living things, events, and social relationships *existents*. These constitute everything that exists in the created order and each has a structural principle, constituted by the entire array of modal aspects.

110. Strauss, *Philosophy*, 141; Schuurman, *Technological World*.

environment.¹¹¹ Human relations become directed toward the common end of productivity and efficiency.¹¹² At the expense of patient well-being, the latter is all too common in medicine today. Ellul, like Gerrit Glas more recently, cautions against the dualistic influence of modal reduction. This is exemplified by many contemporary cognitive scientists who reduce mental function to a mental substance as well as by the monistic reduction of non-substantive aspects of human existence to the biological or physical ways of being.¹¹³

It is also very important to understand the philosophical framework of human personhood as concentrated in the human heart, the core of humanness that constitutes the religious personality of human beings. This religious core of the human self, however, is nothing in itself. It only has meaning in relationship to God the creator, to other human beings, and to the totality of created reality.¹¹⁴ This relating is truly covenantal in nature if derived from a biblical understanding of relationship that is driven by the command of love. I agree with Stafleu who argues that philosophical ethics is a component of philosophical anthropology that is concerned with the normativity of human actions.¹¹⁵ However, I think human anthropology also involves giving substance to the moral agent and to identifying direction to moral activity.

A covenantal ethic operates at this level in all relationships and in all kinds of individual and communal relational settings. Specific expression of the ethical aspect develops in different relational associations, including medicine. Andre Troost distinguishes philosophical ethics from ethics as a special aspect with its own science. He considers the study of neighborly love between human beings to be a special science of ethics while philosophical ethics or praxeology concerns the human ethos.¹¹⁶ The latter is a religious-ethical mentality that transcends sciences, is a part of human anthropology, and is closely tied to the human relationship with God. This relatedness of human beings will be discussed in detail in the next chapter.

I agree with this distinction between philosophical ethics and the ethical modal aspect of human existence. While I also generally agree with Strauss's analysis of human personality, I think that he is too restrictive

---

111. Ellul, *Technological Society*, 78–79.
112. Ibid., 355.
113. Glas, "Churchland, Kandel, and Dooyeweerd," 164.
114. Strauss, *Philosophy*, 132–36.
115. Stafleu, "Philosophical Ethics," 25–26.
116. Troost, *The Christian Ethos*, 1–6.

PART TWO: A Modest Proposal for a Biblical Covenantal Biomedical Ethic

in his conceptualization of the human embryo. His concerns about experimenting with them are limited to their philosophical and structural mode of existence. He speaks of an embryo as "the minimal enkaptic structural whole of a person as a human being" and fears the disruption to its functioning, biotically and as a whole, by experimental manipulations.[117] However, this perception of the embryo fails to address whether and how the lack of or reduced expression of social, relational, psychical, and other higher modal aspects affects the status of the human embryo. This is regrettable because acknowledgment of the creationally grounded special status of *imago Dei* can provide a biblical justification for accepting a human embryo as a fully, albeit very vulnerable, human being requiring nurturing and care despite its inability to fully function modally in all ways.

Like Dooyeweerd, W. Norris Clarke highlights the relational character of human personhood, calling it "a primordial dimension of every real being, inseparable from its substantiality."[118] Alistair McFadyen applies this to health practice, arguing that person-centered care deals with a relational person, keeping the social, spiritual, and other dimensions embodied in such a concept. As such, distortions of persons will distort relationships and vice versa.[119] Both the moral worth of the person and the network of relationships that comprise each personal existence must be appreciated.[120]

In the next chapter, I will explore the persons and relationships that constitute medical encounters in practice. I will show how a covenantal ethic can help to secure a disposition focused on patient care. Its selfless character guards against the temptations of self-indulgence made possible by the ever-dynamic proliferation and techno-formative unfolding of medical relationships. As shown previously in chapter 5, Cassel, Nisker, Coffey, and others have also appealed to a covenantal understanding of medicine and its relationships, but often not through appeal to a biblical notion.[121] However, their appeals reflect normative relational needs and demands that touch the consciences of all human beings.[122] Such normative

---

117. Strauss, *Philosophy*, 141.
118. Clarke, *One and the Many*, 135–37.
119. McFadyen, *Bound to Sin*.
120. McArdle, *Relational Health Care*, 193.
121. Cassel, "Patient-Physician Covenant"; Nisker, "A Covenantal Model"; Coffey, "The Nurse-Patient Relationship."
122. This reality is noted by Paul in Rom 2:14–15, "requirements of the law are written on their hearts, their consciences also bear witness."

needs reflect creational law that impresses itself on all human beings, despite the distorting effects of sin on our perceptions of that law. In Wolters's words, human unavoidable appreciation of creation law is like "the finger of the sovereign Creator engraving reminders of his norms upon human sensibilities."[123] In this sense, the covenant theme seems to resonate at the most fundamental level at which all human beings exist and function.

---

123. Wolters, *Creation Regained*, 29.

7

Envisioning Medicine within a Covenantal Ethic

A practical theology of health care based on relationality contests decisions about life based on rigid and abstract determinations of either a legal or biological character. The moral discernment it envisages presupposes an unfolding search for meaning within an ultimate and theological conviction of human destiny as sharing the very life of God.[1]

—Patrick McArdle (2008)

PRINCIPLISM AND MEDICAL PRACTICE: SOME CONCERNS

Relationships between caregivers and patients are central to medicine. Increased attention has been given recently to the structure and dynamic within and among medical relationships. Richard Zaner writes that the illness of the patient, *homo patiens*, is the hub of a web of medical relationships.[2] This person bears a burden of distress, pain, and/or anxiety that alters relationships with others, at the same time forcing the creation of new relationships involving caregiver specialists. The patient is the centre of a centripetal force, modulated by a vulnerability that pulls others toward him or her as novel medical encounters are established.[3] Zaner

---

1. McArdle, *Relational Health Care*, 151.
2. Zaner, "Encountering the Other."
3. Ibid., 29–30; Zaner, "Illness and the Other."

sees this vulnerability as a power to alter the patient's life. It can be either a power *for* the patient, *over* the patient (paternalism), or *with* the patient.[4]

The caregiver-patient relationship is bidirectional. The caregiver has always had the duty of care but patients may have duties to the caregiver as well. James Nelson offers a corrective to patient-centered models, cautioning against "moral immunity" for patients.[5] The contemporary emphasis on patient autonomy and uncoerced decision-making may wrongly translate patient vulnerability into freedom from obligations and duties. Instead, patients have an explicit or implicit commitment to be truthful, compliant with a mutually agreed-upon care plan, and forthcoming with information that will be helpful in decision-making.[6]

I agree with Nelson that commitments to duties improve shared health care planning, making patients more empowered moral decision-makers and less servile recipients of beneficence. Dependency on and duties owed to others support the development of virtuous dispositions that should characterize all participants in covenantal relationships.[7] From a Christian perspective, these should reflect the gracious giving, forgiving, and commitment of God toward humankind as well as the required humility and obedience that constitutes a biblical understanding of the right relationship between God and human beings.

Relatively few Christians have written on the effect of principlism on medical practice. As mentioned previously, Pellegrino has comprehensively critiqued principlism. Two noteworthy contributions of his recontextualization of the four principles are the addition of the overarching biblical principle of love that should guide patient care and the replacement of autonomy with beneficence as the dominant principle. However, some Christians have been more critical. Theologian Brian Brock and physician John Wyatt have recently presented principlism as a distorting influence on the normative role of physicians in health care. In their view, principlism fails to provide satisfactory solutions to difficult cases while disempowering physicians. This results from a methodology in which solutions to ethical problems are assumed to be self-evident through a common morality, while scruples of conscience are systematically overruled.[8]

---

4. Ibid.

5. Nelson, "Duties to Patients," 201–6. This may be particularly problematic in more paternalistic perceptions of the physician–patient relationship.

6. Ibid., 211. Nelson also feels that patients should avoid situations of caregiver vulnerability that risk distorting the relationship.

7. Ibid., 213.

8. Brock and Wyatt, "Physician," 159.

Part Two: A Modest Proposal for a Biblical Covenantal Biomedical Ethic

Brock and Wyatt provide their own interpretation of the basic premises of principlism. The method of deliberation involves repeated discussions intended to dissolve or move aside deep moral differences. These differences are often perceived as obstructive personal prejudices and biases rather than as values and beliefs that can improve the moral fabric of society. Contemporary medical professionalism encourages the separation of personal moral values from more generic societal values reputedly found in the common morality.[9] Physicians often assume a mediating role, balancing different perspectives among moral participants. In so doing, they argue, physicians are asked to "submit their powers of judgment and their conscience to a refashioning which denies the importance of their very particularity, especially the appeal to the transcendent."[10] In principlism, virtue becomes the internalization of professional and ethical standards created by a minimalist, common-morality framework.

According to Brock and Wyatt, legislators, pharmaceutical companies, and hospital administrators try to minimize physician protests about corporate or institutional self-service by keeping them focused on their patient care responsibilities. Such institutional stakeholders of medicine contend that principlism allows for the expression of individual, conscience-driven, and sometimes religious caregiver views in order to relieve the stress of possessing such "marginal" views. In reality, however, these views eventually are marginalized for the sake of collective agreement in policy-making settings. In this regard, Brock and Wyatt refer to the insights of Jacques Ellul and George Grant who unmask the bureaucratizing of dissent that suppresses the grievances of the less empowered members of society. At the level of the patient-caregiver relationship, however, patient views often prevail over the consciences of physicians for the sake of patient autonomy.[11] In its attempt to establish "liberal pluralist equipoise" (their term for reflective equilibrium), principlism tries to create a method of resolving perceived moral problems that devalues the basic grounds of the moral systems from which it claims to draw its legitimacy.[12] Brock

9. Landis, "Physician Distinguish Thyself." This point was taken up in chapter 5 in an analysis of David Landis's model of distinct physician selves that can conflict when identifying physician covenantal responsibilities.

10. Brock and Wyatt, "Physician," 161.

11. Ibid., 162. Brock and Wyatt refer to the insights of Jacques Ellul (*Technological Society*, 354–58) and George Grant (*Lament of a Nation*) into the bureaucratizing of dissent in an effort to suppress the grievances of the less empowered members of society. Ellul speaks of the "technique" of human relations in which human relating is maintained for the sake of the common end of maximum productivity.

12. Ibid., 163. Citing MacIntyre (*After Virtue*, 2), they argue that principlism

and Wyatt argue against moral compromise that requires taking positions against moral conscience for the sake of finding middle ground. A working conscience can only be maintained by resisting perpetuating systems that run counter to one's conscience.[13]

I share the concerns of Brock and Wyatt and laud their exposure of the unbiblical nature of the basic tenets of principlism, particularly its method of inducing compromise among participants under the pretext of common rational persuasion. From a Reformed Christian viewpoint, becoming a formative voice in the public forum should not mean giving up the beliefs of one's conscience or those of one's community of faith. Doing so promotes a minimalist public morality and subverts the missional nature of contributing biblically inspired insights into public dialogue. Principlism's willingness to hear voices from diverse traditions and belief systems hides its ultimate objective: persuading the compromise of beliefs for the sake of solutions that can be reduced to often groundless and weakly justifiable common denominators.[14] However, I also think that physicians also take some responsibility by opposing corporate and institutional self-interest in health care where patient care is compromised for the sake of efficiency and fiscal frugality.

COVENANTAL ETHICS, CHRISTIAN SOCIAL PHILOSOPHY, AND MEDICINE

Insights of Dooyeweerd's Social Philosophy

In addition to his anthropological insights mentioned above, Dooyeweerd has developed a complex philosophical framework for understanding normative social relationships.[15] Its basic concepts can be applied to medicine and will be articulated in this section. Political scientist Jonathan Chaplin has recently provided constructive reconceptualizations of Dooye-

---

consists of simulacra of morality wherein the language of morality is used but in which its comprehension is largely if not entirely lost.

13. O'Donovan, *Desire of the Nations*, particularly 215–17; O'Donovan, *Resurrection and Moral Order*, 96; Bonhoeffer, *Ethics*.

14. Brock and Wyatt, "Physician," 156. Brock and Wyatt apply some of their arguments using the example of a case of a young mother who is pregnant with a fetus known genetically to have Down's Syndrome. Arguments for and against abortion of a fetus with Down's Syndrome are given, but no recommendation is made for a particular position.

15. Dooyeweerd, *New Critique*, vol. 3.

weerd's insights into societal relationships. Dooyeweerd's philosophy and Chaplin's reinterpretations are significant advances toward a Christian understanding of relationships that can form a helpful framework of a biblical understanding of relationships in medicine.[16] Chaplin suggests that the covenant theme can contribute to a normative understanding of creational unfolding over time. This has relevance for gaining a normative perspective on the increasingly complex network of relationships in medical practices. In Dooyeweerd's philosophy, human relationships are seen as individual entities. Like individual living things, non-living objects, or events, each relationship has a normative structure that includes a plurality of ontologically grounded, irreducible dimensions or aspects.[17] Each aspect is irreducibly sovereign relative to other aspects. Every relationship exists and is acted out through these aspects in different ways over time, depending on the nature of the relationship, its interrelationship with other relationships, and its historico-cultural context.

Dooyeweerd develops this notion of sovereign, basic ways of existing in response to non-biblical reductions of various aspects of life prevalent in secular worldviews. Human responsibilities toward envisioning and living out these aspects of life are expressed through norms. Ethical norms are rules of conduct that guide responsible human choices regarding good and evil, virtues and vices, etc. For Christians, the overarching ethical norm is obedience to the call from God to act for the good of others as exemplified by God's commands and actions in Scripture.

According to Dooyeweerd, social structures are relatively fixed components of the created order, while the human responses to such structures differ and can change over time.[18] Chaplin rightly challenges this static notion of invariant social structures,[19] suggesting that it stifles the concept of cultural unfolding in history or "cultural disclosure."[20] Chaplin suggests that this process of cultural unfolding could be better reconceived with a focus on human flourishing. Invariant structural norms or laws become normative imperatives, grounded in and directed to the human person.

---

16. Chaplin, *Herman Dooyeweerd*.

17. Ibid., 55–57; Dooyeweerd, *New Critique*, vol. 1, 2–3. These include faith, ethical, juridical, aesthetic, economic, social, lingual, historical, logical, psychic, biotic physical, kinematic, spatial, and numerical aspects of reality.

18. Chaplin, *Herman Dooyeweerd*, 62–63.

19. Wolterstorff (*Until Justice*, 62–63) also disagrees with Dooyeweerd's claim that social structures are bound by invariant principles.

20. Chaplin, *Herman Dooyeweerd*, 72–79; Dooyeweerd, *New Critique*, vol. 2, 181–92.

As human needs and demands arise during cultural unfolding over time, structural principles of relationships are applied to new social relationships. Chaplin cites Jan Dengerink who argues that different qualified human activities come to expression in differentiated structures, each of which must recognize a normative structure inherent in the creation order that matches the normative structure of the relevant human activity.[21] As applied to medicine, for example, the need for new specialized medical expertise may demand a new caregiver role, such as a nurse practitioner, whose unique skill set can best meet certain needs through this new caregiver-patient relationship.

Another conceptual problem with Dooyeweerd's cultural unfolding or disclosure process concerns the role of the historical aspect in understanding social relationships. Organized professional communities such as those found in medicine are distinguished from natural ones such as the family and marriage.[22] Dooyeweerd claims that all organizational communities are founded on the historical aspect (i.e., they arise primarily out of a historical context) but are qualified by some other aspect (in the case of medicine, this is the ethical or care aspect). Calvin Seerveld, Chaplin, and others have suggested that the historical aspect is too all-embracing (i.e., transmodal) to function as the founding aspect for these communities. Seerveld has suggested that "technical, formative control" better suits the founding function of organizational communities, a corrective with which I fully agree.[23] This aspect better reflects new knowledge and the human functional differentiation that often follows.

Dooyeweerd also develops a typology of social relationships, the two main types being interlacements and interlinkages, or organized communities.[24] The distinctions between these types will be discussed later in this

---

21. Chaplin, *Herman Dooyeweerd*, 107.

22. Ibid., 124–25. Dooyeweerd's typology further distinguishes voluntary from institutional communities, of which medical relationships in a practice would be voluntary. Chaplin adds a distinction of governance among voluntary communities. *Associatory* associations lack authority distinctions among participants, whereas *authoritarian* ones have inherent authority distinctions between participants. Certain medical relationships in a practice, such as those involving primary or specialized caregivers and a patient, seem to fit the latter type whereas relationships between caregivers or between caregivers and external institutions better fit the former.

23. Seerveld, "Dooyeweerd's Legacy," 76 n. 60.

24. Dooyeweerd, *New Critique*, vol. 3, 653–93; Chaplin, *Herman Dooyeweerd*, 112 n. 5, 278. Chaplin credits the term "interlinkages" to Bernard Zylstra, which is a synonym for Dooyeweerd's terms "interindividual and intercommunal relationships." Chaplin prefers the term "communal relationships," explaining the term from

Part Two: A Modest Proposal for a Biblical Covenantal Biomedical Ethic

chapter in the context of medicine. The normative functioning of these relational interactions is affected by the direction inherent in the basic beliefs of the participants, leading to either enrichment or distortion within the relational matrix as interpreted through Scripture. Dooyeweerd's social philosophy supplies a theoretical framework for envisioning the basic structures of social relationships regardless of the religious perspective of participants. The normativity of this framework is grounded in Dooyeweerd's attentiveness to scripturally derived insights in reaction to the conceptual errors of sociological individualism and universalism, both of which have their own non-biblical groundmotives.[25]

Dooyeweerd claims that humankind needs a biblical view of the radical spiritual solidarity in which "mankind in its spiritual root transcends the temporal order with its diversity of social structures."[26] This is needed in order to avoid absolutizing human relationships at either communal or interindividual social extremes. However, Chaplin feels that such a supratemporal appeal to a community of those in confessional relationship with God is not necessary to avoid absolutizing communal relationships. Agreeing with Chaplin, it is my view that a covenantal view of relationality would help non-believers to gain insight into the normative structures of human relationships, even though the full meaning of such structures can only be appreciated in light of the covenantal relationship between God and human beings. Only when understood in this way can each individual person and specific community be seen most meaningfully in its own unique integrity and in its unique relationships with other persons and communities.[27]

I would now like to explore how this Christian philosophical framework can be extremely helpful in developing a normative understanding of medical relationships.

Covenantal Ethics and a Christian Philosophy of Medical Practice

Henk Jochemsen and others have applied the structural and directional concepts of Dooyeweerd's social philosophy to medical practice.[28] Jo-

---

a covenantal viewpoint that stresses the purposeful intent of such associations and contrasting it with an instrumentalist view typical of individualistic liberal thought.

25. Chaplin, *Herman Dooyeweerd*, 151–52.
26. Ibid., 154; Dooyeweerd, *New Critique*, vol. 3, 169.
27. Chaplin, *Herman Dooyeweerd*, 154–55.
28. Jochemsen, "Normative Practices."

chemsen notes that Christians such as MacIntyre, Taylor, and Dooyeweerd believe that meaning is at the core of reality. Reality has inherent value that is independent of its usefulness to human beings. The alternative view, that existence precedes meaning, is a dominant view of contemporary applied ethics, including principlism. The latter view stresses the quality of instrumental thinking while meaning is derived from specific ethical situations.[29] Meaning becomes a construct of the activity of human individuals and human collectives. Moral conduct is judged in terms of rights and duties. Such applied ethics relies on mid-level principles while showing disinterest in underlying worldviews in order to claim universal relevance and applicability. It is embedded in an ethos of neutrality that ignores the influences of religious belief. Principlism is an ethical framework through which advocates of this "worldview without a worldview" engage in ethical deliberation.

Jochemsen and others have developed the Normative Reflective Practitioner model, whereby medical relationships are seen as historically conditioned, coherent forms of socially established human activity, not voluntary relations between free rational subjects seeking mutual self-interests.[30] Like Pellegrino's philosophy of medicine, this model acknowledges the core of medical practice as the principle of care, the expression of the ethical aspect encompassing benevolence and beneficence.[31] Jochemsen, in the spirit of the critiques of Seerveld and Chaplin, proposes that the founding aspect of medicine, the historical aspect, "can best be understood as the formative or technical aspect" of medical practice.[32] Constitutive rules of this so-called techno-formative aspect prescribe the activities that give the practice its particular content. Rules of other, conditioning aspects (e.g., social, economic, psychic, etc.) formulate conditions under which a competent performance of a practice takes place. Compliance with these rules is guided by the normative principle of the qualifying or ethical aspect.

In medical practice, social structures can open up at different levels of practice in response to human formative activity. This might be expressed by a change in a physician's management of a particular medical problem

---

29. Ibid., 97–102. In elaborating on this predominant view, Jochemsen speaks of the application of abstract ethical principles and the use of disengaged reason for determining the ethical correctness of human action, a clear reference to principlism.

30. Jochemsen, "Normative Practices," 103. He acknowledges that this model has been developed and used by others as well (97 n. 3).

31. Ibid., 105.

32. Ibid.

Part Two: A Modest Proposal for a Biblical Covenantal Biomedical Ethic

due to a new treatment or new diagnostic tool. Over time, technical improvements or improved understanding of disease processes can also result in a differentiation of professional functions resulting in new relationships and new practices. For example, nurse practitioners may take on some responsibilities previously assumed by physicians and may include taking more time for better empathic communication and more attention to patient needs. Such nurses may care for patients independently or under the distant supervision of physicians. Such new relationships with patients have their own sovereignty, yet they also communicate with others caring for the same patient. In addition, subspecialists might be asked to develop a relationship with that patient in order to offer expertise beyond that of the referring physician. A growing complex web of relationships develops in response to techno-formative differentiation.

Dooyeweerd's relational types can be helpful here, but with some improved reconceptualizations suggested by Chaplin. For medicine, the most important of such types is enkaptic interlacement.[33] Dooyeweerd distinguishes this type from other relationships, in part by the subservience of one party to another in the interlacement relationship. Chaplin has suggested that enkaptic interlacements should be considered a special category of intercommunal relationships or "interlinkages," as he prefers to call them, a subcategory characterized by relative permanence, intimacy, and proximity in the relationship.[34] However, he later suggests that interlinkages be reconceived as interdependencies among parties.[35] In so doing, he seems to replace Dooyeweerd's distinction of subservience of one party relative to another with equality of all parties with recognized mutual support and interdependence. This can be applied to relationships involving persons, institutions, or both. It recognizes basic human relationality and service to each other out of mutual need. Some relationships in medical practice are more dependent than independent, though all are in some way interdependent. Consequently, maintaining Dooyeweerd's distinction has merit for understanding relational differences within the whole network of medical practice relationships. Dooyeweerd's concept of enkaptic interlacement may better serve to describe the patient-caregiver relationship, given the component of subservient dependence on the part of patients with respect to their health needs, while interlinkage of equal parties may better describe intercaregiver relationships.

33. Chaplin, *Herman Dooyeweerd*, 67–70; 130–38.
34. Ibid., 134.
35. Ibid., 285.

Envisioning Medicine within a Covenantal Ethic

The physician and the patient are each sovereign individuality structures or spheres that exist in all modal aspects, being equal before God as image-bearing human beings. The patient, however, chooses to perform an enkaptic function with the physician. That function is to gain help and expertise from the physician. Here, enkaptic means that the physician and patient are independent and equal individuals. However, the patient requests help from a *subservient position of need*, a position determined by illness and vulnerability. This distinction of inequality by virtue of need is based on the techno-formative knowledge and power advantage of the caregiver versus the needy and vulnerable patient. The physician, however, also needs the patient in order to fulfill her calling to serve the needy and vulnerable. In this sense, this functional subservience typifies all medical relationships involving a caregiver and patient. While most of these relationships are dyadic, some are triadic, such as in the case of a patient with cognitive disability who may require a fully capacitated and trusted other person to assist in communication and decision-making with the caregiver.[36]

In medical practice, a relational network develops around each patient who seeks care. Each patient may develop a relationship not only with a primary care physician, but also with other types of caregivers for different situations requiring special expertise. In addition, relationships form between different caregivers, between specific caregivers and health care institutions, and between institutions. Relationships between caregivers might be seen as interlinkages in the practice setting but also as voluntary associations when considering mutual professional needs. Either way, each relationship has its own distinct structural principle and is equal to others so that one is not functionally subservient to another.[37] Caregiver participants are interdependent in that their livelihood and vocational callings depend on patient referrals. For example, a referring primary caregiver may seek help for a patient with a particular need while a specialist may accept the challenge of providing help and service that is not available from the referring caregiver.

Each relationship is also interrelated with other relationships. For example, a patient-primary care physician relationship can be interlinked (or interdependent, according to Chaplin's terminology) with a relationship between a physiotherapist and the same patient. Within each relationship is an enkaptic interlacement between individuals, an interlacement

36. Adelman et al., "Physician-Elderly Patient-Companion"; Jecker, "Role."
37. Chaplin, *Herman Dooyeweerd*, 133.

defined by internal enkaptic functional subservience based on patient needs. Yet, each relationship can also be seen as part of an interdependency of relationships in which one serves the others through the distinct expertise being offered and implemented but all having a unified focus on the overall needs of the same patient.

Recently, new professional care specialists such as nurse practitioners and physician assistants have evolved, assuming some responsibilities once reserved only for physicians. These professionals add new complexities and challenges to patient care as the size of caregiver teams and practices increase. Challenges include maintaining optimal inter-team communications and improved adherence to obligations within other relationships outside of medical practice. Similarly, patients need to adapt and relate meaningfully to more caregivers, adding to these challenges. Each relationship involving a patient must be linked by the common ethical *telos* of care to help that patient. A covenantal ethic is well-suited to balance those relationships around that central *telos* than is an ethic that focuses primarily on ethical principles.

In the applying the Normative Reflective Practitioner model to medical practice, Jochemsen describes a regulative (directional) side, actuated through attitudes, motivations, and beliefs of practice that reflect worldview and presuppositional beliefs.[38] A biblical covenantal ethical framework would apply to this side of their model. It would also give specific content to the expression of the qualifying ethical aspect of medical practice in each relational component of medical care. With this model, the created order is viewed from the same worldview perspective. Medical practice can be understood as social relationships constituted under the realization of normative social principles, while human social interactions and activities in the practice are guided by a covenantal ethic of caring. Together, they capture the relational richness of practice while being attentive to the particular ways of functioning within the relational complex that constitutes medical practice. Covenantal ethics enriches the elements of the normative structure of medical practice as outlined by Hoogland and Jochemsen.[39]

Chaplin introduces the term "covenantal voluntarism" to describe voluntary, non-hierarchical social engagement in which human activities are seen as vocations, callings, or human responses to God's invitation to

---

38. Jochemsen, "Normative Practices," 106–8.
39. Hoogland and Jochemsen, "Professional Autonomy," 463–72.

Envisioning Medicine within a Covenantal Ethic

community service.[40] This captures well the idea of covenantal service to fellow human beings in need while at the same time it links the origin of that service to God's divine covenantal invitation at creation. Covenantal voluntarism can also apply to the network of relationships in medical practice mentioned above. The notion of a covenantal commitment to others in different functional capacities can give cohesive meaning to relationships and can "keep the multiple parts of the social body functioning in harmony."[41] Working out the expression of religious motif(s) and worldview(s) of participants in medical practice will determine the ethical depth and direction of those committed to harmony within the practice.

Practice as a Covenantal Relational Network

The requirement of professional competence through the adherence to constitutive rules is also part of the fiduciary aspect of a covenantal relationship between a caregiver and patient. According to Jochemsen, these rules are derived from normative principles that are at the core of irreducible aspects of reality.[42] However, while medical practices encompass all aspects of reality, its aspect-expressing constitutive rules do not always function in the same way in all relational activities within practices. Connected with this, the internal goods of medical practice demarcate the standards and goals necessary for meeting medical needs. In keeping with its own internal goods, medical practice is qualified by the ethical aspect expressed through the normative *principle of benevolence or caring*. That practice takes place using the web of relationships in the medical encounter, the focus of which is the needy patient. The constitutive rules, in turn, are influenced by a regulative framework that flows from the worldview and faith commitment of the practitioner.

In this sense, an ethic of covenant is not restricted to the qualifying ethical aspect of the practice but is also an overarching ethic or *ethos* that integrates and directs our actions within relationship with others.[43] This *ethos* is grounded in a faith commitment. Each relationship or network of

40. Chaplin, *Herman Dooyeweerd*, 142.
41. Ibid., 286.
42. Dooyeweerd, *New Critique*; Jochemsen, "Normative Practices," 104–8.
43. Stafleu, "Philosophical Ethics," 25; Troost, *Christian Ethos*, 108–13. As mentioned earlier, Troost uses the term *ethos* to connote characteristics of human nature including the depth-dimension of human action and relationality. Ethos encompasses a basic attitude toward life, integrating, directing, and forming our dispositions while orienting our concrete acts and actions.

PART TWO: A Modest Proposal for a Biblical Covenantal Biomedical Ethic

relationships has a regulative framework that determines the regulative rules, including dispositions and obligations that accompany a covenantal commitment. Structurally, the various social, ethical, economic, and other aspects of the reality of the medical encounter are operative at all times but are regulated by the disposition and direction that are guided by the worldview of the caregivers.[44]

Administrative and corporate participants in the relational matrix of medical practice should also be disposed to a covenantal ethic. Working closely with clinicians, hospital administrators should adopt service policies that minimize medical risk and maximize care for patients in hospital and attending outpatient clinics. Fiscal considerations should be subservient to patient needs, sometimes necessitating increased fund raising or, in government-funded health care systems, fervent appeals directly to funding authorities. The health of caregivers is also critical but often insufficiently considered. Work hours and conditions should engender long-term caregiver enthusiasm, satisfaction, and balance with personal relationships outside of the practice.

A covenantal ethic can also serve global health care by encouraging the sharing of resources to meet global health needs, particularly for economically challenged communities and countries. For example, the Interfaith Center on Corporate Responsibility (ICCR) develops ethically motivated investment choices through shareholder activism at corporate shareholder meetings, including pharmaceutical companies.[45] An example of specific corporate efforts to contribute meaningfully to societies with the most urgent need of care is Avant Immuni-therapeutics. This company directs profits generated from developed regions toward subsidizing therapies in developing countries. As chair of the Biotechnology Industry Organization's subcommittee on global health, the company's Chief Executive Officer is positioned to modify corporate profit-making behavior in light of religiously informed values.[46]

There is evidence that the steady increase in women physicians has fostered necessary reflection on normative relational limits to duties and responsibilities within medical practice. Fears of a physician supply crisis have arisen as more women have entered medical practice and chosen part-time practice in order to fulfill family roles of motherhood or care

---

44. Hoogland and Jochemsen, "Professional Autonomy," 468–72.
45. Cahill, *Theological Bioethics*, 66; Robinson, "Doing Good," 343.
46. Brower, "Finding Biomedicines," 3; Cahill, *Theological Bioethics*, 68.

for elderly parents.[47] McMurray and colleagues have suggested various creative strategies to ensure that physicians responsible for aging parents, children, or sick family members participate in the full spectrum of professional medical activities. These include distance telecommunications for meetings and educational activities, improved use of flexible working groups for decision-making and on-call coverage, and even explicit reward structures for physicians who work part-time.[48]

Despite the expressed concerns that part-time practice may result in poorer patient care, a recent study of a practice model designed for part-time practitioners shows no reduction in four patient outcomes and better outcomes in the areas of diabetes patient management and cancer-screening rates.[49] Encouraged by such studies, health care planners in the Netherlands are developing work models that better enable part-time professional patient care. Early reports suggest that such models can add flexibility and can improve both the flow and delivery of care, provided there is cooperative acceptance of such models by administrative, caregiver, and patient stakeholders.[50]

At the heart of a biblical covenantal ethic is the ordering principle of agape love and the love-command that flows from it. As O'Donovan points out, this love-command interprets the application of other principles to moral situations and decisions. It is universally applicable for all human relationships, takes all other commands or moral principles under its umbrella, and takes priority over other principles, particularly when other principles are in conflict.[51]

One can also envision the multiple relationships within the clinical encounter as expressions of the pluriformity of the created order. O'Donovan defines this pluriformity as "a capacity of different things to transpire and succeed one another within a total framework of intelligibility that allows

---

47. Jacobson, Nguyen, and Kimball, "Gender and Parenting." In this study of dermatologists, women worked fewer hours in general but spent more time with patients compared to males who spent more time in surgery. In addition, women more frequently reduced their hours because their spouse also worked, and parenting women physicians worked fewer hours than parenting male counterparts.

48. McMurray et al., "Women in Medicine."

49. Parkerton et al., "Effect of Part-time Practice."

50. Molema et al., "Healthcare System Design."

51. O'Donovan, *Resurrection and Moral Order*, 200–3. A major critique of principlism is its inability to give moral grounds for prioritizing different principles in different situations.

Part Two: A Modest Proposal for a Biblical Covenantal Biomedical Ethic

for their generic relationships to be understood."[52] In a biblical covenantal framework, such pluriformity manifests as the church, marriage, family, school, corporations, etc., all existing alongside each other before the face of God.[53] Pervasive sin requires the guidance of community-led interpretations of Scripture to ensure that such new roles and relationships recognize and maintain their normative structure and creational purpose.

For Pellegrino, the healing relationship is internal to medicine and is the ordering principle of other principles.[54] He considers other perceptions of medicine's core, such as a body of knowledge,[55] an end (for instance, the goal of wholeness or well-functioning),[56] or the patient-physician encounter,[57] as too socially and culturally contingent. Only the need for healing is constant. Human illness and the human response to it constitute the clinical reality of the healing relationship.[58] Pellegrino's concept of healing has covenantal overtones, covering the broad spectrum of care from curative therapy to the amelioration of suffering and providing comfort in the face of predictably incurable disease.[59] This broad *telos* provides full interhuman expression of God's gracious care within his covenant with humankind.

William F. May has explored a more explicitly covenantal model for medicine. Like Pellegrino, May focuses on the act of healing. He distinguishes the physician's covenant and a medical covenant between society at large and its citizens. In the United States, the latter alludes to a health care system that is wanting in the care of its citizens.[60] At the personal level, May sees healing as the striving for wholeness, even in the face of incurability and approaching death.[61] Pellegrino elaborates extensively on the patient-physician relationship but speaks much less

52. Ibid., 189.

53. Wolters, *Creation Regained*, 89, 99, 109.

54. Pellegrino, "Healing Relationship," 154.

55. Seldin ("Boundaries of Medicine") considers medicine as applied biology.

56. Kass, "Regarding the End." For Pellegrino ("Healing Relationship," 159), the weakness of Kass's philosophical framework is the indefinite conception of health.

57. Siegler, "Doctor-Patient Encounter." Pellegrino ("Healing Relationship," 160) is concerned that Siegler's approach fails to define clinical medicine. Its emphasis is on the process of the clinical relationship, while not articulating the essence of the relationship.

58. Pellegrino, "Healing Relationship," 162.

59. Ibid., 163.

60. May, *Testing the Medical Covenant*, 1–12.

61. May, *Physician's Covenant*, 131.

Envisioning Medicine within a Covenantal Ethic

about other medical relationships within medical practice.[62] May, on the other hand, is more attentive to others in the medical encounter. He emphasizes character and virtue as distinguishing foci of a medical covenantal ethic that determine the moral identity of nurses, chaplains, and social workers as well as physicians. So equipped, they can take on the full burden of making moral judgments. May's covenantal model also requires professional covenantal obligations to hold peers ethically accountable for their actions toward patients.[63] Such obligations should override self-serving "codes of silence" among caregivers regarding ethical infractions committed by peers.

In Joseph Allen's covenantal language, the inclusive covenant established by God with humankind at creation provides guidance for the obligations and responsibilities inherent in special covenant relationships among human beings.[64] In medicine, the distinct structural principles and normative roles of relational participants must be explored in order to define the borders and limits of each special covenant relationship. In my view, the biblical covenantal model described here and conceived in the context of the Normative Reflective Practitioner model, extends the formative work of both Pellegrino and May. This model incorporates the ethical core of medicine and the importance of a virtuous, covenantal disposition. However, it also envisions medicine as a relational network involving a wide variety of caregivers and institutions. It provides a comprehensive understanding of medicine at its foundational levels. Pillars of a biblical covenantal model for medicine include 1) the overarching principle of covenantal love, 2) the ethical core aspect that qualifies the nature of medical relationships and their normative interrelational interactions, and 3) the outworking of these relationships in the context of a practice of medical care.

Within medicine, each relationship must operate with the ultimate goal of meeting patient needs through care and healing. Physicians must give appropriate credit to the insights of nurses, physiotherapists, and social workers, who have their own enkaptic relationship with patients and are equally valuable contributors to patient well-being. Each relationship is distinguished by technical and communicative skills. A covenantal ethic gives biblical meaning to the maintenance of competence when delivering

62. Pellegrino, "Toward a Reconstruction," 42–45.
63. May, *Physician's Covenant*, 134–35.
64. For Allen (*Love and Conflict*, 39–45), inclusive covenant refers to that between God and all of humankind from creation, whereas special covenants are those between human beings.

primary or specialized care.[65] Within a covenant ethic, one must maintain a mindfulness of one's own self and needs and of the cultivation of relationships outside of medicine, aspects not well addressed by Pellegrino and May. Such self-attentiveness helps caregivers to resist burying themselves in "the bottomless needs of others."[66] Feminist sensitivities to the risk of losing one's self through fulfilling the needs of others apply to medical caregivers as well.[67]

A COVENANTAL ETHIC FOR MORAL STRANGERS IN MEDICINE

In a biblical covenantal model, the overarching framework of relationality not only gives support to the radically corrective analysis of Levinas regarding the foundations of philosophy but also provides a transcendent source and eschatological hope. The covenant framework reacquaints us with a language of duty suppressed in a culture obsessed with a language of rights. May's distinction between covenant and contractual relations parallels this duty/rights tension in contemporary Western society. Campbell and Lustig argue that caring professions express traditions of duty that are embedded in particular, religiously rooted visions of the good that is intrinsic to those practices, thus adding a richness of moral content to them.[68] They see an increasing interest among secular philosophers to "reclaim an adequate account of persons in society by adding the language of duties to that of rights."[69]

Michael Horton shows how a theology of covenant avoids both an unbiblical dualism between creator and creature, heaven and earth, etc. as well as a monistic construct of collapsing dualities.[70] Overcoming estrangement of others, he argues, is achieved when meeting the stranger is envisioned through an ontology of genuine difference and an epistemology of the external word, both grounded in a theology of covenant.

---

65. May, *Physician's Covenant*, 134; Jochemsen, "Normative Practices." Both May and Jochemsen emphasize the importance of maintaining technical competence as a measure of good practices. I think May's approach embeds this more in a framework of covenantal obligation and fidelity.

66. Langerak, "Duties to Others," 106.

67. Beach, "Covenantal Ethics," 107–49.

68. Campbell and Lustig, "Call to Respond," ix.

69. Ibid.

70. Horton, "Participation and Covenant," 115–20.

A "covenant love" that permeates the created order generates an ethic wherein the covenant becomes the site where strangers can meet.[71] A biblical covenantal ethic manifests as God's undeserved gifts of creation covenant and Christ's sacrifice on the cross.[72] It is a universal condition of dependency that binds all human beings and draws them to each other in a unity of dependency. For the Christian, *agape* love engenders the sense of gratitude for deliverance in Christ, manifesting in duties required of each other and of the community.

May considers this act of duty to others in response to divine, undeserved gift-giving as a fundamental aspect of a covenantal ethic. He contrasts this with the "conceit of philanthropy," an inherent pretension of self-sufficiency bred from a contractual model of medical relationships.[73] In fact, physicians and other caregivers are constrained by the receipt of prior gifts such as education, financial support, social privilege, and past patient offerings for research purposes. In the context of biblical covenantal ethics, gift-giving loses its tendency for expectant reciprocation, refocusing on grateful responsiveness. In the specific context of a medical care relationship, a covenantal ethic tempers the power of the caregiver through greater receptivity to the gift of providing care to the one in need.[74] Campbell suggests that both covenantal and care ethic paradigms "seek to affirm and retain a form of giftness of human relationships while also incorporating equality and dignity through revealing our common experience of dependency."[75]

---

71. Gunton, *Triune Creator*, 26; Horton, "Participation and Covenant," 120. Significantly, Horton argues that one implication of a covenantal approach is the reconceptualization of divine presence and absence as being ethical and relational in nature, not primarily ontological. This allows for a direct justificatory link between the human relationship with God and our relationships with strangers. The recognition of the stranger becomes an ethical enterprise in both cases.

72. Ibid., 191. C. S. Lewis (*Four Loves*) calls this "gift-love," being universal and indiscriminate in scope yet self-giving and personalized in motive, while creative and reconciling in action.

73. May, *Physician's Covenant*, 114; Campbell, "Gifts and Caring," 190.

74. Noddings, *Caring*, 72–74. Nell Noddings sees the caregiver-patient relationship as one of reciprocal dependency. Unlike a biblical covenantal conception of the relationship, however, there is no referral back to the divine-human relationship for moral authority, justification, and guidance. Rather, the motive for caring without inherent expectation of reciprocation comes from the memory of prior acts of caring.

75. Campbell, "Gifts and Caring," 193–94. This clearly resonates with the covenantal ethic and Normative Reflective Practitioner model presented earlier. It also recalls Chaplin's suggestion that relational interlinkages be seen more normatively as interdependencies of relational participants.

PART TWO: A Modest Proposal for a Biblical Covenantal Biomedical Ethic

Medical encounters often involve participants who have fundamentally different moral beliefs. For Engelhardt, such "moral strangers" are "acting out of fundamentally divergent moral commitments."[76] In *The Foundations of Christian Bioethics*, he develops his vision of medical care as it applies to his own Eastern Orthodox moral community.[77] Begrudgingly, he accepts the larger societal moral framework that looks for agreement on common endeavors among individuals with diverse moral differences who are moral strangers.[78] This framework is morally minimalist and primarily procedural in nature. It is necessitated, Engelhardt claims, by the failure of both the Enlightenment and Roman Catholic traditions to give firm grounding to a societal morality that is heavily influenced by a strong faith in reason.[79] Moral strangers can only be bound by permission, formally granted by mutual, common consent.[80]

John Arras contends that in postmodern individualism and pluralism everyone exists as moral strangers in moral isolation. Public morality is reduced to individual autonomy and resistance to coercion in order to achieve minimal uniformity of values in a normatively splintered world. One's only clear moral duty becomes respect for the autonomous choices of others.[81] However, the perception of such autonomous isolation can lead to some interesting consequences, whether perceived as voluntary autonomy from others in society or forced isolation from a larger societal group. For example, gays and lesbians in the 1980's claimed that their exclusion from the social contract by society gave them the right to access to drugs under investigation of HIV/AIDS before they were approved by society's regulatory process.[82]

---

76. Engelhardt, *Bioethics and Secular Humanism*, xiii.
77. Engelhardt, *Foundations of Christian Bioethics*.
78. Engelhardt, "Four Principles," 243.
79. Campbell and Lustig, "Call to Respond," xvi.
80. Engelhardt, "Four Principles," 241.

81. Arras, "Principles and Particularity." This is in agreement with Engelhardt's principle of permission that dominates secular bioethics.

82. Ibid., 13–15. This declaration of rights to unapproved but promising treatments outside of clinical trials is part of a larger ethical issue involving future HIV/AIDS patients. What is inappropriately neglected with this perspective is the negative impact of this approach on the drug development process. Allowing large-scale access of promising but unapproved drugs would potentially slow the progress of clinical studies, slow the approval time for drugs that have been shown through such studies to be effective, and thus deprive some future patients of their clinical benefit.

James Tubbs's distinction between stranger and non-stranger is more nuanced than that presented by Engelhardt. Family members and close friends may be *moral* strangers but are usually not *relational* strangers.[83] He begins with the assumption that an encounter with any other self is, to some degree, an encounter with a stranger. He borrows Thomas Ogletree's description of hospitality to the stranger as the overarching metaphor of the moral life. Tubbs agrees with Ramsey who sees God's righteous attending to Israel's needs in their covenantal relationship as the measure of rightness within human relationships. This righteous attending by God demanded that Israel respond with grateful obedience, which included sensitivity to the needs of the aliens living among them just as God provided for their needs while aliens in Egypt.[84]

I agree that our postmodern culture has led to moral alienation that can impede the development of trusting relationships in medicine. Principlism in particular fosters such alienation by failing to acknowledge the importance of moral beliefs and values for care options and decisions. A biblical perspective concerning the importance of strangers for our own faith communities shows how a covenantal ethic can give meaning to medical relationships among strangers.

Hans Boersma observes that reflections on hospitality by postmodern philosophers such as Derrida and Levinas carry a sense of transcendence but stop short of identifying a transcendent warrant of our human responsibility for hospitality.[85] While Derrida desires to grant unconditional hospitality to everyone, he sees this as an unachievable goal, devoid of messianic and eschatological promise. He calls the hospitality of this world "hospitality narcissism" in that it always has strings of self-love attached. With no God to usher in the messianic future perfection of creation, Derrida sees pure hospitality as a perpetual mirage.[86]

By contrast, Simon Steer sees human hospitality as a reflection of God's hospitable heart underwritten by his perfect hospitality through Jesus Christ.[87] Tubbs suggests that estrangement is overcome among believers because in Christ the old distinctions that made us strangers are no longer relevant.[88] However, in our not-yet-perfected world, Christians

83. Tubbs, "Theology," 39–40.
84. Ibid., 41.
85. Boersma, *Violence*, 27.
86. Ibid., 34–37.
87. Steer, "Eating Bread," 40.
88. Gal 3:28.

Part Two: A Modest Proposal for a Biblical Covenantal Biomedical Ethic

also must remain mindful of God's care of his people Israel when they were aliens in Egypt. This experience gives Christians insight into the heart of the alien, a connectedness that must translate into a sensitivity and sympathy for their needs. This shared awareness of alienation binds human beings through God's demonstrated grace to his own covenanted people.[89] Tubbs reminds us that the needy stranger might best be regarded as if he or she were of heavenly origin, given that there are scriptural precedents for angels disguising as strangers.[90] Similarly, Christ teaches that hospitality to strangers will be credited to his followers as though they were tending to Christ himself.[91] In medicine, a biblical covenantal ethic should reach out to strangers out of a common sense of alienation and vulnerability shared by all human beings. Its missional mandate is to reveal our mutual vulnerability and dependency on God's grace through Christ.

Is there a "natural" discernment through which human beings can relate to strangers normatively outside of scriptural revelation? In the pagan Greek tradition, Asklepeions were places of healing where physicians were expected to cure with moral courage and proper moral attitude. They were open to anyone regardless of social status, race, or wealth.[92] The potential for self-gratification and gain from the inherent power of the physician over the patient was recognized and to be resisted. Zaner contrasts this with the myth of Gyges who took full advantage of his power position to overcome others for self-gain. With these two opposing themes of Greek mythology serving as justification for dispositional choices, why would an ancient Greek physician choose helping others over self-interest, given his power position? Zaner's answer is that the compelling nature of the vulnerable and sick evokes a moral sense that turns the power imbalance on its head. That exposure of vulnerability and the muting of animation in illness are strangely commanding and compelling.[93] Conversations are probing and exploratory in nature, textured by uncertainties.[94]

Drawing on reinterpretations of natural law after Vatican II, Roman Catholic Richard McCormick identifies a relational tendency or sociality

---

89. Hunter, *To Change the World*, 243–46. In his presentation of a theology of faithful presence, James Davison Hunter stresses the biblical directive to be fully present to those who are not within the community of faith. "To welcome the stranger—those outside of the community of faith—is to welcome Christ."

90. Heb 13:2.

91. Matt 25:40.

92. Edelstein, *Ancient Medicine*, 344.

93. Zaner, "Encountering the Other," 29–30.

94. Ibid., 32.

that affects his understanding of human personhood. He considers relational ability and potential to be above life itself. That is, a not-yet-developed relational ability, as in the case of an embryo or a loss of relational ability toward others, prevents the preservation of biological life from being worthwhile to the individual.[95] However, McCormick still retains the traditional Thomist notion that faith in God motivates individuals to obey the natural moral law that is common to all human beings. While that common moral law allows for engagement with moral strangers, later in his career McCormick focuses more on ensuring that his religious commitment truly shapes his perspective, motivations, and process of reasoning with a Christian depth not evident in secular reasoning.[96]

Sharon Welch and others explore the advantages of understanding an intercommunity dimension of the concept of the moral stranger.[97] Internal moral truth-seeking within communities, she argues, is unable to identify clearly its own forms of injustice in moral and social discourse and practice. Instead, Welch advocates for a *communicative ethic* that provides for a sharing of community-defined meaning and values *between* communities through an openness that fosters a willingness to change. She feels that recognition of particularities and differences can introduce new ways of understanding truth if there is a commitment to solidarity. The goal is to shape and expand moral consciousness by means of learning from strangers so that such strangers become our teachers.[98] While reminiscent of principlism's process of determining morality by consensus, it is also very different in that community-specific values and meaning are used to enrich the search for greater understanding of the moral perspective of others. A biblical covenantal ethic is supportive of intercommunity interactions as suggested by Welch, testing the validity of the community's basic beliefs as well as the strength of commitment to those beliefs. In my view, for those professing to live out a Christian worldview, such testing should be welcomed at two community levels. Christian denominational communities should seek to learn from each other, while these communities should also share beliefs with non-Christian communities.

Both mutual learning and appreciation for the basic beliefs of others help to refine one's own basis beliefs as well as improve one's communication skills when engaging those with basic beliefs of similar conviction.

---

95. Cahill, "On Richard McCormick," 92.
96. McCormick, *Critical Calling*, 193.
97. Tubbs, "Theology," 51; Welch, *A Feminist Ethic*.
98. Welch, *A Feminist Ethic*, 122–37.

Part Two: A Modest Proposal for a Biblical Covenantal Biomedical Ethic

More broadly, a community truthful to itself and its moral authority will carefully reflect on the moral worthiness of their own beliefs when confronted with persuasive moral challenges from other communities. Implementing such a communicative ethic in medicine would likely enrich practice engagement, drawing on the insights and wisdom of various faith traditions toward policies that might better serve humankind. When engaging those of non-Christian faith beliefs, the idea that all of humankind is bound covenantally, based on common vulnerability and need, can be an attractive starter for dialogue regarding bioethical issues. Covenantal relating requires preparedness for such encounters; it requires knowledge of basic religious teachings of Islam, Judaism, Hinduism, pagan Greek or neo-pagan (i.e., secular) beliefs, and Christian teaching. Understanding of such beliefs along with a disposition of respect for those beliefs can give practitioners common cause for optimizing patient care.

When appropriate, opportunity should be taken to give testimony to the full meaning of covenant relating through its scriptural grounding in the creational covenant with God. Emphasizing the common vulnerability of all human beings and their equal value before God could encourage more interest in gaining mutual understanding and a valuation of views from diverse traditions without a sense of proselytizing or coercion. With the increasing number of medical relationships based on more specialized expertise, the greater differentiation of care presents challenges including the risks of further fragmenting care due to greater miscommunication or the dehumanization of caregivers or patients. For example, patients can be linguistically and conceptually reduced to their illness ("Let's go see the myocardial infarction in room 6." or "How did the stroke in room 5, bed 2 do last night?").[99] Avoiding linguistic reductionism requires constant awareness of the dehumanizing effect of such linguistic shorthand along with respectful communications skills. Patients should feel covenantally cared for while receiving the benefits of all available skills and expertise by all members of the medical team.

As the network of multiple care relationships grows, it becomes increasingly critical that each caregiver perceives when misinformation is given or when a failure to provide information has occurred. For example, a patient who has had a complete resection of all visible traces of her breast cancer will often be referred by the surgeon to an oncologist for consideration of additional treatment to reduce the risk of cancer recurrence.

---

99. Such reductive language is common in a culture of expediency and acronymic reductionism.

Certain features of the resected tumor may suggest a high likelihood that residual cancer cells were left behind, leading to a high risk of recurrence and a recommendation for additional risk-reducing systemic preventative therapy (i.e., chemotherapy and/or hormone therapy). Since recurrence of the disease is treatable but usually incurable, optimal communication between the patient and each of her physicians as well as between the physicians themselves (family physician, surgeon, radiation oncologist, medical oncologist) is critical. Only with such optimal communication can a treatment plan be developed that best balances benefits and risks and that can be started in a timely fashion before any residual cells have time to replicate and develop resistance to systemic treatment.

Such interrelational communication can be further complicated by relational triads as mentioned previously. A *preferred triad* may involve a fully competent patient, supporting other, and caregiver to maximize patient understanding through the more objective interpretive ears of the supporting other. All three parties can discuss proposed care plans together but the supporting other can also help the patient to better understand what was said after leaving the presence of the caregiver. By contrast, an *essential triad* is necessitated by patient undercapacity or incapacity. An elderly patient with early dementia may need a trusted supporting person to act as mediator, interpreter, and/or pure surrogate in discussions with caregivers. Another common example is the essential triad of parent, child, and caregiver.[100]

Adelman and colleagues have identified different coalitions within such relational triads involving elderly patients.[101] Distinctions based on the power distribution within the relationship can involve 1) a patient and supporting person coalition struck to ensure caregiver attention to the elderly patient's needs, 2) dialogue and decision-making between a supporting person and caregiver wherein the patient is virtually ignored, and 3) a coalition of patient and caregiver against the supporting person. Regarding the second relationship, supporting family members may believe they know what is best for their elderly loved one, regardless of expressed patient preferences.[102] Such an attitude among supporting family

---

100. With adolescents, the distinction between a preferred and an essential triad can be blurred, since determining the decision-making capability for this age group can be very difficult.

101. Adelman et al., "Physician-Elderly Patient-Companion."

102. This can occur when an elderly patient appears fully competent in the eyes of the caregiver but is claimed to be incompetent by supporting persons. Such discordance may reflect underlying mistrust or self-interest on the part of the supporting

members may also result in the third relationship, where both caregiver and patient know that the patient is competent but must resist the claims of family members to the contrary. In a covenantal ethic, the last two scenarios should be consciously avoided. The caregiver has the power and responsibility to keep the focus on the well-being of the patient over the preferences of others.

In a covenantal ethical framework, all parties should understand who will be responsible for what aspects of care. An oncologist assumes responsibility for the administration and supervision of active anticancer treatment and may not address aspects of care unrelated to the cancer or its treatment. In this way, primary care physicians stay directly involved in the patient's care and the specialist can concentrate on cancer-related needs. Some aspects of care responsibilities should be formally discussed and responsibilities assigned or clearly assumed by different care providers and by patient supporters. If a symptom raises the suspicion of tumor recurrence, whom should the patient notify, and which caregiver has the duty to follow-up with tests designed to rule out non-cancer causes? Who is responsible for delivering bad news and its implications to the patient if cancer recurrence or progression is found on clinical assessment after treatment? How should changing circumstances reconfigure those interprofessional relationships relative to the patient-caregiver relationships? How can the patient's duty to maintain medication compliance be monitored and its importance conveyed to the patient in a way that is empathetic without appearing paternalistic or intimidating?

If a covenantal ethic is practiced, optimal communications will be sought, errors or deficiencies of one party will be corrected by others on the team, and all parties will cooperatively strive to meet the health care needs of the afflicted person. Those from faith communities will also strive to use their faith beliefs to strengthen relational bonds, correct injustices or incompetence, and keep the focus on meeting the needs of the vulnerable and afflicted. Differences in faith beliefs should be shared as sources of wisdom from each tradition rather than as impediments to care, for the sake of both current and future patient needs.

I have presented the grounding, basic structure, and direction for a biblical covenantal ethic as it applies to biomedical ethics and the medical practice encounter. The articulation and implementation of its ethical

---

persons, leading to formal third-party determinations of patient competence or even charges of caregiver incompetence. However, embedded cultural mores can also promote paternalistic, protective dispositions that encourage withholding information and empowering family members to make critical decisions for patients.

framework is rooted in a Reformed Christian interpretation of Scripture wherein the theme of covenant is central to an understanding of Christian living. This framework gives relational meaning to Christian worldview and Christian social philosophy that resists individualistic and universalistic perceptions of human interrelating with other human beings and with other aspects of the created order.

Habermas's response to the question "Why be ethical?" involves a procedural solution strikingly similar to the rational process of principlism and its Rawlsian origins.[103] His procedural path to true modernity lacks substantive motivation and appreciation for the devastating influence of sin, which is self-seeking rather than other-seeking. Sin cannot be translated into merely human inadequacy requiring change as suggested by Sturm.[104] It must be recognized as human disobedience to divine grace and authority, without which the full meaning of covenantal human relationships is lost.[105] Similarly, Habermas replaces striving for the good life by way of obedience to Christ with a communicatively agreed-upon proceduralism, a derivative of which is the principles-guided rational consensus of principlism.[106]

I have argued that a covenantal ethic properly envisions the caring purpose of medicine and recognizes sovereign and functionally distinct relationships that must interrelate with steadfast focus on meeting patient needs within medical practice. Maintaining this focus entails adherence to caregiver and patient duties and responsibilities. In a biblical covenantal ethic, individuals are equal members of humankind in the eyes of God. Each person has inherent value and direct accountability to God, all the while seeking fulfillment in life with help from a covenanting community of believers. Human health is under God's providential care, maintained by way of human communal activity. While God calls each human being by name to service for him, the expression of that calling is accomplished

---

103. Barrigar, "'Thick' Christian Discourse," 295–97.

104. Sturm, "Contextual and Covenant." See chapter 5.

105. Ibid., 286–96. For Habermas, the universal basis of human communication requires validity claims of truth, rightness, and sincerity. Chris Barrigar argues that Habermas ignores the reality of "insincere" communication as another universal human characteristic, one rooted in our sinful nature. The attitudes and dispositions derived from this human selfishness do not come from contingent historical conditions alone as Habermas suggests but from our sinful nature.

106. Habermas, *Between Facts and Norms*, 277.

Part Two: A Modest Proposal for a Biblical Covenantal Biomedical Ethic

in community where God's shalom and the presence of the Holy Spirit is sought.[107]

In the next and final chapter, I will reconceptualize the nature and validity of the four principles of principlism in light of this biblical covenantal ethic.

---

107. Mouw, *God Who Commands*, 52–54.

8

The Four Principles Revisited

The four principles should not be abandoned. Rather, they need to be re-defined and grounded in the reality of the doctor-patient relationship. This grounding can provide a standard against which the fundamental conceptual problem of conflict among prima facie principles can be resolved. This approach is also more congenial than "principlism" to enrichment by moral insights from a variety of non-principle-based ethical perspectives.[1]

—Edmund Pellegrino (1994)

CONTRASTING PRINCIPLISM AND A BIBLICAL COVENANTAL ETHIC

A BIBLICAL COVENANTAL ETHIC puts relationships at the forefront of the biomedical enterprise. The common-morality idea and the derivative principles of principlism are not to be ignored as merely mythical or as a figment of a nominalist imagination. Principles such as respect for persons, beneficence, and justice were identified by the Belmont Commission after many hours of intense thought by bioethicists, philosophers, theologians, and physicians with a diversity of background beliefs. Given their popular support, the longevity of these elements of principlism needs to be understood, to be re-evaluated, re-envisioned, and renewed through the spectacles of a biblical covenantal framework for human moral activity.

---

1. Pellegrino, "Four Principles," 353.

PART TWO: A Modest Proposal for a Biblical Covenantal Biomedical Ethic

As previously argued, the four principles of principlism lack a well-grounded source of meaning and moral authority that is beyond the faculty of reason. With some exceptions, many Christians have accepted these four principles without attempting to critically appraise their basic assumptions and beliefs or to establish their merit from a Christian worldview, philosophical, and ethical perspective. Notable exceptions are Edmund Pellegrino and William F. May, who envision biomedical ethics in a *more* relational framework in light of the Word of God as interpreted in their respective faith traditions.

As the quote above indicates, Pellegrino is dissatisfied with principlism as presented and promoted by James Childress and Tom Beauchamp. He acknowledges on the one hand that their version of principles-based ethics "unquestionably advanced the quality of ethical decision-making at the bedside."[2] It has provided a *lingua franca* for communication among those with divergent and often incommensurable moral presuppositions.[3] However, he concludes that medicine should be grounded in "the reality of the doctor-patient relationship." Is this sufficient for a Christian? How is his approach more "congenial" toward one's perception of biomedical ethics, as he suggests in the quote given above? Pellegrino is not clear about the particulars of this congeniality. The reality of this relationship is not self-referential, nor is it self-evident. His statement sounds uncomfortably close to the self-evident nature of the common morality of principlism. I would counterclaim that medicine is qualified by the principle of care as an expression of the ethical aspect of our created being in response to human health care needs. When its relationships are understood within a biblical covenantal ethical framework, medicine is ultimately grounded in *agape* love as revealed by God. Furthermore, biomedical ethics is concretely worked out through multiple relationships involving needy patients. Multiple caregivers may be involved, creating interrelating relationships whose *telos* remains focused on the care of the patient.

Pellegrino advocates for reimaging the four principles within a classic virtue ethic that is synthesized with and grounded in the Roman Catholic Thomist tradition. These virtues give greater substantive moral capacity to the moral agent who brings the four principles into bioethical reflection. In this tradition, supernatural virtues give direction through biblical

---

2. Ibid., 360. In addition, "Its utility must not be lost in the current zeal for replacing it with alternative approaches which have their own inherent difficulties."

3. Ibid.

revelation, and the virtue of love or charity binds morality in general, including all other principles. The principle of love is firmly grounded in the Word of God. This is in contrast to principlism, wherein no single unifying principle or concept is claimed. However, Pellegrino rightly perceives that the principle of autonomy has maintained dominance among the principles since their first formal inception in the Belmont Report. This is not surprising given that the Belmont Commission was constituted to protect human research subjects from unethical treatment. This dominance is also an expression of the individualism of American society, which emphasizes individual rights and freedoms, often at the expense of appreciating normative relationality in medicine. In response, Pellegrino favors retention of the principles but elevates the principle of beneficence to become the core principle for medicine and medical practice. Transformed into a virtue, beneficence best captures care for the needy, which in turn is driven by the overarching principle of love as taught in Scripture.

As mentioned previously, May's ethical framework contrasts with Pellegrino's virtue-laden ethic regarding its central positioning of the biblical theme of covenant. He grounds his ethic in the covenant relationship between the creator and humanity as a special creature chosen for special service at creation. It is this covenant from which all relationships between human beings derive direction and develop normative content. Like Pellegrino, May reconceptualizes the principle of autonomy but in covenantal relational terms. The individual is still responsible and accountable but within a necessary relational matrix that includes the divine and other human beings.

Pellegrino's philosophy of medicine and May's covenantal ethic would be perceived by Beauchamp and Childress as private moralities that function outside of the common morality. As mentioned in chapter 1, in principlism such private moralities exist *alongside* the common morality. They are often distinguished by their core religious beliefs, which are excluded from serious consideration if they are perceived to clash with claimed views of the common morality.[4] However, in my view, Beauchamp and Childress also fail to note that being *alongside* private moralities exposes the common morality as merely another private, albeit perhaps widely promoted and accepted, moral viewpoint! Their morality is "common" only by virtue of voluntary agreement to minimal moral claims. Interestingly, they do not rule out the possibility that some individuals might be members of both the common morality and of a so-called pri-

---

4. Beauchamp and Childress, *Principles of Biomedical Ethics*, 5th ed., 403.

Part Two: A Modest Proposal for a Biblical Covenantal Biomedical Ethic

vate morality. However, such dual membership requires full acceptance of the basic beliefs of the common morality, though they are unclear as to the spectrum of such moral beliefs.

Beauchamp and Childress concede that the common morality may not have *total* authoritative moral force and that they cannot necessarily claim the validity of its authority in all of its content. In a recent edition of their book *Principles of Biomedical Ethics*, they attempt to further develop the basis for this common morality. They admit that providing substantive evidence for a universal common morality is a "nuanced problem." Beauchamp and Childress follow up with a disclaimer that the common morality has no authoritative grounding in pure reason, rationality, or natural law.[5] Instead, its starting point is in ordinary, shared moral beliefs on which morally serious individuals agree. The authoritative reasons for those beliefs apparently need not be known to fellow members of the common morality.

Regarding the justification of universal norms within their common morality, they try to show that different ethical theories (e.g., Kantian, utilitarian, and rights-based theories) provide some theoretical justification of the norms of the common morality due to the convergence of action-guided norms supported by those theories.[6] However, when they identify specific moral vices such as dishonesty and lack of integrity, they declare that these "seem necessarily excluded from the domain of the morally acceptable" because they lead to lying and the punishment of the innocent.[7] These vices seem to be self-evidently immoral given that no moral authority is claimed outside of consensus among those aspiring to the common morality. This leaves a small set of norms floating free of any moral authority other than consensus agreement for any actions generated from such a framework. Such consensus lacking moral authority may lead to the vacuous nominalism predicted by Plantinga mentioned in chapters 1 and 4 in response to Rorty's suggestion that truth is what one's peers allow one to get away with.[8]

---

5. Ibid. Beauchamp and Childress, *Principles of Biomedical Ethics*. 6th ed., 4, 392.

6. Beauchamp and Childress, *Principles of Biomedical Ethics*. 6th ed., 361–63. Here the authors muster the support of utilitarian Richard Brandt in their claim that primary ethical obligations cross ethical theories despite significant differences in moral justification. This, they claim, reflects common acceptance of the principles of the common morality as pretheoretical presuppositions. These differences in moral justification are deemed secondary to the convergence and consensus agreement about the principles.

7. Ibid., 395.

8. Louthan, "On Religion," 179–80.

This discussion is relevant to the justification of nonmaleficence as a distinct principle in principlism. In the Belmont Report, nonmaleficence was not considered a principle independent from beneficence. Its independent standing in principlism seems to reflect the minimalist requirements for beneficence that contrasts sharply with the biblical notion of giving to others through *agape* love. (This contrast will be shown more fully later in this chapter in a discussion about the parable of the Good Samaritan as explicated by Beauchamp and Childress in *Principles*.) As mentioned in chapter 1, nonmaleficence is usually expressed as "do no harm." For those promoting the common morality, it seems to serve as a unifying moral default in a morality where any expectation of beneficent actions that carry risk of self-sacrifice may offend some adherents to the common morality. In order not to risk such offence, Beauchamp and Childress relegate self-sacrificing levels of beneficence to private, religiously and culturally contingent moralities of specific moral communities. This is a key distinction from a biblical covenantal ethic whereby covenantal love carries a relational expectation of self-sacrifice if deemed necessary to fulfill the covenantal obligations.

From a Christian viewpoint, there is merit in exploring the relationship between the universal common-morality claim of Beauchamp and Childress and the Apostle Paul's suggestion of a "natural" disposition to act in accordance with God's law. Paul suggested that non-Christians may act morally appropriately as required by that law, despite being ignorant of the law.[9] Beauchamp and Childress themselves deny such a link in their denial that common morality has any basis in natural law.[10] In Romans 2:11–16, Paul writes that those who refuse the truth and follow evil will perish under God's judgment. Unlike the Jews who know the law and the truth but refuse to follow them, the Gentiles are a law unto themselves. The requirements of God's law are written on their hearts and consciences so they are not blameless.

The interpretations of these verses vary considerably. For example, C. E. B. Cranfield argues that "Gentiles" here refers to Christian Gentiles; thus, the passage would mean that the Christian Gentiles acquired God's law upon their conversion, even though they were not raised in the law as were their Jewish Christian brothers and sisters.[11] John A. T. Robinson interprets Paul's teaching here as purely Stoic; conscience is common

---

9. Rom 2:13–16.
10. Beauchamp and Childress, *Principles of Biomedical Ethics*. 6th ed., 387.
11. Cranfield, *Romans*, 50–51.

PART TWO: A Modest Proposal for a Biblical Covenantal Biomedical Ethic

moral knowledge and Paul "allows for 'nature' being a good thing."[12] While this interpretation has a "common morality" flavor reminiscent of principlism, Robinson insists that a link to a natural law idea is needed, albeit a watered-down version.

James Dunn, on the other hand, arguing according to the structure of the Greek text, concludes that Paul's intention is to present a broad statement of a more open-ended principle of moral conduct that goes well beyond Jewish particularity. The law given to Israel, says Dunn, is the law for all human beings. Gentiles are capable of doing the work of the law through an inward dependence on God and moral self-doubt and searching.[13] However, while knowledge of the law is not necessary, this capability is still achieved by knowledge of God through the surrounding creation and by an aversion to immoral living, which becomes more fully evident and expressed by the touch of the Holy Spirit.[14] I agree with Dunn that Paul is alluding to an innate sense of moral sensitivity against immoral living among the Gentiles, yet this sense is incomplete owing to its failure to appreciate covenantal obedience to God. Paul later says that no one will be declared righteous in God's sight by observing the law; rather, the law makes us conscious of sin.[15] Paul seems to suggest that innocence by ignorance is a moral default for those unaware of the law and that such pagans should not be considered evildoers as would those who do know the law and violate it.

Righteousness from God comes through faith in Jesus Christ. Those who believe are justified by his grace through Christ's redemptive sacrifice and resurrection.[16] Hence, moral rightness for Christians will be fundamentally different in meaning and authoritative source from the righteousness of those who do not believe, even if moral actions of unbelievers mimic the righteous actions of believers. What is particularly important

---

12. Robinson, *Wrestling with Romans*, 27–28.

13. In chapter 6, I describe a covenantal anthropology centered on human beings as image-bearers of God from the beginning of creation. Human dependence on God is an integral part of this covenantal anthropology within a biblical covenantal ethic. Furthermore, human relationships can be construed as interdependencies as suggested by Hoekema (*Created*) and by Chaplin (*Herman Dooyeweerd*) in his reconsideration of Dooyeweerd's relational typology.

14. Dunn, *Romans* 1–8, 98–107. D. Stuart Briscoe (*Communicator's Commentary*, 63) agrees that Paul is addressing Gentiles here, giving credit to those "who had such sensitivity to what they know of God that their consciences were keen and alert and in touch with reality."

15. Rom 3:20.

16. Rom 3:21–24.

is what is in the heart of the moral agent. What is the intention of such righteous action? Principlism is wholly inadequate for justifying righteous action because it lacks an authoritative moral anchor for the proper relationship of the moral agent to God as revealed in Scripture. Principlism tries to look forward and fears looking back to a grounding that may offend. As Derrida suggests in his critique of Levinas's relational orientation to philosophical enquiry, human beings are a common humanity linked by a common plight.[17] From a Christian perspective, that common plight is covenant breaking against God. A biblical covenantal ethic provides a more meaningful relational framework for identifying and correcting this plight through repentance and renewal. It is the historical, ontological, and covenantal nature of this common plight that needs to be more clearly worked out for biomedical ethics.

While a biblical covenantal ethic offends some, it will be attractive to others, owing to its claim of relational restoration within a common narrative of human relationships since the beginning of time. Sin has distorted but not destroyed that covenant. In Christ, covenant relations are restored, albeit thus far imperfectly, in anticipation of the covenant perfection that will come when Christ returns. The building of a renewed ethical framework that overcomes the deficiencies of principlism begins with a biblically grounded covenantal ethic realized through a Christian worldview "which allows for a God of creation and justice" while resisting the influence of sinful distortion.[18] In such a framework, human beings are "given the mandate of looking after creation, of bringing order to God's world, of establishing and maintaining communities."[19] The expanding openness inherent in postmodern pluralist thought can be an opportunity for Christian missional witnessing to be expressed, heard, and perhaps accepted and practiced in biomedical ethics. A biblical covenantal ethic can become the vehicle for such a missional witness.

In the remainder of this chapter, I will present the four principles and pillars of principlism as contextualized through the spectacles of a biblical covenantal ethic. Each principle, as defined and promoted by Beauchamp and Childress, is reviewed in chapter 1. In the following sections, each principle will be interpreted in light of a covenantal ethical framework. In such an ethic, an ordering principle of *agape* love encompasses these

---

17. Derrida, "Violence and Metaphysics," 79–153.
18. Wright, *Surprised by Hope*, 80.
19. Ibid., 212.

Part Two: A Modest Proposal for a Biblical Covenantal Biomedical Ethic

principles so that their relevance is clarified but their significance is reconceptualized in light of the covenantal relationships in medicine.

RESPECT FOR PERSONS WITHIN A COVENANTAL ETHIC

Beauchamp and Childress promote the application of this principle for many health care situations including medical research and medical practice. The preferences of the human subject or patient dominate this principle and are expressed in terms of freedom, liberty, and self-expression. This is an outgrowth of the Western liberal emphasis on individualism and has been adopted as a corrective to the historical paternalism embedded in medical practice. This individualism inadequately accounts for relationships, often emphasizing the potentially coercive dangers of relationships. Rooted in a postmodern worldview, each individual becomes the final arbiter of his or her own moral judgments. Any collective agreement on moral right or wrong comes from reasoning that leads to permissive consensus.

A biblical covenantal framework grounds patient freedom and respect in our ontic status as image-bearers of God the creator. This grounding subverts individualistic notions of respect for other persons. Personhood is acknowledged as meaningful only in the context of relationships with God, other human beings, and the rest of creation. Expressed in the South African concept of *ubuntu*, human beings are not truly human when conceived as individuals but only in relation to other human beings.[20] Within a biblical covenantal concept of personhood, however, each human being is uniquely accountable to God for thoughts and actions involving any interaction with other individuals or objects in the cosmos. A Christian philosophy should acknowledge these distinct structures of individuality as well as the relationality that human beings establish. Human volition is truly free when exercised through faithful obedience and subservience to God and his commands.[21]

---

20. Moore, *Being Me*. See chapter 5.

21. Christ declares in John 8:32 that those who become his disciples through belief in and living out his teachings will know the truth and that truth will set them free. In 2 Cor 3:12–18, the apostle Paul speaks of this freedom in covenantal terms. Those who turn to Christ experience a release from the veil of ignorance that covered their minds and hearts under the old covenant and gain freedom in Christ under the new covenant through the power of the Holy Spirit. In Rom 8:18–21, Paul speaks of such freedom in Christ in terms of the entire cosmos. At Christ's return, "the creation itself

The Four Principles Revisited

As mentioned previously, Pellegrino has rightly identified the dominance of human autonomy over other principles in principlism but has not provided an in-depth critique of the notion. Rather, he dethrones autonomy and enthrones beneficence as the dominant principle of his philosophy of medicine. With this and the introduction of love as an overarching guiding principle, he provides a normative response to principlism that provides a firm foundation for a covenantal ethic as well. It also resonates with O'Donovan's idea of the love-command of God that has a universal all-inclusiveness but is not the sole criterion by which all moral decisions are resolved. The normative "differentiated pluriformity of the moral field" in the created order must be confronted as reality.[22] Pellegrino is not always clear in his distinction between the principle of beneficence as care and the love-command of God. Nonetheless, he must be credited with keeping beneficence as the focus and core of medicine while keeping love as the insight that gives meaning to the moral principles and rules that help with specific moral situations. It is this conceptualization of the overarching love-command and beneficence that underlies a covenantal ethic.

I also agree with O'Donovan's understanding of the relation between reason and God's commands that cuts through Pellegrino's Thomist elevation of rationality. O'Donovan cautions against rationalist and voluntarist traditions, both of which can degenerate into a secular humanism. He suggests that human beings must show trusting and hopeful obedience to God in seeking to grasp God's actions as a coherent whole. While the rationalist tradition "was not wrong to promise an ultimate scrutability in the divine purpose," its Achilles's heel is its tendency to move forward toward a premature fulfillment via a reductive immanentism.[23]

However, Pellegrino's premise that "we are able to reach accommodation with the well-rehearsed principles of modern bioethics, since they make sense in a secular, pluralistic environment" is problematic for a

---

will be liberated from its bondage to decay and brought into the glorious freedom of the children of God."

22. O'Donovan, *Resurrection and Moral Order*, 202–3. He responds to situationalist suggestions that such an overarching primacy of love can reduce moral decision making to the simplest of terms. This opens the door to a relativism that ignores the particulars of love's outworking in moral life.

23. Ibid., 132–36. For the Christian, there must be hope for the day when God's action can be grasped as a coherent whole. This is a manifestation of faith as "the assurance of things hoped for, the conviction of things not seen" (Heb 11:1).

Part Two: A Modest Proposal for a Biblical Covenantal Biomedical Ethic

covenantal ethic.[24] A biblical covenantal ethic acknowledges the existence of principlism and, like Engelhardt, accepts its use by bioethicists of different traditions and beliefs. However, in my view, a covenantal ethic keeps in sharp focus the relational context of a Christian ethical perspective while providing biblically grounded reasons for views offered in public dialogue. Agreement can occur despite very diverse background beliefs that originate from very different sources of justification.

For Christians, the most important aspect of moral reflection is deriving dispositions and positions that are justified through biblical teaching and grounded in accountability to God. Scripture teaches that God, unlike the fickle and untrustworthy gods of pagan Greece, will always remain fully committed to the covenantal relationship with the human agent. Without such grounding and a divine-human model of relationality, moral dialogue and deliberation by autonomous individuals becomes merely agreement by permission, lacking any moral content that can be justified outside of individual preferences and values. Autonomy as pure individual will and choice, outside of any relational context, is a false autonomy that is wrongly directed. Autonomy in its fullest, normative sense involves freedom to obediently think and act as servants of Christ.

Charles Taylor insightfully and rightly notes that minimizing suffering is an outworking of the modern notion of human autonomy.[25] It is a consequence of the loss of belief that human beings play any role in a larger cosmic moral order and related divine history. Revulsion for suffering of any kind is a utilitarian response to a perception of human suffering as always needless. In a biblical covenantal ethic, suffering such as disease-related pain should still be alleviated where humanly possible. But it can be more normatively understood and addressed if perceived as a test of perseverance and learning provided by God for purposes about which we may have little or no knowledge.

In principlism, the tyranny of autonomy results on a power struggle wherein autonomy is the right and power of one party over another. In paternalism, the caregiver holds and exercises the power, including the right to persuade reluctant patients to pursue treatments that are perceived by the caregiver to be medically essential. Soft paternalism *for the patient's own good* is considered the moral high ground.[26] Here Beauchamp and Childress align with Mark Siegler, who believes that the physician has the

---

24. Pellegrino and Thomasma, *Christian Virtues*, 135.
25. Taylor, *Sources of the Self*, 12–13.
26. Ibid., 95.

The Four Principles Revisited

duty to define health, while Carol Whitbeck counters that the definition might better be made by the suffering patient.[27] Within a covenantal ethic, in the case of terminally ill children, both caregiver and family should resist the tendency, derived from the liberal idea of autonomy, to be preoccupied with family privacy and child rights.[28] They should prioritize, instead, decisions concerning what treatment is appropriate, or not, for terminally ill children and maximize the use of medical resources for children exposed to potentially lethal but preventative illnesses.[29]

A biblical covenantal ethic forms a worldview that reinterprets autonomy through transcendent grounding. The inequality between a caregiver's greater knowledge and power and a patient's vulnerability are transformed from an autonomy power struggle to caring concern for healing. Through covenantal relationships in medicine, those who are caring and compassionate work to communicate through metaphors that enrich patient narratives of struggles with illness. Seen as narrative, our present is affected by the persons with whom we interacted in the past and who are intimately involved in the direction of our future. In this covenantal framework, the self does not autonomously concern itself only with the present in isolation from others. It has a self-defining image. That image is enduring over time and reflects our relationship to God, though in different forms and ways at different times in our lives. We are not multiple selves as suggested by David Landis earlier. We are not consecutive persons as suggested by Derek Parfit, wherein we are different persons as adolescents with a different self-consciousness from that which we possess when we are older.[30] Our childhood cannot be repudiated and our future cannot be projected in isolation from those with whom we share our past and present. We live throughout our lives under God's gracious covenantal promises, never losing sight of our relationship with and effect on others with whom we interact.

---

27. Pellegrino, "Healing Relationship," 161; Siegler, "Doctor-Patient Encounter," 627–44; Whitbeck, "Theory of Health"; and Fabrega, "Concepts of Disease."

28. Miller, *Children*, 123–25.

29. Cahill, *Theological Bioethics*, 33.

30. Locke, *Essay*; Parfit, *Reasons and Persons*; Taylor, *Sources of the Self*, 49, 50. John Locke saw human personal identity as a matter of self-awareness, its only constitutive element. Viewed in this reduced form, the self lacks constitutive elements of engagement with other humans or with God. This opens the possibility of perceived multiple persons with no relational constitutive elements.

Part Two: A Modest Proposal for a Biblical Covenantal Biomedical Ethic

BENEFICENCE/NONMALEFICENCE WITHIN A COVENANTAL ETHIC

Beauchamp and Childress distinguish beneficence from nonmaleficence by highlighting the greater moral demand of the former. Beneficence involves active, positive action toward helping others rather than simply refraining from harmful acts.[31] They further distinguish different types of beneficence. While positive beneficence requires the provision of benefits to others, the utility principle requires the balance of benefits and liabilities in order to strive for the best overall result as an extension of positive beneficence. In addition, they contrast the virtue of benevolence and non-obligatory ideals of beneficence.[32] They consider the distinction between ordinary and extraordinary acts to be morally irrelevant, preferring the distinction between obligatory versus optional as determined by the balance of benefits and risks.[33] However, regarding obligatory and heroic acts, they are careful to minimize positive obligations toward others, suggesting that self-sacrificing or even self-effacing actions should be considered ideals to be admired rather than morally obligatory.[34]

In my view, minimalist obligations to others are expected as a condition of common morality. To be nonmaleficent, to simply "do no harm," avoids association with even minimally sacrificial, positive obligations inherent in many faith traditions. From a covenantal ethical perspective, the principles of beneficence and nonmaleficence fall on a continuum of ethical obligations whose grounding is in one's relationship to God. Nonmaleficence is not a prescription for covenantal helping or caring but a codal and legal warning to not harm, with an implicit "or else" as a warning of punishment. It is analogous to the Decalogue if the latter is understood as primarily a code, emphasizing what not to do in relation to God and fellow human beings. By contrast, the directives of the new covenant require unconditional beneficence as a fulfillment of the old covenant stated in the Summary of the Law.[35]

---

31. Beauchamp and Childress, *Principles of Biomedical Ethics*, 5th ed., 113–58. These authors devote an entire chapter to nonmaleficence but much of its content deals with active withholding or withdrawing of treatment, double effect concerns, and distinguishing ordinary from heroic treatment.
32. Ibid., 165–66.
33. Ibid., 123–25.
34. Ibid., 45–47; 167–70.
35. Matt 22:37–39; Lev 19:18; Deut 6:5.

The Four Principles Revisited

A division between beneficence and nonmaleficence as presented by Beauchamp and Childress is understandable, given the worldview from which principlism justifies its structural elements. Since moral positions are based on rationally formulated consensus and given that no moral authority is the model for love or beneficence, nonmaleficence becomes the lowest common denominator for moral relating to others. However, this minimum standard of ethical relating is, in my view, an unbiblical justification for relating to others. This position is in agreement with Engelhardt, who considers nonmaleficence as unhelpful and morally insufficient on its own as a guide for moral decision-making and for determining morally appropriate behavior toward others.[36] The principle of permission fails to bind moral strangers and prevents them from sharing deep and divergent moral beliefs. Pellegrino almost discounts nonmaleficence as a distinct principle, considering it a legal default for the minimal protection of all, regardless of any relational ties.[37] However, he does not go far enough in revealing the basic postmodern beliefs that leave nonmaleficence, and principlism in general, morally wanting as a moral framework.

Beauchamp and Childress try to clarify the distinction between minimal beneficence to all other persons versus special beneficence, which is linked to the nature of the relationship between the beneficent agent and the recipient. To expect someone to have the same obligation of beneficence to one's family members as anyone else is "both overly romantic and impractical."[38] They give contemporary examples of bioethicists whom they consider too generous in their moral requirements for beneficence (e.g., Peter A. Singer), but they also chastise those whom they consider too lax or too ambiguous.[39]

Interestingly, Beauchamp and Childress relate in some detail the biblical story of the Good Samaritan as an example of problematic beneficence.[40] They suggest that "common interpretations" view the Samaritan's beneficence to the injured man as an ideal rather than as a moral obligation and thus constitute part of particular moralities rather than the common morality. This view contrasts sharply with Charles Taylor's interpretation. For Taylor, the Samaritan's actions express an altruistic ideal for practicing Christians, attainable through the transformation of one's will by the grace

---

36. Engelhardt, "Four Principles," 138.
37. Pellegrino, "Four Principles," 363.
38. Beauchamp and Childress, *Principles of Biomedical Ethics*, 5th ed., 169.
39. Ibid., 169–70.
40. Ibid., 167.

PART TWO: A Modest Proposal for a Biblical Covenantal Biomedical Ethic

of God.[41] Without such morally transforming grounding, Beauchamp and Childress seem frustrated, confessing that "it is therefore doubtful that ethical theory or practical deliberation can set precise, determinate conditions for beneficence."[42] Without an overarching principle, such as *agape* love, they are reduced to presenting several moral rules in an attempt to prescribe moral specificity without providing the moral grounds for such specificity. In restoring the relational focus that is lost in principlism, a biblical covenantal ethical framework establishes beneficent intention and action upon the needy for God's sake, through Christ, as being the true message of the parable of the Good Samaritan.

Jesus presents the parable in response to a question from an "expert in the law" who seeks the way to inherit eternal life. He knows the teaching to "Love the Lord your God with all your heart . . . soul . . . strength and . . . mind and, Love your neighbor as yourself."[43] But he "tests" Jesus on the question: whom should he consider to be his neighbor? The key characters in the parable represent two groups in local society that hated one another and that refrained even from verbal contact. To the Jew, the Samaritan was a half-breed Gentile who perverted Jewish law and customs with pagan inclusions. The racial and national identity of the victim is not given. The priest and the Levite represent two leadership groups in Jewish society whose legalistic view of righteousness focused on righteous acts. Pursuit of these acts not only did not require them to deal with the unclean but compelled them to avoid the man as if he was dead rather than help him if he were alive. By contrast, the Samaritan provides initial aid as well as provisions for future care, even though the victim is a stranger and possibly an enemy.[44]

After presenting the parable, Jesus asks whom the legal expert thinks should be considered his neighbor. When he acknowledges that only the Samaritan shows mercy to the beaten man, Jesus simply instructs him to do likewise. Beauchamp and Childress question whether the Samaritan's act exceeds ordinary morality without explicitly offering their own view.[45] It would be difficult if not impossible to require such ideal moral behav-

---

41. Taylor, *Sources of the Self*, 21–22.
42. Ibid., 173.
43. Luke 10:27.
44. May (*Physician's Covenant*, 123–24) stresses that contractual arrangements determine only what is required and are in this sense minimalist. Covenants, on the other hand, obligates the more powerful party to accept some responsibility over the vulnerable party and therefore strive for what is just rather than only what is required.
45. Beauchamp and Childress, *Principles of Biomedical Ethics*, 5th ed., 167.

ior as part of their common-morality concept. Expressions of love and generosity to strangers or even enemies seem extraordinary and too demanding for the common morality of principlism. By contrast, Pellegrino considers love to be the ordering principle for all other moral principles, giving reference to Augustine who considers love to be the ordering virtue of the Christian life.[46]

For Pellegrino love is the key to resolving conflicts between *prima facie* principles. While this perception of love in this context risks the characterization of love as a process for conflict resolution, Pellegrino consistently advocates for love as the disposition and wisdom to address difficult ethical problems without resorting to reduction to simple statements of principle that lack moral grounding. O'Donovan considers the love-command in the Summary of the Law to be supreme among the *principles of order*, referring particularly to the created order. But he uses the term as an *overarching* principle for all dispositions and actions toward the created order.[47] It has a universal inclusiveness, captured in the Good Samaritan story as Jesus's command to show mercy to the needy. O'Donovan also considers the text of Hosea 6:6 ("I desire mercy, and not sacrifice") to be a principle of order. Generally, he sees ordering principles as "more significant than mere procedural rules-for-applying-rules. They will provide insight into what the rules are really about."[48]

However, Pellegrino also uses the term "ordering principle." In renaming the principle of beneficence as "beneficence-in-trust," he calls this the ordering principle among ethical principles. He grounds this principle in the humanity of the persons interacting in the medical relationship. At first glance, this dual use of "ordering principle" seems to reflect his Thomistic dualism: while love is the greatest of the supernatural virtues, beneficence-in-trust is the greatest of the recognized temporal moral principles. However, I think this distinction can also be conceived as two distinct manifestations of love in a Christian covenantal ethic in the framework of the Christian philosophy of Dooyeweerd discussed earlier in chapter 7. That is, love can be understood as the ethical core for relating to the whole created order in general, while beneficence-in-trust is the ethical qualifying aspect of medical practice specifically. The biblical principle of love serves as a cosmic principle that grounds the central ethical principle of beneficence in medical relationships.

46. Pellegrino and Thomasma, *Christian Virtues*, 19, 109.
47. O'Donovan, *Resurrection and Moral Order*, 200–3.
48. Ibid., 203.

Part Two: A Modest Proposal for a Biblical Covenantal Biomedical Ethic

BENEFICENCE IN BALANCE: PRINCIPLES, PERSONHOOD, AND NON-MEDICAL RELATIONS

A biblical covenantal ethical framework encourages beneficent action for caregivers entrusted with the care of the needy. Care is offered empathically and competently. Minimal limits on care are not carefully calculated. However, care also cannot be offered without limits and boundaries that allow for fulfilling other obligations pledged in non-medical relationships. In addition, within medicine such a framework does not focus intently on the patient-physician relationship alone. It understands the importance of other relationships, those within a relational web that encompasses the patient in need. In a covenantal ethic, the patient's well-being is not limited to physiological and physical needs but also encompasses emotional, spiritual, and other needs.

May's intense focus on covenant relationships includes the indebtedness of physicians both to patients and to society, creating an obligation of general beneficence to them. This need and indebtedness is described as "a reciprocity of giving and receiving" and is an integral part of May's covenantal ethic for medicine.[49] However, in my view, reciprocation should not be a necessary and expected outcome. The scriptural mandate to help others and to show mercy must remain in the foreground. That commitment should be the guiding principle for all caregivers and supporting others, including professionals and the supporting friends, family, and faith community. This mix of voluntary relationships in addition to natural associations such as family, marriage, etc. requires careful attention to commitments in time and relational energy. New voluntary relationships based on patient needs must learn the commitments and relational priorities already established. They must promote the strengths that natural and previously established voluntary relationships provide while working to correct relational stresses that may add to patient suffering. This is part of the covenantal ethic of relational priority and balance that accompanies the biblical notion of responsibility and commitment.

I agree with Pellegrino that the relationships between the principles must be radically altered and this is the case with a covenantal ethic as well. Beneficence is the moral foundation of any concept of human autonomy. It is relational by definition, not individualistic. However, I do not think that nonmaleficence should be retained as a distinct principle. Rather, it should be an implicit aspect of beneficence that, if considered

---

49. May, "Code, Covenant," 33.

isolated from beneficence, merely represents the failure to fulfill obligations of beneficence.

Finally, it must be remembered that any true understanding of beneficence, whether it be as the overarching ethic toward the whole created order or as the qualifying and guiding aspect of medicine, is inexorably embedded in an anthropology grounded in God's love for us. Only when perceived in this way can personal suffering, pain, and death acquire meaning and reflect true human dignity.[50] Pellegrino and Thomasma speak of Christian physicians having a mission to serve the whole of society through their expressions of competence, compassion, and caring as well as through their true knowledge of the ends and purposes of human life. Our very existence as human persons is jeopardized outside of a Christian anthropology.[51] Included in that anthropology is a caring for human beings at all stages of life. Beneficence within a covenantal ethic can be particularly helpful in reflecting on two important issues in biomedical ethics: protecting the unborn at all stages of development and guiding decisions involving the treatment of terminally ill patients.

The moral status of the unborn has been a concern since ancient times. Contraception, abortion, and infanticide were widely practiced by the ancient Greeks and Romans.[52] Paul Carrick cites preferences to practice contraception rather than abortion within those ancient cultures, but contraceptive measures were unreliable. Even so, many other reasons have been cited for carrying out abortion or infanticide. Some were very personal, such as avoiding poverty, preference for male rather than female children, and concealing adultery. Other reasons were more utilitarian and societal, such as keeping the population down, selecting only the fittest to survive for a healthier society, and preferring males in order to keep the economy and military strong.[53]

Philosophy had a very different relationship to medicine in ancient times. Medicine was a distinct discipline from about the fifth century BC onward, and philosophers would often draw on medical analogies in their arguments about ethical prescriptions.[54] However, philosophers often

---

50. Pellegrino and Thomasma, *Christian Virtues*, 149.

51. Ibid.

52. Carrick, *Medical Ethics*, 115–38.

53. Ibid., 117–18.

54. Jaeger, "Aristotle's Use of Medicine," 54–61. Werner Jaeger argues that Aristotle, son of a physician, liberally used medical terms and concepts to demonstrate details of his ethical system.

considered physicians to be vocational rivals.[55] Regarding the moral status of the unborn, divergent beliefs existed between and among these professional groups.[56] The Pythagoreans, for instance, condemn the abortion of unborn, soul-possessing humans and animals. They believed that from conception animals possess animate souls while humans have rational ones. For Aristotle, soul and body are intimately related in all living things and living things possess different types of souls based on different worth and value. By contrast, Plato taught that the soul comes into the body from outside at the time of birth.[57] Aristotle believed that the zygote has a nutritive soul like plants. Later, at forty days for males and ninety days for females, the sensitive soul is acquired by the unborn fetus. Only when the unborn acquires the rational soul, perhaps sometime in the second trimester, is the fetus protected from abortion.[58] As pantheists, the Stoics envision a world-soul from which each human being derives a portion, the essence of which is the vital breath (*psyche* or soul). As a result, the fetus is not considered human in the biological or moral sense. Once born, however, the soul is biologically present but remains morally incomplete. Only at puberty is full rational capacity reached. Consequently, at birth and through childhood a person does not have full moral rights but has some degree of moral worth by virtue of the natural ability to become a rational being.[59]

For some formative ancient philosophical schools, particularly those of Aristotle and the Stoics, human worth is not intrinsic to every human being. In fact, there is no sense of the importance of the individual. In general, beneficence is restricted to expressing the virtues and to not harming others. Sacrificing one's own happiness or life for the sake of someone else is considered absurd. They do not advocate protection of the weak and vulnerable.[60] Human dignity is tied inexorably to *arête*, or human virtue and excellence.[61] Within their pantheistic world order, Stoics are indifferent to suffering. For them, human life is not worth living without spiritual peace of mind pursued through living life rightly. This is achieved

55. Carrick, *Medical Ethics*, 22. According to Carrick, physicians could describe how one might recover or preserve one's health while only the philosophers could prescribe whether and when one should try to recover or preserve one's health.

56. Ibid., 125–38; Ferngren, *Medicine & Health Care*, 29.

57. Carrick, *Medical Ethics*, 127.

58. Ibid., 132.

59. Ibid., 134–35.

60. Ferngren, *Medicine & Health Care*, 96–97.

61. Ibid., 95.

The Four Principles Revisited

by learning how to live according to the four cardinal virtues of wisdom, courage, justice, and self-control.[62]

Prior to Christianity, the Jewish people could not represent Yahweh in pictorial images. Rather, human beings were called the image-bearers of Yahweh because they reflected the creator by their being and nature. Human beings were seen as a unity of soul and flesh that could not be separated. In contrast to Greco-Roman thought in the surrounding culture, Jewish anthropology gave human beings, including their bodies, intrinsic value by virtue of their status as image-bearers of God. As a result, infanticide, child sacrifice, and abortion were not a part of Israelite culture, except among those who fell into idolatry and adopted such practices from the surrounding pagan nations.[63]

David Novak argues that this special God-reflecting status began at creation in both Jewish and Christian traditions. He notes that some Jewish theologians going back at least as far as Philo in the first century identified this image-bearing with possessing reason. Both Plato and the Stoics taught that reason distinguishes animals from humans and links humans to the gods. Such an ontology and anthropology, however, is insufficient for grounding an ethic for all of humankind. If reason is considered a quality and capability that humans develop rather than an ontic core that identifies humanity, unborn, severely mentally incapacitated, and comatose humans would become non-persons.

As mentioned in chapter 6, Novak argues that all human beings including unbelievers can be understood as image-bearers of God.[64] Such an appreciation of the image of God would acknowledge a natural appreciation of something outside of ourselves, an extratemporal aspect or connection that is even appreciated by unbelieving human beings not exposed to revelation. As a concrete example, human beings can name things of the world around them but their own name must come from outside of this world.[65] Novak ties in the notion of human value with this transcendent connection. All human beings have full worth because God is concerned

---

62. Carrick, *Medical Ethics*, 134.

63. Ferngren *Medicine & Health Care*, 97–98.

64. Novak, "Human Person," 48. Novak claims it is plausible that the origin of the Hebrew word for "image," *tselem*, is derived from the word *tsel*, which means "shadow" and that such a word can be applied to unbelievers who are capable of appreciating God but some negative sense.

65. Ibid., 49. In a remarkable statement, Novak states, "No matter how much humans might share with the other creatures in the world, they are always *in* the world, but never truly *of* it" (emphasis in original).

for us. Human dignity can also be construed as our inner desire to seek out God.[66] Novak suggests that "the image of God is shown in the needy voices of humans one to another, whose authority is because they are the objects of divine concern."[67]

With the coming of Christ, human relationships change forever. At creation, God offered a covenant relationship with humankind as an expression of *agape* love. Despite human failure to maintain obedient obligations to that covenant, God has repeatedly shown his faithfulness to that covenant. Yet his love takes on a new soteriological and eschatological emphasis with the Incarnation, the suffering and death of Jesus, and his Resurrection. As a result of this, the Christian message links love toward all other human beings with God's love for us.[68]

This radical departure from pagan concepts of human value and relationships had four major consequences for Greco-Roman culture. Firstly, beyond civic philanthropy on behalf of the community as a whole, Christian love teaches personal concern for the needy as an outgrowth of *agape*. Such concern is universal, being extended to all human beings, believers and unbelievers, neighbors and enemies. This breaks with the Jewish focus on their community and refocuses instead on Israel's original mandate to be a light unto all the nations. Secondly, every human being has intrinsic value by virtue of being an image-bearer of God. Such intrinsic value is bestowed on the unborn as well as reflected in the condemnations of abortion as violating God's handiwork.[69] Thirdly, the idea of human beings as image-bearers of God suggests a new concept of personhood in Christ. Christ expands the concept of person beyond the Jewish concept of a person as an integration of body and soul, further opposing the dualistic Manichean and Gnostic philosophies of ancient times. In the Christian community, all are valued parts of the body of Christ, whether Jew or Gentile, slave or free, male or female, replacing the polis ideal in which citizens

---

66. Ibid., 50.

67. Ibid., 52.

68. 1 John 4:19: "We love because first he loved us."

69. Lindemann, "Do Not Let," 253–71 and Noonan, Jr., "Almost Absolute Value," 7–18. Such intrinsic value is reflected in such very early Christian works as the *Didache*, the Apocalypse of Peter, and references by Tertullian to abortion as homicide. Jones (*The Soul and the Embryo*, 57) notes that absolute condemnations of abortion were consistently noted until the late fourth century. Only after that time, under the influence of Philo and others, was lesser value assigned to the unformed fetus and lesser condemnation and punishment given.

were variably valued according to class, gender, wealth, and health state.[70] Finally, care for the poor and needy is a hallmark of Christian expression of love toward fellow human beings. Just as Christ relieves our suffering through his suffering and death on a cross, so we must give relief to the poor and oppressed.

Thus, the unborn can be ascribed value and worth as human beings within a covenantal ethic by means of their gift as image-bearers of God. Their inability to fully reciprocate relationships with other human beings does not negate their worth as humans; rather, their vulnerability cries out to other human beings for support and nurturing. Such nurturing is another expression of the relationship between God and humankind. Like an abandoned, helpless fetus or newborn infant, humankind loses its meaning and full value outside of its relationship with God. Just as God extends his undeserving love to us as completely vulnerable creatures, so parents must take responsibility to nurture the unborn as an obligatory expression of *agape* love.

By this example, one can see how both the relational character and intrinsic moral value of human beings are confirmed in a covenantal ethic that keeps in its sights the relationship between humankind and God the creator. The ordering principle of love authorizes and justifies beneficence to guide the care for the unborn as fully human in their own right. There is no moral trump of maternal autonomous preference over fetal survival. There is an obligatory caring and nurturing demand for all parents of the unborn. This begins with the responsibility of a mother to safely nourish and nurture her unborn charge and protect her from physical and emotional harm. Abortion out of convenience or willful neglect of a mother's own health is not an option. It is Stoic, not biblical, to consider the abortion of ultrasonically visualized, deformed fetuses as an act of reason because such an unborn child may not be able to acquire the virtues necessary for a good life. This view fails to see the intrinsic value of all the unborn as gifts from God to be raised up in a community of caring human beings.

A covenantal ethic can also be helpful in properly balancing the priority of different aspects of care. In keeping the focus on relational aspects of care, time is taken and sensitive dialogue is enacted to address the immediate needs of a person on life support and the grieving family. The economics of continuing life support for a critically ill patient should be a secondary concern. However, the knowledge that other patients either are, or soon will be, in need of the same equipment should be an incentive to

---

70. 1 Cor 12:5.

address directly the utility or futility of continuing life support, sensitively considering cultural and religious values. In a hospital ward or intensive care setting, emotions run high among both family and medical care staff.

Ward supervisors and hospital administrators are usually not involved in situations where religious views clash with medical staff views regarding whether or not a particular patient should be maintained on life support. Even if medical staff and family members are members of the same religious faith, major differences can lead to major conflict. In situations where life support systems will be considered in a patient with incurable disease, the earlier that end-of-life support issues are discussed, the more time is available to air and work out differences. Such differences in attitudes regarding whether or not life support should be instituted or under what particular circumstances it should be initiated may involve key family members, the patient and staff, or among staff members. Such situations must be managed with extraordinary sensitivity and knowledge of other traditions represented in the dialogue.

INTERPRETATIONS OF JUSTICE AND LOVE

Beauchamp and Childress present their principle of justice as a group of principles in the common morality, though little space is devoted to the components of this group. They distinguish a formal principle of justice from material ones.[71] Appealing to Aristotle's minimal formal requirement for justice, they argue that equals must be treated equally and unequals treated unequally. Material principles of justice specify characteristics earmarked for equal treatment. They speak, for example, of the principle of need as a requirement without which harm to the person in question could result. In characteristic minimalist terms, they declare that "Presumably our obligations are limited to fundamental needs."[72] Regarding six material principles of distributive justice, they accept them all after failing to find an objection to any of them. Then they reiterate a common theme of principlism as "a plausible thesis": that each material principle represents a *prima facie* obligation, the moral weight of which is contingent on context and situation. They endorse a qualified egalitarianism whereby citizens are given equal treatment except when unequal treatment may benefit those in greater need. They contend that principles of justice mandate attention to medical utility or to maximizing patient welfare.

71. Beauchamp and Childress, *Principles of Biomedical Ethics*, 5th ed., 226–30.
72. Ibid., 228.

The Four Principles Revisited

As noted in chapter 1, Beauchamp and Childress decry health care inequalities in the United States but, unfortunately, choose not to explore the underlying philosophies or worldviews behind such a societal imbalance. They simply blame the insurers and legislators. They claim to witness an emerging social consensus that all citizens should be able to secure (or are entitled to) equitable access to health care in the United States. However the recent debates of very divergent views regarding health care reform bear witness that such a consensus is emerging ever so slowly, if at all. Consistent with their method of choosing parts of existing theories without claiming a new, if not composite, theory of their own, Beauchamp and Childress note that definitions of unfair opportunities and unfortunate status in life vary among those who adhere to different theories.

Different theories of justice influence policy preferences regarding the setting of priorities for the rationing of limited resources. When Beauchamp and Childress render their own preferences, for example in the case of health care plans, they identify aspects of several existing plans that have utility and that promote some form of egalitarian justice. They then declare in broad strokes that "the best plan is likely to be the one that most coherently promotes both values [of utility and justice] and that insists on universal access to a decent minimum of health care." They appeal to four objectives toward the development of a coherent health care system: avoid obstructing access to decent minimal health care, develop acceptable incentives for physicians and consumers/patients, have a fair system of rationing that supports decent minimal care for all, and develop an incremental, minimally disruptive implementation plan.[73]

While they claim that each theory of justice offers a philosophical reconstruction of a valid perspective on moral living, each one is insufficient for dealing with the range and diversity of life. Rather than presenting their own perception of an alternative, comprehensive theory, they simply accept societal diversity as a challenge to societal consensus.[74] While implying that social consensus in the United States is not within reach, they do not link the piecemeal health care system that has evolved in that society with the multiple ideologies rooted within it. In other words, they fail to analyze the foundational differences between views within American society. As noted previously, their concept of justice has no presuppositional roots and no philosophical orientation other than an egalitarian tendency. In short, they fail to acknowledge that the underlying individualism of

---

73. Ibid., 262.
74. Ibid., 272.

PART TWO: A Modest Proposal for a Biblical Covenantal Biomedical Ethic

American society impedes progress toward the sacrifice and selflessness that mark a covenantal and more communal approach to health care.

Critics of the principle of justice often respond by recontexualizing this principle in a specific ethical theory or framework, in an attempt to provide missing moral content. R. H. Nicholson argues that the principle of justice in principlism is only helpful for individuals of like status in a particular society. He notes that principlism has developed within a particular societal context and that this limits its usefulness to relatively minor ethical problems.[75] Feminist critics focus on discrimination or unequal treatment based on gender. An example of such injustices includes the burdens put on women who are unpaid caregivers of family members for whom institutional care is not available or deemed not needed by hospitals.[76]

Peter Kasenene gives credibility to the importance of context for understanding the principle of justice. From his African perspective, justice is foremost a social affair; individual and communal welfare are intertwined. He presents a case of a woman seeking help at a local hospital for symptoms of pre-eclampsia. Her husband and relatives decide to take her to a traditional healer against medical advice but, at least outwardly, with her consent. She deteriorates and requires intensive care. Should she now forfeit the right to care, asks Kasenene, because of previous non-compliance? In his view, in this tribal setting, the patient and her family can be perceived as having a covenantal duty to be compliant with medical advice and treatment such that negligence in accepting that duty should have retributive consequences. He sees this as weighing the principle of distributive justice against beneficence.[77]

Quite different views may also be expressed within the same religious tradition. Writing from an Islamic perspective, Zaki Hasan speaks almost apologetically of combining justice and goodness into a more primitive concept. He considers the manifestations of righteousness (as equated with goodness), including faithfulness and sincerity towards oneself, as not useful for medical ethics! Muslims, he claims, share with Christians and Jews the idea that acting beneficently is imitating God. However, he also believes that justice is determined in given situations by the patient and the physician. Both, he feels, should follow the tenets of the Greek physician Galen by stressing moderation, liberation from passions, and

75. Nicholson, "Limitations," 270–71.
76. Cook, "Feminism," 203.
77. Kasenene, "African Ethical Theory," 186–87, 190–91.

seeking the Aristolelian mean.[78] By contrast, Muslim physician G. I. Serour focuses more directly on the Quran's directives and ideas, noting that injustice may result in punishment after death and that justice must be meted out in both personal and societal contexts.[79]

According to R. E. Florida, Buddhist ethics makes no specific reference to justice. While friends are considered on an egalitarian footing, other relationships involve reciprocal duties and obligations among individuals with higher or lower ranking. Florida notes that medical relationships are not explicitly mentioned in Buddhist writings, but extrapolates that the physician would likely have a paternal role and the patient a subservient one. However, he notes that Buddhist thought does include an obligation for the higher or wealthier person to care for those less fortunate.[80] For Avraham Steinberg, justice is a restricted notion in current biomedical settings. Most discussion and deliberation focus on distributive justice as fair economic distributions of goods and services. He distinguishes this from justice in traditional Jewish thought wherein justice is closely linked with mercy, grace, truth, trust, fairness, and charity. In critique, Steinberg argues that distributive justice as conceived in contemporary biomedical ethics is more procedural in focusing on how to do thinking whereas justice from a Jewish perspective is more substantive in focusing on the nature and quality of human life.[81] Furthermore, Jewish justice is linked to the commands of God, and humans fulfill the meaning and purpose of justice by acting according to God's law and to the guidance of wise interpreters of those laws who imitate Godly justice in their lives.[82] Steinberg stresses the command in the book of Deuteronomy to be generous to the poor and to the needy.[83]

For Beauchamp and Childress, as well as for Daniels and Sabin, the principle of justice involves equal access and opportunity. These are determined based on *reasonableness*. In their pursuit of fair equality of opportunity in health care, Daniels and Sabin express empathy for those with religious views. They admit that even reasonable people differ in their religious views such that finding terms of fair cooperation that are accepted as reasonable by all can be very difficult. Still, they seek not to alienate a

78. Zaki Hasan, "Islam," 100–1.
79. Serour, "Islam," 83–84.
80. Florida, "Buddhism," 110–12.
81. Steinberg, "Jewish Perspective," 71–72.
82. As presented in Psalm 119:137–44.
83. Deut 15:11.

Part Two: A Modest Proposal for a Biblical Covenantal Biomedical Ethic

minority that cannot agree with the majority on religious grounds. They appeal to a process (deliberative democracy) whereby the majority's preference rests on a rationale that eventually even the minority can view as legitimate.[84] Many theologians and other scholars have explored the relationship between justice and *agape* love. Views on the relationship vary widely among theologians and ethicists, as systematically presented by Gene Outka.[85] For instance, Joseph Fletcher considers justice and *agape* love to be synonymous; more precisely, justice is simply love distributed.[86] Because each situation of moral choice is multifaceted, involving multiple claimants, justice becomes love coping with situations demanding distribution of some kind. However, he also says love is utilitarianism. The principle of justice is completely independent of beneficence, given that the former deals with the manner by which beneficence or the quantity of good over evil is distributed.[87] Elsewhere, Fletcher says that justice can override beneficence if it allows goods to be distributed more equally.

Reinhold Niebuhr and Emil Brunner consider justice to be a necessary but insufficient requirement for love. For Niebuhr, the law of love fulfills all other laws but does not abrogate the laws of justice, just as Christ's death and resurrection fulfill the Mosaic law but do not abolish it. For Brunner, justice is a precondition of love. Love applies to personal ethics but cannot be made intelligible in relations between collectives in which case it is replaced by justice.[88] Anders Nygren distinguishes justice as appraisal of worth from *agape* love as bestowal of worth. According to him, in the New Testament, *agape* is gratuitous impartial benevolence. However, Nygren also puts distance between justice and *agape* love. He considers *agape* to be justice blind; that is, love supplants justice. Gerard Gilleman describes justice as assuring the minimum of charitable relations, applying largely to goods, possessions, and services rendered. Char-

---

84. Daniels and Sabin, *Setting Limits Fairly*, 36. In his debate with Robert Audi (*Religion in the Public Square*, 160), Wolterstorff articulates this tension of accepting legitimate differences in views or positions and accepting to obey or implement the positions of others as an Augustinian point of view. That is, to be coerced to obey a law or policy that one opposes but acquiesces to, unless it is truly appalling, is an acceptable form of political decision-making in this sin-corrupted world, as long as full opportunity is given to present one's reasons for one's own position, genuinely and in full. This would allow religious reasons to prevail without the need to translate them into secular terms that may change the meaning of those reasons.

85. Outka, *Agape*.
86. Fletcher, *Situation Ethics*, 87.
87. Frankena, *Ethics*, 37.
88. Outka, *Agape*, 78–82.

ity, on the other hand, is much richer and more complex through human communication that makes parties aware of each other's inner lives. This is strikingly similar in analogy to Habermas's distinction between secular and religious positions in the public square. Whereas secularists seek common goods such as money, security, or leisure time, devoted religious persons seek "goods of salvation." Conflicts over such existential values may be irreconcilable even among religious citizens. For Habermas, these can only be resolved through compromise that requires "being politicized against the background of a jointly assumed consensus on constitutional principles."[89] In my view, in striving for "goods of salvation," *agape* love gets at a different level of caring and welfare for others than does justice. The latter is a necessary result of our sinful world and nature, while *agape* love provides a dispositional respite from "vindictive instincts" that pervade efforts to achieve justice.[90]

Despite these differences, these various Christian views of justice and agape love consistently see the relationship between *agape* love and justice as achievable expressions of beneficence. This contrasts with the concept put forward by Beauchamp and Childress in which *agape* is to be admired as an ideal but not realistically expected or even achievable. According to proponents of principlism, justice strives for what is deserved, though the criterion to judge what is deserving eludes them. Fair treatment for Beauchamp and Childress involves equalizing opportunities such as access to health care in order to develop coherence and stability. As well, they use utilitarian views to prioritize resources for those who will more likely benefit from treatment and thus serve the greater good of society. They are egalitarian in their effort to equalize medical utility before permitting access to scare health care resources on the basis of chance or queuing.[91]

Some ethicists, including Christians, have tried to argue for a generic justice and even generic *agape* love concept, exclusive of its Christian moorings. Gregory Vlastos tries to rationalize a case for egalitarian justice without appealing to theological doctrines. He argues that persons have irreducible value but does so without revealing by what moral authority he makes such a claim. Furthermore, he states that each person's wellbeing should be given the same weight as that of another person.[92] This, however, is not justification but an argument for normative content. Kai

---

89. Habermas, *Between Naturalism and Religion*, 135.
90. Outka, *Agape*, 84–85.
91. Beauchamp and Childress, *Principles of Biomedical Ethics*, 5th ed., 271.
92. Vlastos, "Justice and Equality," 70.

Part Two: A Modest Proposal for a Biblical Covenantal Biomedical Ethic

Nielsen counter-argues that different persons with the same values can have experiences whose intrinsic values are not the same. According to Nielsen, it is not the logic of moral discourse or some conceptual necessity but Vlastos's Christian commitment that does not allow him to grade human beings as more superior or inferior to another.[93]

Outka examines whether there exists some common core of native moral insight that all human beings share or some common standards to which anyone can appeal.[94] It is sometimes assumed that some moral principles may be justified through appeals to natural law, the golden rule, phenomenology, and, perhaps most frequently, justice itself. For Outka, justice can be considered a moral principle and thus an action guide if it is prescriptive, universalizable, and overriding/final/authoritative. He includes an important additional criterion: Frankena's conditions of relationality (i.e., relations between individuals) and the consideration of the effects of one's action on others from the perspective of those others.[95] However, Outka also notes that certain religious background beliefs regarding a "full-dress" theological idea of *agape* and justice cannot be included in a humanist version of *agape* and justice. Such beliefs embody the intrinsic goodness of communion with God and the belief that the irreducible value of each person is linked with being a creature of God.[96]

Outka rightly insists that a relationship with God includes an anthropology that is interdependent with that relationship. Humanists and other non-Christians can envision aspects of *agape* love but without the professed relational tie to God; such evidence of *agape* can only be appreciated as moral fragments of a fallen world. However, while Outka argues that any possible atheistic *agape* rests on a guarantee that the needs of others will be met, in my view true *agape* must encompass a full understanding of redemptive history and the eschatological hope that *agape* carries. While doing justice is a reflection of God's love, it is tainted by sin and a natural human disposition toward just-deserving rather than a desire to sacrifice for others. The arguments that true *agape* can be experienced by humanists or secularists are weak and, like the law, can be seen as a discovered but incomplete inclination to pay equal respect to the other.

In the new covenant, Christ expects his followers to go beyond a temporal practice of justice. Selfless regard for another without expectation

---

93. Nielsen, "Skepticism and Human Rights," 586.
94. Outka, *Agape*, 196.
95. Ibid.
96. Outka, *Agape*, 205–6.

The Four Principles Revisited

of reward follows the model of the Good Samaritan and is an expectation rather than an ideal to be revered yet not sought after in real life. For reasons such as this, during bioethical discussions and deliberations, Christians should put forward religious views backed by religious reasons. As Weithman notes, Robert Audi's requirement for religious citizens to back up their religious views with secular notions that have secular motivations will not work.[97] Similarly, Wolterstorff argues that even legislative representatives might best serve their constituents by using their religious beliefs, not alone, but in light of other views of constituents. In the end, however, such representatives might best serve as purveyors of wisdom. As Wolterstorff puts it:

> The representative must decide as she judges best—after gleaning what wisdom she can from her constituents, and anyone else. Her decision will have to be in the light of all that she believes, including her religion or irreligion, as the case may be. She runs the risk of being removed from office the next time around. But that is the risk any representative takes who sees her role not as one who follows political polls but as one who exercises political wisdom.[98]

JUSTICE AS PERCEIVED WITHIN A BIBLICAL COVENANTAL ETHIC

In a covenantal ethic, beneficence is the core aspect or principle of health care that recontextualizes justice as a derivative of love and, thus, as inherently self-sacrificing. Beauchamp and Childress provide an example of the implications of a failure to appreciate the necessary relational link between *agape* love, beneficence, and a divine/human covenant. For them, supererogatory action is an ideal, while justice falls in the realm of the humanly possible and expected obligations to others. *Agape* love does not play a practical role in their idea of justice or in living the moral life of the common morality. Rather, a human being should never be expected to

---

97. Weithman (*Religion and the Obligations of Citizenship*, 152–60) provides an excellent response to Audi's contention that religious persons who integrate their faith into their daily lives must abstain from supporting a law or public policy if they cannot provide evidence of motivation by adequate secular reasons. Because Audi treats such motivation as a principle of virtue, it is "incompatible with aspiring to the integrationist ideal" (155).

98. Audi and Wolterstorff, *Religion in the Public Square*, 118–19.

Part Two: A Modest Proposal for a Biblical Covenantal Biomedical Ethic

give up one's rights or life for someone else. They should decide what is morally expected by consensus and be consistent in practicing such consensus justice.

Wolterstorff has recently argued for a Christian account of "justice as rights." His Christian concept of justice can be linked to the principle of respect for persons and integrates well into a covenantal ethic because it is grounded in respect for human worth. Unlike respect for persons as an autonomy principle defined by Beauchamp and Childress, this respect for the worth of human beings is grounded in the ontic status of image-bearers of God. Wolterstorff is careful, however, to distance his idea of *imago Dei* from that of theologians such as Barth or Buber, who link it with an I-thou relationship. Christian right-order theorists, who he argues do not hold human worth to be morally basic, require rational capacities to anchor human rights. Secular concepts of human rights have similar requirements for capacity, though some secular scholars like Raymond Gaita can see the impossibility of grounding rights in capacity and thus can still give human rights to the unborn and those with dementia.[99] Wolterstorff's justice as rights theory is covenantal in nature because natural human rights are not only inherent rights based on our ontic status as image-bearers of God. They also require the worth-imparting relation of human beings to God. That relation is rooted on being loved by God, and being loved by God bestows worth.[100] Like the concept of justice understood by Outka and Frankena, justice as rights is defined by its basic relational nature. This relational basis for justice links it with beneficence and with respect for persons.

Agape love alone does not constitute an ethic.[101] Guides for application are needed to implement love. Justice implements love toward others. Human beings have worth or value, not as a constitutive property but as a status conferred by God in unmerited grace and shared by all human beings.[102] Islam and Judaism may also endorse such a theory of justice as natural human rights because of their religious resources for grounding such a theory. However, secular perspectives fail to find a valid grounding for such human rights. In addition to including individual human beings as having natural rights, he argues that social entities, such as voluntary

---

99. Wolterstorff, *Justice*, 324–25; Gaita, *Common Humanity*, 5, 23–24.

100. A provision of human worth also credited previously to David Novak in chapter 6.

101. Wolterstorff, *Justice*, 107.

102. Kierkegaard (*Works of Love*) agrees that every other human being is one's neighbor based on the equality of all human beings before God.

organizations, acquire rights. This is particularly relevant for medicine and its relationships.[103] For these reasons, Wolterstorff's concept of justice as rights fits well within a biblical covenantal ethic as applied to medicine.

From a biblical covenantal perspective, justice involves the pursuit of prioritized care for the most needy as well as fair treatment for those of perceived equal need.[104] However, a covenantal ethic also stresses the need for understanding and learning the reasons why some receive care ahead of others. Patients should be given the opportunity to give up their place for fellow human beings in greater need when awaiting treatment. They have their own immediate needs but should understand how important it is to consider the needs of fellow citizens out of a sense of giving of themselves. However, caregivers also have the responsibility to provide the reasons why waiting may be necessary, even if it is not considered detrimental to overall health outcome of the patients waiting for treatment. The ultimate meaning of such willingness gets at the very nature of what it is to be human beings.

A covenantal ethic encompasses a multidimensional perspective of love and justice wherein human sacrificial giving not only reflects ongoing divine grace. It is also a further eschatological step in time toward the final day, when such giving will be unimpeded by self-serving sin and all moral ambiguity will pass away.[105] Divine love provides explicit backing by requiring human beings to conform to loving what and whom God loves, done through an injunction to love one's neighbor. In humanist ethics, there is no supreme exemplar, no teleology, on the cosmic end of times. Instead, there are many options for the good life but none that is the greatest good.[106]

---

103. However, one must be note that Wolterstorff's concept of voluntary organizations may be less inclusive than Dooyeweerd's concept in his social philosophy, as previously discussed in chapter 7. The latter considers voluntary organizations to be those that are not natural, such as marriage and family relations.

104. Wolterstorff, *Justice*, 117; Isa 58:6-7; Luke 4:17-21. Wolterstorff notes that Jesus incorporated into his message the Old Testament prophetic sensibility to injustice by giving priority to the vulnerable lowly ones, identified as the widows, the orphans, the poor, and the resident aliens.

105. Outka, *Agape*, 181.

106. Ibid., 194.

Epilogue

The End of the Beginning

PRINCIPLES-BASED ETHICS AND BIBLICAL covenantal ethics both claim elements of moral commonality, which makes them attractive as generalizable frameworks for ethics. However, covenantal ethics has a more valid claim due to its creational, cosmic, and divine grounding. Principlism claims that a common morality is derived from human experience and history, distilled into a universally shared product reflective of its roots in modernity. For Beauchamp and Childress, the common morality transcends culture, while particular moralities are limited in acceptance and practice to specific cultures.[1] The common morality comprises moral beliefs rather than moral standards and is historically expressed through theories of common morality. At the same time, however, Beauchamp and Childress claim that *their* theory of common morality does not form lower-level ethical theories. Instead, they pick and choose elements from existing ethical theories to build their own concept of a common morality. They repudiate any extratemporal authority from which their most fundamental moral beliefs might be derived and claim that the authority of norms in their common morality comes from consensus. Ultimately, belief in the rightness of moral judgments lies in one's faith in the common capacity of reason to derive the norms of a common morality.

For Beauchamp and Childress, private or particular moralities, such as those derived from Protestant traditions, are simply different ways of creating guidelines and procedures from abstract starting points of the common morality. However, they admit that striving for overall coherence among competing resolutions of ethical reasoning may not always pick

---

1. Beauchamp and Childress, *Principles of Biomedical Ethics*, 6th ed., 3–4.

out a unique set of justifiable moral beliefs. In such a case, more than one set of beliefs may be justifiable. This is because specification and input from competing particular moralities often resist optimal coherence and moral consensus.[2] For example, Beauchamp and Childress would consider a biblical covenantal ethic to be a private and particular morality because of its grounding in Scripture and adherence to beliefs derived from Scripture. Yet, this covenantal ethic is not particular in the sense that it is rooted in a covenantal relationship between *all* of humankind and Yahweh that was established at creation. Rather, it is "common" or "universal" in the sense that *every human being* is bestowed with an inherent status as an image-bearer of Yahweh, and all interhuman relationships draw their deepest moral meaning from that original divine-human relationship. Only a state of inherent and inherited unfaithfulness adversely affects that covenant relationship and consequently all of creation as well.

From such a covenantal perspective, principlism's claim that adherence to its common morality over other, more particular moralities is invalid. It can justifiably lay claim to its use as a common language, but the meaning and use of its terms are biased by presuppositional and prelogical beliefs that participants carry from their own traditions. That said, in reality, *principlism is itself a particular morality*. Its basic faith in reason—its basic belief about the source of moral truth—defines it as a religious ethic; reason becomes its source of moral authority. This basic faith breeds its own particularity. As a result, its moral validity should be allowed expression with equal status among other particular moral communities. It not only should be judged against the claims of all other particular moral frameworks but is also deserving of no greater privilege in the postmodern public forum of moral reflection.

Neither the common morality of principlism nor a biblical covenantal ethic is rooted in scientifically provable premises. Beauchamp and Childress try to reduce the common morality to the hypothesis that all persons committed to morality adhere to standards that they call the common morality. However, rather than proceeding to prove their case, they awkwardly acknowledge that their common-morality theory not always "gets this morality just right or that it extends the common morality in just the right ways." They further acknowledge that in attempting to build on this common morality, they cannot always "validly claim its authority at every level of our account."[3] Such cryptic suggestions of uncertainty in

2. Ibid., 388.
3. Ibid., 4.

moral authority and fallibility of interpretation attest to their inability to claim moral authority outside of human moral thinking and action alone. For the principlist, this fallibility is attributed to ignorance, inexperience, and historico-situational contingencies. For the Christian, it goes to the very nature of sin as the root of distorted human nature. Similarly, biblical covenantal ethics does not seek its moral authority or wisdom in the scientific method but nor does it rely on reason as a source of moral truth. It professes a faith in God, as revealed in Scripture, that guides moral reflection and decisions. As such, rationality is a faculty that assists in reflection but that requires directional guidance from a basic faith commitment to a standard of moral truth. Put another way, both deductive and inductive thinking are components of weighing the evidence, but spirits of our age and culture fundamentally influence our interpretation of the evidence.

Like the common-morality theory of principlism, the covenant with God, human relationships, and the created order are part of history. According to principlism, norms of the common morality develop from historically contingent content, the moral authority of which arises from human rational consensus. On the other hand, within a biblical covenantal ethic, history is the unfolding story of Yahweh's interaction with human beings and creation. History and culture do not determine what constitutes moral beliefs held by all human beings. Rather, they witness the interaction between Yahweh and his created creatures and structures. Thus, morality is defined by our response to Yahweh's revelation of himself. From that response are derived obligations to him and to the creation for which we have been entrusted care. As well, biblical teaching indicates that Yahweh desires human beings to live life rightly, despite their repeated unfaithfulness to him. He enables creational structures to remain intact despite the encroachment of sin and the resulting distorted state of affairs. Human beings can still recognize these structures and their importance but can only imperfectly and incompletely work normatively with them without a fully restored relationship with Yahweh. As a result, the identification of general moral principles and moral agreement is possible. However, the meaning of morality and moral decisions in biomedical ethics as normative moral dispositions and actions is only fully envisioned and realized through the moral authority of God and his Word and in a right relationship with him and fellow human beings.

Lisa Cahill rightly emphasizes the importance of persuasion in the confrontation between different basic value systems in public bioethical discourse. She adds participatory discourse to the other ethical, policy, prophetic, and narrative modes of discourse through which theology engages society.[4] The persuasive value of such a discourse comes from its intellectual coherence and its allusion to shared concerns and goals, expressed through relationships constituted by empathy and a perceived interdependence of participants. Currently, she argues, much of theological bioethics concedes the discussion to those who define it in policy-discourse terms. In response, theological ethics should stand its ground in its own language and strive to have a subversive or revolutionary impact on the "other religions" such as science, liberalism, and the market.[5] She treats these as distinct forces that might be seen conceptually as flowing from a worldview out of which science and market forces are molded. The potential positive impact of theological imagery and themes in public settings should not be underestimated. They can spark the emotions and imaginations of other discussion partners and can be provocative in a transformative way.[6] In fact, Cahill suggests that religious symbolism, grounded in particular communities with particular moralities, "can also mediate a sensibility of transcendence and ultimacy that is achingly latent in the ethical conflicts, tragedies, and triumphs that are unavoidable in biomedicine."[7] Appeal can also be made to the examples of early Christians who practiced devotion and self-offering to the sick at a time when the pagan culture of the day treated such gestures as foolishness.[8]

Cahill proposes that participatory discourse could be implemented through a framework known as "deliberative" democracy. Such a framework can help to reintroduce theology into bioethics in several ways. This approach seeks consensus but not for its own sake. It seeks ways to agree concerning practices that are compatible with the interest and

---

4. Gustafson, *Varieties of Moral Discourse*; Gustafson, *Intersections*. Gustafson describes these modes of discourse as interconnected, yet each may be accented differently at different times and for different purposes.

5. Cahill, *Theological Bioethics*, 38–39.

6. Ibid., 42.

7. Ibid.

8. Ferngren, *Medicine & Health Care*, 113–23. Gary Ferngren describes the early church's response to the sick as well as its evolution into institutions of care. This response to the sick is in stark contrast to the lack of public hygiene and to the prevalent attitudes that individuals suffering from infectious diseases during outbreaks had to fend for themselves. Plagues and other health endemics were attributable to divine retribution, corrected only through sacrifice and purification. Furthermore, pagan attitudes toward the poor as base and ignoble creatures reduced the poor to passive recipients of their fate. Despite the common practice of blaming Christians for plagues, the latter responded by systematically helping the afflicted.

commitments of all concerned without demanding the abandonment of basic convictions. Those with substantive values bring them to the table in various ways and through a variety of disciplines, including philosophical, theological, political, and economic ones. These disciplines are represented by their own special sciences; theorizing about aspects of reality at work within each science can lead to important and substantive insights for ethics.[9] However, any one aspect and its respective science can be mistakenly given inappropriate prominence, reducing the understanding of other special sciences to the narrow terms and meaning inherent in one, inappropriately dominant, aspect. Deliberative democracy also demands adherence to human interactive values, such as mutual respect, transparency, the recognition of basic obligations, and accountability.[10] It is an iterative process that moves back and forth between particular decisions and ultimate foundations of belief.[11]

According to Beauchamp and Childress, principlism has no single unifying principle or concept. It is not grounded in natural law or pure reason; it is grounded in itself. Rational consensus becomes an end in itself without acknowledgment of the core beliefs that drive the reasons behind deliberations that will determine whether agreement is possible and to what degree. This is radically different from a biblical covenantal ethic, which declares love to be the overarching moral force behind human disposition and action toward other human beings, other creatures, and the creation as a whole. In this context, love is an anthropological imperative that encompasses all of human activity. If possible, moral agreement should come by means of a persuasive presentation of views backed by core beliefs. Convergence of views may occur even where these core beliefs are very different. However, such convergence should not result from linguistic accommodation at the expense of distinctive moral meaning. Rather, moral positions articulated in language that maintains the full meaning of moral reasons should dominate dialogue and lead to the discovery of new insights that will edify the moral understanding of all participating parties. Linguistic commonality should not take precedent over the maintenance of distinctive moral meaning among ethical positions because such commonality risks sinking into linguistic reductionism at the expense of moral meaning.

9. Dooyeweerd, *New Critique*; Chaplin, *Herman Dooyeweerd*, 59.
10. Cahill, *Theological Bioethics*, 50.
11. Gutmann and Thompson, *Democracy and Disagreement*, 3, 79–92.

A biblical covenantal ethic as presented above is well suited for a revival of theological bioethics in the public sphere. Its appeal to a covenantal model of human relationships forms the platform for reflecting on and engaging in practices and policies that can become embedded with values grounded in basic beliefs of any kind. The persuasive power of participants should determine the inclusion or exclusion of such values. For principlists, such persuasion resides in a faith in rational convincibility, using reasons that appeal to a common morality that rests on its own moral authority. For Christians, the power of persuasion relies on the faith and hope that truth will flow from the power of the Holy Spirit rather than from human "words of wisdom" alone. The apostle Paul puts persuasion in its proper place in 1 Corinthians 2:4, 5: "My message and my preaching were not with wise and persuasive words but with a demonstration of the Spirit's power, so that your faith might not rest on men's wisdom but on God's power."

The universal nature of human vulnerability to illness, the desire to maintain health, and the inevitability of death can be expressed as patterns of life that are shared by all of humankind. These can be addressed through mutual understanding of covenant commitments to each other. As shown in chapter 5, appeals to covenantal relating in medicine have come from a diverse collection of medical professionals who claim its validity and moral authority from Christian and non-Christian traditions. In other words, it is a relational starting point of broad appeal. As such, it can form the focus of biomedical ethical dialogue that encourages the preservation of depth and meaning regarding concepts of respect of persons, beneficence, and justice. In my view, covenantal relating provides opportunities for sharing the deepest meaning behind reasons for covenantal inclinations. Biblical grounding in creation and in eschatological hope can be woven into moral discourse to deepen its persuasive tenor as a response to other grounding beliefs that are offered by others.[12] As mentioned, both principlism and a biblical covenantal ethical perspective admit to failure in discerning moral rightness and truth, but they do so for very different reasons. For the principlist, greater experience and more facts improve moral rightness but to no eschatological conclusion. For the Christian, seeking moral rightness is an obligation with a redemptive goal and purpose. It witnesses by working

---

12. Cahill, *Theological Bioethics*, 16. Cahill gives examples where biblical images of theological concepts can be evoked in response to metaphors such as "playing God" or claims that human beings are free because they are co-creators with God. Such metaphors have often been used by those of non-Christian traditions and could be a point of contact requiring qualification through a biblical context.

out the expression of the kingdom of God on earth in anticipation of the perfect morality that will come with Christ's return.

The journey leading up to this book has been a Christian response to the encroachment of non-Christian, primarily secular thought into the field of biomedical ethics and its root causes. The modernist and postmodern roots of principlism have been overtly exposed, as have been its structural and conceptual insufficiencies as a conceptual framework for guiding ethical thinking, conduction, and living. Principlism fails to adequately recognize the relational character of medicine and the complexities of its interhuman relationships that medicate ethical expression. It also ignores the trustworthy, extratemporal rule of the triune God, whose creational covenant with humankind defines us as special and cherished creatures. Only through acknowledgment of and obedience to this rule can human beings understand and live out the full meaning of biomedical ethics for medicine in contemporary society.

I have shown that a biblical covenantal ethic provides greater moral depth of understanding regarding human moral reflection and responsibility in medicine compared with principles-based ethics. Non-Christians have also appealed to a covenantal ethic out of concern that medical care often moves away from its normative focus of meeting patient needs, sometimes seeking ends of self-interest or utilitarian efficiency at the expense of patient care. The next major challenge is to explore means of communication and improved understanding that persuade both Christians and non-Christians to develop covenantal relationships in medicine, relationships that serve the needs of both caregivers and patients. Such improved understanding is particularly promising between Christian, Islamic, and Jewish traditions where covenantal relating is a common central religious theme. Indeed, this common theme among these traditions reflects covenantal caring for each other as vulnerable beings that has been a characteristic of human nature from the beginning of time. In addition, Christians must identify opportunities to witness to the fullest meaning of covenantal relating by relational expressions of Christian love that reflect the self-less giving of God through his covenant with humankind, as taught in Scripture.

Appendix

The Hippocratic Oath

I swear by Apollo Physician and Asclepius and Hygieia and Panaceia and all the gods and goddesses, making them my witnesses, that I will fulfill according to my ability and judgment this oath and this covenant:

To hold him who has taught me this art as equal to my parents and to live my life in partnership with him, and if he is in need of money to give him a share of mine, and to regard his offspring as equal to my brothers in male lineage and to teach them this art—if they desire to learn it—without fee and covenant; to give a share of precepts and oral instruction and all the other learning to my sons and to the sons of him who has instructed me and to pupils who have signed the covenant and have taken an oath according to the medical law, but no one else.

I will apply dietetic measures for the benefit of the sick according to my ability and judgment; I will keep them from harm and injustice.

I will neither give a deadly drug to anybody who asked for it, nor will I make a suggestion to this effect. Similarly I will not give to a woman an abortive remedy. In purity and holiness I will guard my life and my art.

I will not use the knife, not even on sufferers from stone, but will withdraw in favor of such men as are engaged in this work.

Whatever houses I may visit, I will come for the benefit of the sick, remaining free of all intentional injustice, of all mischief and in particular of sexual relations with both female and male persons, be they free or slaves.

What I may see or hear in the course of the treatment or even outside of the treatment in regard to the life of men, which on no account one must spread abroad, I will keep to myself, holding such things shameful to be spoken about.

Appendix

If I fulfill this oath and do not violate it, may it be granted to me to enjoy life and art, being honored with fame among all men for all time to come; if I transgress it and swear falsely, may the opposite of all this be my lot.[1]

---

1. Edelstein, *Ancient Medicine*, 6.

Bibliography

Adelman, Ronald D., et al. "The Physician-Elderly Patient-Companion Triad in the Medical Encounter: The Development of a Conceptual Framework and Research Agenda." *The Gerontologist* 27 (1987) 729–34.

Allen, Barbara. *Tocqueville, Covenant, and the Democratic Revolution: Harmonizing Earth with Heaven.* Lanham, MD: Lexington, 2005.

Allen, Joseph L. *Love and Conflict: A Covenantal Model of Christian Ethics.* Nashville: Abingdon, 1984.

Annas, Julia. *The Morality of Happiness.* Oxford: Oxford University Press, 1993.

Aquinas, Saint Thomas. *Questiones Disputatae de Veritate.* Edited by Joseph Kenny. Translated by Robert W. Schmidt. Chicago: Regnery, 1954.

Arras, John D. "Principles and Particularity: The Roles of Cases in Bioethics." *Indiana Law Journal* 69 (1994) 983–1014.

———. "Taking Rights Seriously? The Decline of Duties in a Rights Culture." In *Duties to Others*, edited by Courtney S. Campbell and B. A. Lustig, 3–16. Theology and Medicine 4. Dordrecht: Kluwer Academic, 1994.

Audi, Robert, and N. Wolterstorff. *Religion in the Public Square: The Place of Religious Conviction in Political Debate.* Lanham, MD: Rowman & Littlefield, 1997.

Ayer, Alfred J. *Language, Logic, and the Truth.* New York: Dover, 1936.

Baier, Annette. "Frankena and Hume on Points of View." *Monist* 64 (1981) 342–58.

———. *Postures of the Mind: Essays on Mind and Morals.* Minneapolis: University of Minnesota Press, 1985.

Baier, Kurt. "Ethical Principles and Their Validity." In *The Belmont Report: Ethical Principles and Guidelines for the Protection of Human Subjects of Research.* 2 vols, 5.1–5.46. Washington, DC: U.S. Government Printing Office, 1978.

———. *The Moral Point of View.* Ithaca, NY: Cornell University Press, 1958.

Bailey, James E. "Asklepios: Ancient Hero of Medical Caring." *Annals of Internal Medicine* 124 (1996) 257–63.

Baltzer, Klaus. *The Covenant Formulary: In Old Testament, Jewish, and Early Christian Writings.* Philadelphia: Fortress, 1971.

Barrigar, Chris. "'Thick' Christian Discourse in the Academy: A Case Study with Jurgen Habermas." *Christian Scholar's Review* 34 (2005) 283–308.

Bartholomew, Craig G. "Covenant and Creation: Covenant Overload or Covenantal Deconstruction." *Calvin Theological Journal* 30 (1995) 11–33.

———. "Introduction." In *A Royal Priesthood? The Use of the Bible Ethically and Politically: A Dialogue with Oliver O'Donovan*, edited by Craig Bartholomew et al., 1–45. Scripture and Hermeneutics 3. Grand Rapids: Zondervan, 2002.

———. "A Time for War, and a Time for Peace: Old Testament Wisdom, Creation, and O'Donovan's Theological Ethics." In *A Royal Priesthood? The Use of the Bible*

Bibliography

Ethically and Politically: A Dialogue with Oliver O'Donovan, edited by Craig G. Bartholomew et al. Scripture and Hermeneutics 3. Grand Rapids: Zondervan, 2002.

Bartholomew, Craig G., and Michael W. Goheen. *The Drama of Scripture: Finding Our Place in the Biblical Story*. Grand Rapids: Baker Academic, 2004.

———. "Faith and Philosophy." In *Christian Philosophy: A Systematic and Narrative Introduction*. Grand Rapids: Baker Academic, 2013.

Battle, Michael J. *Reconciliation: The Ubuntu Theology of Desmond Tutu*. Cleveland: Pilgrim, 1997.

Bavinck, Herman. *The Philosophy of Revelation*. Grand Rapids: Baker, 1979.

———. *Reformed Dogmatics*. Edited by John Bolt. 4th ed. Grand Rapids: Baker Academic, 2004.

Beach, George K. "Covenantal Ethics." In *The Life of Choice*, edited by Clark Kucheman, 107–49. Boston: Beacon, 1978.

Beale, Gregory K. *The Temple and the Church's Mission: A Biblical Theology of the Dwelling Place of God*. Leicester: InterVarsity, 2004.

Beauchamp, Tom L. "Distributive Justice and Morally Relevant Differences." In *The Belmont Report: Ethical Principles and Guidelines for the Protection of Human Subjects of Research*. 2 vols., 6.1–6.20. Washington, DC: U.S. Government Printing Office, 1978.

———. "The Failure of Theories of Personhood." In *Personhood and Health Care*, edited by David C. Thomasma et al., 59–69. International Library of Ethics, Law, and the New Medicine 7. Dordrecht: Kluwer Academic, 2001.

Beauchamp, Tom L., and James K. Childress. *Principles of Biomedical Ethics*. 1st ed. Oxford: Oxford University Press, 1979.

———. *Principles of Biomedical Ethics*. 4th ed. Oxford: Oxford University Press, 1994.
———. *Principles of Biomedical Ethics*. 5th ed. Oxford: Oxford University Press, 2001.
———. *Principles of Biomedical Ethics*. 6th ed. Oxford: Oxford University Press, 2009.

Beauchamp, Tom L., and Laurence B. McCullough. *Medical Ethics: The Moral Responsibilities of Physicians*. Englewood Cliffs, NJ: Prentice-Hall, 1984.

Beecher, Henry K. "Ethics and Clinical Research." *New England Journal of Medicine* 274 (1966) 1354–60.

Bellah, Robert N. et al. *Habits of the Heart: Individualism and Commitment in American Life*. New York: Harper and Row, 1986.

Berkhof, Louis. *Systematic Theology*. Grand Rapids: Eerdmans, 1949.

Berkouwer, G. C. *Man the Image of God*. Grand Rapids: Eerdmans, 1962.

———. *Sin*. Grand Rapids: Eerdmans, 1971.

Bertens, Hans. *The Idea of Postmodern: A History*. London: Routledge, 1995.

Betz, Werner. "Zur Geschichte Des Wortes 'Weltanschauung.'" *Schriften der Carl Friedrich von Siemens Stiftung*, 18–28. Frankfurt: Verlag Ullstein, 1980.

Boersma, Hans. *Violence, Hospitality, and the Cross*. Grand Rapids: Baker Academic, 2004.

Bok, Sissela. *Common Values*. Columbia, MO: University of Missouri Press, 1995.

Bonhoeffer, Dietrich. *Ethics*. Edited by Ilse Todt et al. Translated by Reinhard Krauss et al. Minneapolis: Fortress, 2005.

Botha, M. Elaine. *Metaphor and Its Moorings: Studies in the Grounding of Metaphorical Meaning*. Bern: Peter Lang AG, 2007.

Bibliography

Bouma, Hessel et al. *Christian Faith, Health, and Medical Practice.* Grand Rapids: Eerdmans, 1989.

Brandt, Richard, B. *Ethical Theory: The Problems of Normative and Critical Ethics.* Englewood Cliffs, NJ: Prentice-Hall, 1959.

———. *A Theory of the Good and the Right.* Oxford: Clarendon, 1979.

Breck, John, and Lyn Breck. *Stages of Life's Way: Orthodox Thinking on Bioethics.* Crestwood, NY: St. Vladimir's Seminary Press, 2005.

Briscoe, D. Stuart. *The Communicator's Commentary: Romans.* Edited by L. J. Ogilvie. Waco, TX: Word, 1982.

Brock, Brian, and John Wyatt. "The Physician as Political Actor: Late Abortion and the Strictures of Liberal Moral Discourse." *Studies in Christian Ethics* 19 (2006) 153–68.

Brody, Baruch. A. "Liberalism, Communitarianism, and Medical Ethics." *Law & Social Inquiry* 18 (1991) 393–407.

———. "Quality of Scholarship in Bioethics." *Journal of Medicine and Philosophy* 15 (1990) 161–78.

Brothers, Kyle. "Covenant and the Vulnerable Other." *Journal of the American Medical Association* 288 (2002) 1133.

Brower, Vicki. "Finding Biomedicines for Infectious Diseases." *Genetic Engineering News* 23 (2003) 3.

Brown, William P. "Character of the Covenant in the Old Testament: A Theocentric Probe." *The Annual of the Society of Christian Ethics* (1996) 283–93.

Bruggemann, Walter. "The Covenanted Family: A Zone of Humanness." *Journal of Current Social Issues* 14 (1977) 23.

Butler, Joseph. "'Preface' from His *Sermons*." In *British Moralists*, edited by L. A. Selig-Bigge. 2 vols. New York: Dover, 1965.

Cahill, Lisa S. "On Richard McCormick: Reason and Faith in Post-Vatican II Catholic Ethics." In *Theological Voices in Medical Ethics*, edited by Allen Verhey and Stephen E. Lammers, 78–105. Grand Rapids: Eerdmans, 1993.

———. *Theological Bioethics.* Washington, DC: Georgetown University Press, 2005.

Callahan, Daniel. "Bioethics as a Discipline." *Hastings Center Studies* 1 (1973) 66–73.

———. "The Emergence of Bioethics." In *Science, Ethics, and Medicine*, edited by H. Tristram Engelhardt Jr. and Daniel Callahan, x–xxvii. Hastings-on-Hudson, NY: Institute of Society, Ethics, and Life Sciences, 1976.

———. "Religion and the Secularization of Bioethics." *Hastings Center Report (Special Supplement: Theology, Religious Traditions, and Bioethics)* 20 (1990) 2–4.

———. "The Sanctity of Life." *Updating Life and Death: Essays in Ethics and Medicine*, edited by D. R. Cutler, 181–251. Boston: Beacon, 1969.

Calvin, John. *Institutes of the Christian Religion.* Edited by John T. McNeill. Translated by Ford Lewis Battles. Philadelphia: Westminster, 1960.

Camenisch, Paul F. "Paul Ramsey's Task: Some Methodological Clarifications and Questions." In *Love and Society: Essays in the Ethics of Paul Ramsey*, edited by James Johnson and David Smith, 67–89. Missoula, MT: Scholars, 1974.

Cameron, Nigel S. *Life and Death after Hippocrates: The New Medicine.* Wheaton, IL: Crossway, 1991.

Campbell, Courtney S. "Gifts and Caring Duties in Medicine." In *Duties to Others*, edited by Courtney S. Campbell and B. Andrew Lustig, 181–98. Theology and Medicine 4. Dordrecht: Kluwer Academic, 1994.

Bibliography

———. "On James F. Childress: Answering That of God in Every Person." In *Theological Voices in Medical Ethics*, edited by Allen Verhey and Stephen E. Lammers, 127–56. Grand Rapids: Eerdmans, 1993.
Campbell, Courtney S., and B. Andrew Lustig. "A Call to Respond: Duties to Others." In *Duties to Others*, edited by Courtney S. Campbell and B. Andrew Lustig, vii–xvii. Theology and Medicine 4. Dordrecht: Kluwer Academic, 1994.
Canadian Council of Churches. *A Health Care Covenant*. Toronto: Canadian Council of Churches, 2007.
Carrick, Paul. *Medical Ethics in the Ancient World*. Washington, DC: Georgetown University Press: 2001.
Cassel, Christine K. "The Patient-Physician Covenant: An Affirmation of Asklepios." *Annals of Internal Medicine* 124 (1996) 604–6.
Cassell, Eric J. *The Nature of Suffering*. New York: Oxford University Press, 1991.
Cayley, David. *The Rivers North of the Future: The Testament of Ivan Illich*. Toronto: House of Anansi, 2005.
Chaplin, Jonathan. *Herman Dooyeweerd: Christian Philosopher of State and Civil Society*. Notre Dame, IN: University of Notre Dame Press, 2011.
Childress, James. "The Identification of Ethical Principles." In *The Belmont Report: Ethical Principles and Guidelines for the Protection of Human Subjects of Research*. 2 vols. 7.1–7.38. Washington, DC: U.S. Government Printing Office, 1978.
———. *Priorities in Biomedical Ethics*. Philadelphia: Westminster, 1981.
———. "Scripture and Christian Ethics: Some Reflections on the Role of Scripture in Moral Deliberation and Justification." In *Readings in Moral Theology 4: The Use of Scripture in Moral Theology*, edited by Charles E. Curran and Richard A. McCormick, 276–88. Ramsey, NJ: Paulist, 1983.
Chrysostom, John. *Six Books on the Priesthood*. Translated by G. Neville. Crestwood, NY: St. Vladimir's Seminary Press, 1984.
Clarke, W. Norris. *The One and the Many: A Contemporary Thomistic Metaphysics*. Notre Dame, IN: University of Notre Dame Press, 2001.
Clouser, K. Danner. "Bioethics." In *Encyclopedia of Bioethics*, edited by W. T. Reich, 115–27. New York: Free Press, 1978.
———. "Medical Ethics: Some Uses, Abuses, and Limitations." *New England Journal of Medicine* 293 (1975) 384–87.
———. "Veatch, May, and Models: A Critical Review and a New View." In *The Clinical Encounter*, edited by Earl E. Shelp, 89–103. Philosophy and Medicine 14. Dordrecht: D. Reidel, 1983.
Clouser, K. Danner, and Bernard Gert. "A Critique of Principlism." *Journal of Medicine and Philosophy* 15 (1990) 219–36.
Clouser, K. Danner. "Common Morality as an Alternative to Principlism." *Kennedy Institute of Ethics Journal* 5 (1995) 219–36.
Clouser, Roy. *The Myth of Religious Neutrality: An Essay on the Hidden Role of Religious Beliefs in Theories*. Notre Dame, IN: University of Notre Dame Press, 2005.
Cochran, Robert F. "The Bible, Positive Law, and the Legal Academy." In *The Bible and the University*, edited by David L. Jeffrey et al., 161–87. Grand Rapids: Zondervan, 2007.
Coffey, Susan. "The Nurse-Patient Relationship in Cancer Care as a Shared Covenant: A Concept Analysis." *Advances in Nursing Science* 29 (2006) 308–23.
Colish, Marcia L. *Stoicism in Classical Latin Literature*. The Stoic Tradition from Antiquity to the Early Middle Ages 1. Leiden: Brill, 1985.

College of Physicians and Surgeons of Ontario. "Ending the Physician-Patient Relationship." Policy Statement # 3-08, 2008.

Cook, Rebecca J. "Feminism and the Four Principles." In *Principles of Health Care Ethics*, edited by Raanan Gillon, 193-206. New York: Wiley, 1994.

Cranfield, C. E. B. *Romans: A Shorter Commentary*. Grand Rapids: Eerdmans, 1985.

Curran, Charles. E., and Richard A. McCormick. *Natural Law and Theology*. Readings in Moral Theology 7: New York: Paulist, 1991.

Dallmayr, Fred. "The Discourse of Modernity: Hegel, Nietzsche, Heidegger, and Habermas." In *Habermas and the Unfinished Project of Modernity: Critical Essays on "The Philosophical Discourse of Modernity,"* edited by Maurizio P. d'Entreves and Seyla Benhabib, 59-96. Cambridge: MIT Press, 1997.

Daniels, Norman. *Justice and Justification: Reflective Equilibrium in Theory and Practice*. New York: Cambridge University Press, 1996.

———. "Wide Reflective Equilibrium and Theory Acceptance in Ethics." *The Journal of Philosophy* 76:5 (1979) 256-82.

Daniels, Norman, and James E. Sabin. *Setting Limits Fairly: Can We Learn to Share Medical Resources?* Oxford: Oxford University Press, 2002.

Davis, Richard B. "The Principlism Debate: A Critical Overview." *Journal of Medicine and Philosophy* 20 (1995) 85-105.

de Vaux, Roland. *Ancient Israel: Its Life and Institutions*. Grand Rapids: Eerdmans, 1961.

Deane-Drummond, Celia. *Genetics and Christian Ethics*. Cambridge: Cambridge University Press, 2006.

DeGrazia, David. "Moving Forward in Bioethical Theory: Theories, Cases, and Specified Principlism." *Journal of Medicine and Philosophy* 17 (1992) 511-39.

DePaul, Michael R. *Balance and Refinement: Beyond Coherence Models of Moral Inquiry*. London: Routledge, 1993.

Derrida, Jacques. *Of Grammatology*. Translated by G. Sprivak. Baltimore, MD: Johns Hopkins University Press, 1976.

———. "Violence and Metaphysics: An Essay on Emmanuel Levinas." In *Writings and Difference*, edited by Jacques Derrida, 79-153. London: Routledge, 1978.

Devettere, Raymond J. "The Principled Approach: Principles, Rules, and Actions." In *Meta Medical Ethics: The Philosophical Foundations of Bioethics*, edited by Michael A. Grodin, 27-47. Boston Studies in the Philosophy of Science 171. Dordrecht: Kluwer Academic, 1995.

Dilthey, Wilhelm. *Dilthey's Philosophy of Existence: Introduction to Weltanschauunglehre*. New York: Bookman, 1957.

———. *Selected Writings*. Edited by H. P. Rickman. Cambridge: Cambridge University Press, 1976.

Donagan, Alan. *The Theory of Morality*. Chicago: University of Chicago Press, 1977.

Dooyeweerd, Herman. *A New Critique of Theoretical Thought*. Philadelphia: Presbyterian and Reformed, 1969.

———. *Roots of Western Culture: Pagan, Secular, and Christian Options*. Edited by D. F. M. Strauss. Lewiston, NY: Mellen, 2003.

Dumbrell, William J. *Covenant and Creation: An Old Testament Covenantal Theology*. Exeter, UK: Paternoster, 1984.

———. "Paul and Salvation History in Romans 9:30—10:4." In *Out of Egypt: Biblical Theology and Biblical Interpretation*, edited by Craig G. Bartholomew et al., 286-312. Scripture and Hermeneutics 5. Grand Rapids: Zondervan, 2004.

Bibliography

Dunn, James D. G. *Romans 1–8*. Dallas: Word, 1988.
Durham, J. I. *Exodus*. Waco, TX: Word, 1987.
Edelstein, Ludwig. *Ancient Medicine: Selected Papers of Ludwig Edelstein*. Edited by O. Temkin and C. L. Temkin. Baltimore: Johns Hopkins University Press, 1967.
Eichrodt, Walther. *Theology of the Old Testament*. 2 vols. Philadelphia: Westminster, 1961.
Ellul, Jacques. *The Technological Society*. London: Cape, 1964.
Emanuel, Ezekiel J. *The Ends of Human Life: Medical Ethics in a Liberal Polity*. Cambridge, MA: Harvard University Press, 1991.
Emanuel, Ezekiel J., and Linda L. Emanuel. "Four Models of the Physician-Patient Relationship." *Journal of the American Medical Association* 267 (1992) 2221–26.
Engelhardt, Jr., H. Tristram. "Basic Ethical Principles in the Conduct of Biomedical Behavioral Research Involving Human Subjects." In *The Belmont Report: Ethical Principles and Guidelines for the Protection of Human Subjects of Research*, 8.1–8.45. 2 vols. Washington, DC: U.S. Government Printing Office, 1978.
———. *Bioethics and Secular Humanism: The Search for a Common Morality*. London: SCM, 1991.
———. *The Foundations of Bioethics*. 1st ed. New York: Oxford University Press, 1986.
———. *The Foundations of Bioethics*. 2nd ed. New York: Oxford University Press, 1996.
———. *The Foundations of Christian Bioethics*. Lisse: Swets & Zeitlinger, 2000.
———. "The Four Principles of Health Care Ethics and Post-Modernity: Why a Libertarian Interpretation Is Unavoidable." In *Principles of Health Care Ethics*, edited by Raanan Gillon, 135–48. New York: Wiley, 1994.
Evans, Donald. "Paul Ramsey on Exceptionless Moral Rules." In *Love and Society: Essays in the Ethics of Paul Ramsey*, edited by James T. Johnson and David H. Smith, 19–46. Missoula, MT: Scholars, 1974.
Evans, John H. *Playing God? Human Genetic Engineering and the Rationalization of Public Debate*. Chicago: University of Chicago Press, 2002.
Fabrega, Horacio. "Concepts of Disease: Logical Features and Social Implications." *Perspectives in Biology and Medicine* 1 (1973) 538–617.
Ferngren, Gary B. *Medicine & Health Care in Early Christianity*. Baltimore: Johns Hopkins University Press, 2009.
Finnis, John, and Anthony Fisher. "Theology and the Four Principles: a Roman Catholic View I." In *Principles of Health Care Ethics*, edited by Raanan Gillon, 31–44. New York: Wiley, 1994.
Fletcher, Joseph. *Situation Ethics*. Philadelphia: Westminster, 1966.
Florida, R. E. "Buddhism and the Four Principles." In *Principles of Health Care Ethics*, edited by Raanan Gillon, 105–16. New York: Wiley, 1994.
Fox, Renee C. *The Sociology of Medicine: A Participant Observer's View*. Englewood Cliffs, NJ: Prentice-Hall, 1989.
Frank, Arthur. *The Renewal of Generosity: Illness, Medicine, and How to Live*. Chicago, IL: University of Chicago Press, 2004.
Frankena, William. "The Concept of Morality." In *The Definition of Morality*, edited by A. D. M. Walker and G. Wallace. London: Methuen, 1970.
———. *Ethics*. 2nd ed. Englewood Cliffs, NJ: Prentice-Hall, 1973.
Gaita, R. *A Common Humanity: Thinking About Love and Truth and Justice*. 2nd ed. New York: Routledge, 2000.
Gardner, E. Clinton. *Justice and Christian Ethics*. Cambridge: Cambridge University Press, 1995.

Bibliography

Gellman, Marc A. "On Immanuel Jakobvits: Bringing the Ancient World to the Modern World." In *Theological Voices in Medical Ethics*, edited by Allen Verhey and Stephen E. Lammers, 178–208. Grand Rapids: Eerdmans, 1993.

George, Robert P. "Natural Law Ethics." In *A Companion to Philosophy of Religion*, edited by Philip L. Quinn and Charles Taliaferro, 362–65. Oxford: Blackwell, 1997.

Gillon, Raanan. "The Four Principles Revisited—A Reappraisal." In *Principles of Health Care Ethics*, edited by Raanan Gillon, 319–33. New York: Wiley, 1994.

———. "Preface: Medical Ethics and the Four Principles." In *Principles of Health Care Ethics*, edited by Raanan Gillon, xxi–xxxi. New York: Wiley, 1994.

Glas, Gerrit. "Churchland, Kandel, and Dooyeweerd on the Reducibility of Mind States." *Philosophia Reformata* 67 (2002) 148–72.

———. "Ego, Self, and the Body: An Assessment of Dooyeweerd's Philosophical Anthropology." In *Christian Philosophy at the Close of the Twentieth Century: Assessment and Perspective*, edited by Sander Griffioen and B. M. Balk, 67–78. Kampen: Uitgeverij Kok, 1995.

———. "Persons and Their Lives: Reformational Philosophy on Man, Ethics, and Beyond." *Philosophia Reformata* 71 (2006) 31–57.

Glaser, William A. "Medical Care: Social Aspects." In *International Encyclopedia of Social Sciences* 10: 93–100. New York: MacMillan, 1968.

Goheen, Michael. W., and Craig G. Bartholomew. *Living at the Crossroads: An Introduction to Christian Worldview*. Grand Rapids: Baker Academics, 2008.

Grant, George. *Lament of a Nation*. Ottawa: Carleton University Press, 1995.

Greaves, Richard L. "The Origins and Early Development of English Covenant Thought." *The Historian* 31 (1968) 21–35.

Green, Ronald M. "Method in Bioethics: A Troubled Assessment." *Journal of Medicine and Philosophy* 15 (1990) 179–95.

Griffioen, Sander. "The Worldview Approach to Social Theory: Hazards and Benefits." In *Stained Glass: Worldviews and Social Science*, edited by Paul A. Marshall et al., 81–118. Christian Studies Today. Lanham, MD: University Press of America, 1989.

Guardini, Romano. *The World and the Person*. Chicago, IL: Regnery, 1965.

Gunton, Colin. *The Triune Creator: A Historical and Systematic Study*. Grand Rapids: Eerdmans, 1998.

Gustafson, James M. "Context versus Principles: A Misplaced Debate in Christian Ethics." *Harvard Theological Review* 58 (1965) 171–202.

———. *The Contributions of Theology to Medical Ethics*. Milwaukee, WI: Marquette University Press, 1975.

———. *Intersections: Science, Theology, and Ethics*. Cleveland: Pilgrim, 1996.

———. "Theology Confronts Technology and the Life Sciences." *Commonweal* 105 (1978) 386–92.

———. *Varieties of Moral Discourse: Prophetic, Narrative, Ethical, and Policy*. The Stob Lectures 1987–1988. Grand Rapids: Calvin College and Seminary, 1988.

Gutmann, Amy, and Dennis Thompson, *Democracy and Disagreement*. Cambridge, MA: Harvard University Press, 1996.

Habermas, Jürgen. *Between Facts and Norms: Contributions to a Discourse Theory of Law and Democracy*. Cambridge, MA: MIT Press, 1996.

———. *Between Naturalism and Religion: Philosophical Essays*. Cambridge, UK: Polity, 2008.

Bibliography

———. *Der Philosophische Diskurs Der Moderne*. Frankfurt am Main: Suhrkamp Verlag, 1985.

———. *The Philosophical Discourse of Modernity*. Translated by Frederick Lawrence. Introduction by Thomas McCarthy, vi-xvii. Cambridge, MA: MIT Press, 1987.

Habgood, John. "An Anglican View of the Four Principles." In *Principles of Health Care Ethics*, edited by Raanan Gillon, 55-64. New York: Wiley, 1994.

Hagen, Kenneth. "From Testament to Covenant in the Early Sixteenth Century." *Sixteenth Century Journal* 3 (1972) 1-15.

Hahn, Scott W. "Canon, Cult, and Covenant: The Promise of Liturgical Hermeneutics." In *Canon and Biblical Interpretation*, edited by Craig G. Bartholomew et al., 207-35. Scripture and Hermeneutics 7. Grand Rapids: Zondervan, 2006.

———. "Kinship by Covenant: A Biblical Theological Study of Covenant Types and Texts in the Old and New Testaments." PhD diss., UMI Dissertation Services, 1995.

Hare, John. "Can We Be Good Without God? Explorations in Religious Belief and Scholarship." In *Faithful Imagination in the Academy*, edited by Janel M. Curry and Ronald A. Wells, 31-42. New York: Rowman and Littlefield, 2008.

Hare, Richard M. *Freedom and Reason*. Oxford: Clarendon, 1963.

———. "Rawls' Theory of Justice." In *Reading Rawls: Critical Studies on Rawls' "A Theory of Justice,"* edited by Norman Daniels, 81-107. Oxford: Blackwell, 1975.

———. "*In Vitro* Fertilization and the Warnock Report." In *Ethics, Reproduction and Genetic Control*, edited by Ruth F. Chadwick, 71-92. London: Croom Helm, 1987.

Harrison, Christine N. et al. "Bioethics for Clinicians: 9. Involving Children in Decisions." *Canadian Medical Association Journal* 156 (1997) 825-28.

Hauerwas, Stanley. *Against the Nations: War and Survival in a Liberal Society*. Minneapolis: Winston, 1985.

———. "How Christian Ethics Became Medical Ethics: The Case of Paul Ramsey." *Christian Bioethics* 1 (1995) 11-28.

———. *The Peaceable Kingdom*. Notre Dame, IN: University of Notre Dame Press, 1983.

———. "Politics, Vision, and the Common Good." *Crosscurrents* 20 (1970) 399-414.

Hegel, George W. F. *Hegel's Lectures on the History of Philosophy*. London: Routledge, 1892.

———. *Hegel's Philosophy of Right*. London: Oxford University Press, 1967.

———. *Lectures on the Philosophy of Religion*. Berkeley, CA: University of California Press, 1984.

———. *The Philosophy of History*. New York: Dover, 1956.

Hesse, Mary. "How to Be Postmodern without Being Feminist." *The Monist* 77 (1994) 445-61

Hiebert, Paul. *Anthropological Reflections on Missiological Issues*. Grand Rapids: Baker Books, 1994.

Hielema, Syd. "Herman Bavinck's Eschatological Understanding of Redemption." PhD diss., Wycliffe College, Toronto School of Theology, 1998.

Hittinger, Russell. "Theology and Natural Law Theory." *Communio (International Catholic Review)* 17 (1990) 402-08.

Hodge, Charles. *Systematic Theology*. Grand Rapids: Eerdmans, 1940.

Hodges, Herbert A. *Wilhelm Dilthey: An Introduction*. New York: Oxford University Press, 1945.

Hoekema, Anthony A. *Created in God's Image*. Grand Rapids: Eerdmans, 1986.
Hoeksema, Herman. *Reformed Dogmatics*. Grands Rapids: Reformed Free, 1966.
Hoitenga, Dewey J. *Faith and Reason from Plato to Plantinga: An Introduction to Reformed Epistemology*. Albany: State University of New York Press, 1991.
Holmes, Arthur F. *Contours of a World View*. Grand Rapids: Eerdmans, 1983.
———. *The Idea of a Christian College*. Grand Rapids: Eerdmans, 1975.
Holmes, Robert L. "The Limited Relevance of Analytical Ethics to the Problems of Bioethics." *Journal of Medicine and Philosophy* 15 (1990) 143–59.
Hoogland, Jan, and Henk Jochemsen. "Professional Autonomy and the Normative Structure of Medical Practice." *Theoretical Medicine* 21 (2000) 457–75.
Hoose, Bernard. "Theology and the Four Principles: a Roman Catholic View II." In *Principles of Health Care Ethics*, edited by Raanan Gillon, 45–54. New York: Wiley, 1994.
Horsley, Richard A. "The Law of Nature in Philo and Cicero." *Harvard Theological Review* 71 (1978) 35–59.
Horton, Michael S. "Participation and Covenant." In *Radical Orthodoxy and the Reformed Tradition*, edited by James K. A. Smith and James H. Olthuis, 107–32. Grand Rapids: Baker Academic, 2005.
Hughes, Graham. *Worship as Meaning: A Liturgical Theology for Late Modernity*. Cambridge, UK: Cambridge University Press, 2003.
Hume, David. *Enquiry Concerning the Principles of Morals*. Oxford: Oxford University Press, 1998.
Hunter, James D. *To Change the World: The Irony, Tragedy, & Possibility of Christianity in the Late Modern World*. Oxford: Oxford University Press, 2010.
Husserl, Edmund. *Cartesian Meditations: An Introduction to Phenomenology*. The Hague: Martinus Nijhoff, 1973.
———. *Formal and Transcendental Logic*. The Hague: Martinus Nijhoff, 1969.
Iltis, Ana. S. "Bioethics as Methodological Case Resolution: Specification, Specified Principlism, and Casuistry." *Journal of Medicine and Philosophy* 25 (2000) 271–84.
Jacobson, Christine C., J. C. Nguyen, and A. B. Kimball. "Gender and Parenting Significantly Affect Work Hours of Recent Dermatology Program Graduates." *Archives of Dermatology* 140 (2004) 191–96.
Jaeger, Werner. "Aristotle's Use of Medicine as a Model of His Ethics." *Journal of the History of Science* 77 (1957) 54–61.
———. *Early Christianity and the Greek Paideia*. Cambridge, MA: Harvard University Press, 1965.
Jecker, Nancy. "The Role of Intimate Others in Medical Decision Making." In *Aging and Ethics: Philosophical Problems in Gerontology*, edited by Nancy Jecker, 199–216. Clifton, NJ: Humana, 1991.
Jochemsen, Henk. "Normative Practices as an Intermediate between Theoretical Ethics and Morality." *Philosophia Reformata* 71 (2006) 96–112.
Jochemsen, Henk, and Jan van der Stoep. *Different Cultures—One World: Dialogue between Christians and Muslims about Globalizing Technology*. Amsterdam: Rozenberg, 2010.
Jones, David. "The Hippocratic Oath: Its Content and the Limits to Its Adaptation." *Catholic Medical Quarterly* 54 (2003). No pages. Online: http://www.cmq.org.uk/CMQ/2003/hippocratic_oath.htm.
———. *The Soul and the Embryo*. London: Continuum, 2004.

Bibliography

Jones, W. H. S. *The Doctor's Oath*. London: Cambridge University Press, 1924.
Jonsen, Albert R. *The Birth of Bioethics*. Oxford: Oxford University Press, 1998.
———. "Casuistry as Methodology in Clinical Ethics." *Theoretical Medicine* 12 (1991) 295–307.
———. "Clinical Ethics and the Four Principles." In *Principles of Health Care Ethics*, edited by Raanan Gillon, 13–22. New York: Wiley, 1994.
———. *The New Medicine & the Old Ethics*. Cambridge, MA: Harvard University Press, 1990.
Jonsen, Albert R., and Andre Hellegers. "Conceptual Foundations for and Ethics of Medical Care." In *Ethics of Health Care*, edited by Laurence R. Tancredi, 3–20. Washington, DC: National Academy of Sciences, 1974.
Jonsen, Albert R., and Lewis Butler. "Public Ethics and Policy Making." *Hastings Center Report* 5 (1975) 19–31.
Jonsen, Albert R., and Stephen Toulmin. *The Abuse of Casuistry: A History of Moral Reasoning*. Berkeley, CA: University of California Press, 1988.
Justin, Martyr, Saint. *The Writings of Justin Martyr and Athenagoras*. Edited by M. Dodds et al. London: T. & T. Clark, 1909.
Kasenene, Peter. "African Ethical Theory and the Four Principles." In *Principles of Health Care Ethics*, edited by Raanan Gillon, 183–92. New York: Wiley, 1994.
Kass, Leon. "Is There a Medical Ethic: The Hippocratic Oath and Sources of Ethical Medicine." In *Toward a More Natural Science*, 224–46. New York: Free Press, 1985.
———. "Practicing Ethics: Where's the Action?" *Hastings Center Report* 20 (1990) 5–12.
———. "Regarding the End of Medicine and Pursuit of Health." *The Public Interest* 40 (1975) 27–29.
Kelly, David F. *The Emergence of Roman Catholic Medical Ethics in North America: A Historical-Methodological-Bibliographical Study*. New York: Mellen, 1979.
Kelly, George A. *Politics and Religious Consciousness in America*. New Brunswick, NJ: Transaction, 1974.
Kerner, George C. *Revolution in Ethical Theory*. New York: Oxford University Press, 1966.
Kierkegaard, Søren. *Works of Love*. Edited and tranlsated by Howard V. Hong and Edna H. Hong. Princeton, NJ: Princeton University Press, 1995.
Klapwijk, Jacob. "On Worldviews and Philosophy: A Response to Wolters and Olthuis." In *Stained Glass: Worldviews and Social Science*, edited by Paul Marshall, Sander Griffioen, and Richard J. Mouw, 41–55. Lanham, MD: University Press of America, 1989.
Klassen, William. *Covenant and Community*. Grand Rapids: Eerdmans, 1968.
Kline, Meredith. *By Oath Consigned*. Grand Rapids: Eerdmans, 1968.
Kluback, William, and Martin Weinbaum. *Dilthey's Philosophy of Existence: Introduction to Welanschauungslehre*. New York: Bookman, 1957.
Konig, Adrio. "An Outline of a Contemporary Covenant Theology." *Calvin Theological Journal* 29 (1994) 180–89.
Kopelman, Loretta M. "What is Applied about 'Applied' Philosophy?" *Journal of Medicine and Philosophy* 15 (1990) 199–218.
Lammers, Stephen E. "On Stanley Hauerwas: Theology, Medical Ethics, and the Church." In *Theological Voices in Medical Ethics*, edited by Allen Verhey and Stephen E. Lammers, 57–77. Grand Rapids: Eerdmans, 1993.

Landis, David A. "Physician Distinguish Thyself: Conflict and Covenant in a Physician's Moral Development." *Perspectives in Biology and Medicine* 36 (1993) 628–41.

Langerak, Edward. "Duties to Others and Covenantal Ethics." In *Duties to Others*, edited by Courtney S. Campbell and B. Andrew Lustig, 91–108. Theology and Medicine 4. Dordrecht: Kluwer Academic, 1994.

Lebacqz, Karen. "On the Elusive Nature of Respect." In *The Human Embryonic Stem Cell Debate*, edited by Suzanne Holland et al., 149–62. Cambridge: MIT Press, 2001.

Levi, R. B., and D. Drotar. "Health-related Quality of Life in Childhood Cancer." *International Journal of Cancer* 12 (1999) 58–64.

Levinas, Emmanuel. *Otherwise Than Being, or Beyond Essence*. The Hague: Martinus Nijhoff, 1981.

———. *Totality and Infinity*. Pittsburgh: Duquesne University Press, 1969.

Lewis, C. S. *The Four Loves*. New York: Harcourt Brace Jovanovich, 1960.

Li, James T. C. "The Patient-Physician Relationship: Covenant or Contract?" *Mayo Clinic Proceedings* 71 (1996) 917–18.

Lief, H. I., and R. C. Fox. "Training for 'Detached Concern' in Medical Students." In *The Psychological Basis of Medical Practice*, edited by H. I. Lief et al., 12–35. New York: Harper and Row, 1963.

Lillback, Peter A. *The Binding of God: Calvin's Role in the Development of Covenant Theology*. Grand Rapids: Baker Academic, 2001.

———. "The Continuing Conundrum: Calvin and the Conditionality of the Covenant." *Calvin Theological Journal* 29 (1994) 42–74.

Lindemann, Andreas. "'Do Not Let a Woman Destroy the Unborn Baby in Her Belly': Abortion in Ancient Judaism and Christianity." *Studia Theologica* 49 (1995) 253–71.

Little, David, and Sumner B. Twiss. "Basic Terms in the Study of Religion." In *Religion and Morality*, edited by Gene Outka and J. P. Reeder. Garden City, NY: Anchor, 1973.

Locke, John. *An Essay on Human Understanding*. Edited by Peter H. Nidditch. Oxford: Oxford University Press, 1975.

Lockwood, Michael. "The Warnock Report: A Philosophical Appraisal." In *Moral Dilemmas in Modern Medicine*, 155–86. New York: Oxford University Press, 1985.

Louthan, Stephen. "On Religion—A Discussion with Richard Rorty, Alvin Plantinga, and Nicholas Wolterstorff." *Christian Scholar's Review* 26 (1996) 177–83.

Lyotard, Jean-Francois. *The Postmodern Condition: A Report on Knowledge*. Minneapolis: University of Minnesota Press, 1984.

MacIntyre, Alasdair. *After Virtue*. 2nd ed. Notre Dame, IN: University of Notre Dame Press, 1984.

———. "How to Identify Ethical Principles." In *The Belmont Report: Ethical Principles and Guidelines for the Protection of Human Subjects of Research*, 10.1–10.41. Washington, DC: U.S. Government Printing Office, 1978.

———. *Whose Justice? Which Rationality?* Notre Dame, IN: University of Notre Dame Press, 1988.

Marshall, Paul. "Epilogue: Faith and Social Science." In *Stained Glass: Worldviews and Social Science*, edited by Paul Marshall et al., 184–87. Christian Studies Today. Lanham, MD: University Press of America, 1989.

Bibliography

Marty, Martin E. "Medical Ethics and Theology: The Accounting of the Generations." In *Theological Voices in Medical Ethics*, edited by Allen Verhey and Stephen E. Lammers, 239–56. Grand Rapids: Eerdmans, 1993.

May, William F. "Code, Covenant, Contract, or Philanthropy." *Hastings Center Report* 5 (1975) 29–38.

———. *The Physician's Covenant*. Philadelphia: Westminster, 1983.

———. *Testing the Medical Covenant: Active Euthanasia and Health Care Reform*. Grand Rapids: Eerdmans, 1996.

———. "The Virtues in a Professional Setting." In *Medicine and Moral Reasoning*, edited by K. W. M. Fulford et al., 75–90. Cambridge: Cambridge University Press, 1994.

McArdle, Patrick. *Relational Health Care: A Practical Theology of Personhood*. Saarbrucken: VDM Verlag Dr. Muller, 2008.

McCarthy, Dennis J. *Old Testament Covenant: A Survey of Current Opinions*. Atlanta: John Knox, 1972.

———. *Treaty and Covenant*. Rome: Pontifical Biblical Institute, 1978.

McCarthy, Rockne et al. *Society, State, & Schools: A Case for Structural and Confessional Pluralism*. Grand Rapids: Eerdmans, 1981.

McCarthy, Vincent A. *The Phenomenology of Moods in Kierkegaard*. Boston: Nijhoff, 1978.

McCormick, Richard A. "Bioethics in the Public Forum." *Health and Society (Milbank Memorial Fund Quarterly)* 61 (1983) 113–26.

———. *The Critical Calling: Reflections on Moral Dilemmas Since Vatican II*. Washington, DC: Georgetown University Press, 1989.

———. "Does Religious Faith Add to Ethical Perception?" In *Personal Values in Public Policy: Conversations on Government Decision-making*, edited by John C. Haughey, 167–70. New York: Paulist, 1979.

———. "Proxy Consent in the Experimental Situation." In *Love and Society: Essays in the Ethics of Paul Ramsey*, edited by James T. Johnson and David H. Smith, 209–28. Missoula, MT: Scholars, 1974.

McCoy, Charles S. "Johannes Cocceius: Federal Theologian." *Scottish Journal of Theology* 16 (1963) 352–70.

McFadyen, Alistair I. *Bound to Sin: Abuse, Holocaust, and the Christian Doctrine of Sin*. Cambridge, UK: Cambridge University Press, 2000.

McMurray, Julia E. et al. "Women in Medicine: A Four-Nation Comparison." *Journal of the American Medical Women's Association* 57 (2002) 185–90.

Meier, Andreas. "De Geburt de 'Weltanschauung' im 19. Jahrhundert." *Theologische Rundschau* 62 (1997) 414–20.

Meilaender, Gilbert. *Neither Beast nor God: The Dignity of the Human Person*. New York: Encounter, 2009.

———. "Comments of Gilbert Meilaender." *Journal of the Society of Christian Ethics* 24 (2004) 191–95.

———. "On William F. May: Corrected Vision for Medical Ethics." In *Theological Voices in Medical Ethics*, edited by Allen Verhey and Stephen E. Lammers, 106–26. Grand Rapids: Eerdmans, 1993.

———. Review of *The Foundations of Christian Bioethics*, by H. Tristram Engelhardt, Jr. *First Things* (November 2000).

———. *The Theory and Practice of Virtue*. Notre Dame, IN: University of Notre Dame Press, 1984.

Meland, Bernard E. *Fallible Forms and Symbols: Discourses of Method in a Theology of Culture*. Philadelphia: Fortress, 1976.

———. *The Realities of Faith: The Revolution in Cultural Forms*. New York: Oxford University Press, 1962.

Meslin, Eric M. et al. "Principlism and the Ethical Appraisal of Clinical Trials." *Bioethics* 9 (1995) 399–418.

Mill, J. S. *Utilitarianism*. 2nd vol. Indianapolis, IN: Hackett, 2001.

Miller, Richard B. *Children, Ethics, and Modern Medicine*. Bloomington, IN: Indiana University Press, 2003.

Molema, J. J. W. et al. "Healthcare System Design and Parttime Working Doctors." *Health Care Management Science* 10 (2007) 365–71.

Moore, George E. *Principia Ethica*. Cambridge: Cambridge University Press, 1903.

Moore, Peter. *Being Me: What It Means to Be Human*. Chichester, UK: Wiley, 2003.

———. *Enhancing Me: The Hope and Hype of Human Enhancement*. Chichester, UK: Wiley, 2008.

Mount, Eric. *Covenant, Community, and the Common Good: An Interpretation of Christian Ethics*. Cleveland: Pilgrim, 1999.

Mouw, Richard J. *The God Who Commands*. Notre Dame, IN: University of Notre Dame Press, 1990.

Murray, John. "The Adamic Administration." In *Collected Writings of John Murray*. vol. 2, 47–59. Edinburgh: Banner of Truth Trust, 1977.

Naugle, David. *Worldview: The History of a Concept*. Grand Rapids: Eerdmans, 2002.

Nelson, J. L. "Duties to Patients and Their Caregivers." In *Duties to Others*, edited by Courtney S. Campbell and B. Andrew Lustig, 199–214. Theology and Medicine 4. Dordrecht: Kluwer Academic, 1994.

Newbigin, Lesslie. *The Gospel in a Pluralist Society*. Grand Rapids: Eerdmans, 1989.

Nicholson, Ernest W. *God and His People: Covenant and Theology in the Old Testament*. Oxford: Clarendon, 1986.

Nicholson, R. H. "Limitations of the Four Principles." In *Principles of Health Care Ethics*, edited by Raanan Gillon, 267–75. New York: Wiley, 1994.

Niebuhr, H. Richard. *Christ and Culture*. New York: Harper, 1951.

Nielsen, Kai. "On Moral Truth." In *Studies in Moral Philosophy: Essays by David Braybrooke and Others*, edited by Nicholas Rescher, 9–25. American Philosophical Monthly Monograph Series 1. Oxford: Blackwell, 1968.

———. "Skepticism and Human Rights." *The Monist* 52 (1968) 573–94.

Nisker, Jeffrey. "A Covenantal Model for the Medical Educator-Student Relationship: Lessons from the Covenant Model of the Physician-Patient Relationship." *Medical Education* 40 (2006) 502–03.

Noddings, Nel. *Caring: A Feminine Approach to Ethics and Moral Education*. Berkeley, CA: University of California Press, 1984.

Noonan, Jr. John T. "An Almost Absolute Value in History." In *The Morality of Abortion: Legal and Historical Perspectives*, edited by John T. Noonan Jr., 7–18. Cambridge: Harvard University Press, 1970.

Norris, Christopher. *Deconstruction and the "Unfinished Project of Modernity."* New York: Routledge, 2000.

Bibliography

Novak, David. *Covenantal Rights: A Study in Jewish Political Theory*. Princeton: Princeton University Press, 2000.

———. "The Human Person as the Image of God." In *Personhood and Health Care*, edited by David C. Thomasma et al., 43–54. International Library of Ethics, Law, and the New Medicine 7. Dordrecht: Kluwer Academic, 2001.

———. *Jewish-Christian Dialogue*. Oxford: Oxford University Press, 1989.

———. *Law and Theology in Judaism*. New York: Ktav, 1976.

Nozick, Robert. *Anarchy, State, and Utopia*. New York: Basic, 1974.

O'Donovan, Oliver. *Begotten or Made?* Oxford: Oxford University Press, 1984.

———. *The Desire of the Nations: Rediscovering the Roots of Political Theology*. Cambridge: Cambridge University Press, 1996.

———. *Resurrection and Moral Order: An Outline of Evangelical Ethics*. 2nd ed. Grand Rapids: Eerdmans, 1994.

———. *The Ways of Judgment*. Grand Rapids: Eerdmans, 2005.

Olthuis, James H. "The Covenanting Metaphor of the Christian Faith and the Self Psychology of Heinz Kohut." *Studies in Religion* 18 (1989) 313–24.

———. "On Worldviews." In *Stained Glass: Worldviews and Social Science*, edited by Paul Marshall et al., 26–40. Christian Studies Today. Lanham, MD: University Press of America, 1989.

Orr, James. *The Christian View of God and the World*. Grand Rapids: Kregel, 1989.

Orr, Robert D. et al. "Use of the Hippocratic Oath: A Review of Twentieth Century Practice and a Content Analysis of Oaths Administered in Medical Schools in the US and Canada in 1993." *Journal of Clinical Ethics* 8 (1997) 374–85.

Outka, Gene. *Agape*. New Haven, CT: Yale University Press, 1972.

———. "Character, Conduct, and Love Commandment." In *Norm and Context in Christian Ethics*, edited by Gene. H. Outka and Paul Ramsey, 37–66. New York: Scribner, 1968.

Outka, Gene, and Paul Ramsey. *Norm and Context in Christian Ethics*. New York: Scribner, 1968.

Parfit, Derek. *Reasons and Persons*. Oxford: Oxford University Press, 1984.

Parkerton, Patricia H. et al. "Effect of Part-time Practice on Patient Outcomes." *Journal of General Internal Medicine* 18 (2003) 717–24.

Pascal, Blaise. *The Provincial Letters*. Translated by A. J. Krailsheimer. Harmondsworth: Penguin, 1967.

Pearcey, Nancy. *Total Truth: Liberating Christianity From Its Cultural Captivity*. Wheaton, IL: Crossway, 2004.

Pellegrino, Edmund D. "Epilogue: Religion and Bioethical Discourse." In *Jewish and Catholic Bioethics: An Ecumenical Dialogue*, 139–45. Washington, DC: Georgetown University Press, 1999.

———. "The Four Principles and the Doctor-Patient Relationship: The Need for a Better Linkage." In *Principles of Health Care Ethics*, edited by Raanan Gillon, 353–64. New York: Wiley, 1994.

———. "The Healing Relationship: The Architectonics of Clinical Medicine." In *The Clinical Encounter*, edited by Earl E. Shelp, 153–72. Philosophy and Medicine 14. Dordrecht: D. Reidel, 1983.

———. "Philosophy of Medicine: Should it be Teleologically or Socially Construed?" *Kennedy Institute of Ethics Journal* 11 (2001) 169–80.

Bibliography

———. "Toward a Reconstruction of Medical Morality: The Primacy of the Act of Profession and the Fact of Illness." *Journal of Medicine and Philosophy* 4 (1979) 32–56.

———. "What the Philosophy *of* Medicine Is." *Theoretical Medicine and Bioethics* 19 (1998) 315–36.

Pellegrino, Edmund D., and David C. Thomasma. *The Christian Virtues in Medical Practice*. Washington, DC: Georgetown University Press, 1996.

———. *A Philosophical Basis of Medical Practices: Toward a Philosophy and Ethic of the Healing Professions*. New York: Oxford University Press, 1981.

Pieper, Josef. *Belief and Faith*. New York: Pantheon, 1963.

Plantinga, Alvin. "Advice to Christian Philosophers." *Faith and Philosophy* 1 (1984) 253–71.

———. "Reason and Belief in God." In *Faith and Rationality: Reason and Belief in God*, edited by Alvin Plantinga and Nicholas Wolterstorff, 16–93. Notre Dame, IN: University of Notre Dame Press, 1983.

Porter, Jean. *Natural and Divine Law: Reclaiming the Tradition for Christian Ethics*. Grand Rapids: Eerdmans, 1999.

———. "Natural Law as a Scriptural Concept: Theological Reflections on a Medieval Theme." *Theology Today* 59 (2002) 226–43.

Preston, Ronald. H. "The Four Principles and Their Use: The Possibility of Agreement Between Different Faiths and Philosophies." In *Principles of Health Care Ethics*, edited by Raanan Gillon, 23–30. New York: Wiley, 1994.

Preuss, James S. *From Shadow to Promise*. Cambridge, UK: Belknap, 1969.

Ramsey, Paul. *Basic Christian Ethics*. New York: Scribner, 1952.

———. "The Case of the Curious Exception." In *Norm and Context in Christian Ethics*, edited by Gene H. Outka and Paul Ramsey, 67–139. New York: Scribner, 1968.

———. *Christian Ethics and Social Policy*. New York: Scribner, 1958.

———. "Commentary." In *Ethics of Health Care*, edited by Laurence R. Tancredi. Washington, DC: National Academy of Sciences, 1974.

———. *Deeds and Rules in Christian Ethics*. New York: Scribner, 1967.

———. *The Essential Paul Ramsey: A Collection*. Edited by William Werpehowski and Stephen D. Crocco. New Haven, CT: Yale University Press, 1994.

———. *Ethics at the Edge of Life*. New Haven, CT: Yale University Press, 1978.

———. "The Indignity of 'Death with Dignity.'" *The Hastings Center Studies* 2 (1974) 47–62.

———. *The Patient as Person*. New Haven, CT: Yale University Press, 1970.

———. "Shall We 'Reproduce'? I. The Medical Ethics in In Vitro Fertilization." *Journal of the American Medical Association* 220 (1972a) 1346–50.

———. "Shall We 'Reproduce'? II. Rejoiners and Future Forecast." *Journal of the American Medical Association* 220 (1972b) 1480–85.

Ratzinger, Joseph. *Many Religions—One Covenant*. San Francisco: Ignatius, 1999.

———. *The Spirit of the Liturgy*. San Francisco: Ignatius, 2000.

Rawls, John. "The Idea of Public Reason Revisited." *The University of Chicago Law Review* 64 (1997) 765–807.

———. "The Independence of Moral Theory." *Proceedings and Addressed of the American Philosophical Association* 48 (1974–1975) 5–22.

———. *Political Liberalism*. Expanded edition. New York: Columbia University Press, 2005.

Bibliography

———. *A Theory of Justice*. Cambridge: Harvard University Press, 1971.
Richardson, Henry S. "Specifying, Balancing, and Interpreting Bioethical Principles." *Journal of Medicine and Philosophy* 25 (2000) 285–307.
———. "Specifying Norms as a Way to Resolve Concrete Ethical Problems." *Philosophy and Public Affairs* 19 (1990) 279–310.
Ridderbos, Herman N. *The Coming of the Kingdom*. Philadelphia: Presbyterian and Reformed, 1969.
———. *The Epistle of Paul to the Churches of Galatia*. Grand Rapids: Eerdmans, 1953.
Robertson, O. Palmer. *The Christ and the Covenants*. Grand Rapids: Baker, 1980.
Robinson, John A. T. *Wrestling with Romans*. Philadelphia: Westminster, 1979.
Robinson, Lynn D. "Doing Good and Doing Well: Shareholder Activism, Responsible Investment, and Mainline Protestantism." In *The Quiet Hand of God: Faith-Based Activism and the Public Role of Mainline Protestantism*, edited by Robert Wuthnow and John H. Evans, 343–63. Berkeley, CA: University of California Press, 2002.
Rorty, Richard. *Contingency, Irony, and Solidarity*. Cambridge: Cambridge University Press, 1989.
Rose, Margaret. *The Post-Modern and the Post-Industrial: A Critical Analysis*. Cambridge, UK: Cambridge University Press, 1991.
Ross, William D. *The Foundations of Ethics*. Oxford, UK: Clarendon, 1939.
———. *The Right and the Good*. Oxford, UK: Clarendon, 1930. Reprint, Indianapolis, IN: Hackett, 1988.
Rudnick, Abraham. "A Meta-ethical Critique of Care Ethics." *Theoretical Medicine* 22 (2001) 505–17.
Rusthoven, James J. "Are Human Embryos One of Us? An Exploration of Personhood." *Pro Rege* 36 (2007) 8–17.
———. "Book Review—Medicine, Religion, and Health: Where Science and Spirituality Meet by Harold Koenig." *Perspectives in Science and the Christian Faith* 61 (2009) 127.
Rutten, Thomas. "Receptions of the Hippocratic Oath in the Renaissance: The Prohibition of Abortion as a Case Study in Reception." *The Journal of the History of Medicine* 51 (1996) 456–83.
Ryan, Kenneth J. et al. *The Belmont Report: Ethical Principles and Guidelines for the Protection of Human Subjects of Research*. National Institutes of Health, 1979.
Schaeffer, Francis A. *The Complete Works of Francis Schaeffer*. 2nd ed. 5 vols. Wheaton, IL: Crossway, 1982.
Schmemann, Alexander. *For the Life of the World: Sacraments and Orthodoxy*. 2nd ed. Crestwood, NY: St. Vladimir's Seminary Press, 1973.
Schuurman, Egbert. "The Challenge of Islam's Critique of Technology." *Perspectives in Science and the Christian Faith* 60 (2008) 75–83.
———. *The Technological World Picture and the Ethics of Responsibility: Struggles in the Ethics of Technology*. Dordt: Dordt College Press, 2005.
Seerveld, Calvin G. "Dooyeweerd's Legacy for Aesthetics: Modal Law Theory." In *The Legacy of Herman Dooyeweerd: Reflection on Critical Philosophy in the Christian Tradition*, edited by C. T. McIntire, 41–80. Lanham, MD: University Press of America, 1985.
Segal, Alan F. *Rebecca's Children*. Cambridge, MA: Harvard University Press, 1986.
Seldin, Donald. "The Boundaries of Medicine." *Transactions of the Association of American Physicians* 94 (1981) 75–86.

Serour, G. I. "Islam and the Four Principles." In *Principles of Health Care Ethics*, edited by Raanan Gillon, 75–92. New York: Wiley, 1994.

Siegler, Mark. "The Doctor-Patient Encounter and Its Relationship to Health and Disease." In *Concepts of Health and Disease: Interdisciplinary Perspectives*, edited by Arthur Caplan et al., 627–44. Reading, MA: Addison-Wesley, 1981.

Silberfeld, Michel. "Vulnerable Persons: Measuring Moral Capacity." In *The Variables of Moral Capacity*, edited by David C. Thomasma and David N. Weisstub, 203–15. International Library of Ethics, Law, and the New Medicine 21. Dordrecht: Kluwer Academic, 2004.

Singer, Peter. "Sidgwick and Reflective Equilibrium." *Monist* 58 (1974) 490–517.

Sire, James W. *Naming the Elephant: Worldview as a Concept*. Downers Grove, IL: InterVarsity, 2004.

———. *The Universe Next Door: A Basic Worldview Catalogue*. 4th ed. Downers Grove, IL: Intervarsity, 2004.

Smith, David H. "On Paul Ramsey: A Covenant-Centered Ethic for Medicine." In *Theological Voices in Medical Ethics*, edited by Allen Verhey and Stephen E. Lammers, 7–29. Grand Rapids: Eerdmans, 1993.

Smith, James K. A. *Desiring the Kingdom: Worship, Worldview, and Cultural Formation*. Grand Rapids: Baker Academic, 2009.

———. "Introduction: Reverberations." In *Radical Orthodoxy and the Reformed Tradition: Creation, Covenant, and Participation*, edited by James K. A. Smith and James H. Olthius, 15–21. Grand Rapids: Baker Academic, 2005.

———. "Little Story about Metanarratives: Lyotard, Religion, and Postmodernism Revisited." *Faith and Philosophy* 18 (2001) 353–68.

———. *Who's Afraid of Postmodernism? Taking Derrida, Lyotard, and Foucault to Church*. Grand Rapids: Baker Academic, 2006.

Somerville, Margaret. *The Ethical Imagination: Journeys of the Human Spirit*. Montreal: McGill-Queen's University Press, 2009.

Spicker, Stuart. F., and H. Tristram Engelhardt, Jr. *Philosophical Medical Ethics: Its Nature and Significance*. Dordrecht: Reidel, 1977.

Spykman, Gordon. *Reformational Theology: A New Paradigm for Doing Dogmatics*. Grand Rapids: Eerdmans, 1992.

Stafleu, M. D. "Philosophical Ethics and the So-called Ethical Aspect." *Philosophia Reformata* 72 (2007) 21–33.

Steer, Simon M. "Eating Bread in the Kingdom of God: The Foodways of Jesus in the Gospel of Luke." PhD diss., Westminster Theological Seminary, 2002.

Steinberg, Avraham. "A Jewish Perspective on the Four Principles." In *Principles of Health Care Ethics*, edited by Raanan Gillon, 65–74. New York: Wiley, 1994.

Stevenson, Charles L. *Ethics and Language*. New Haven, CT: Yale University Press, 1944.

Stevenson, Kenneth. *Covenant of Grace Renewed: A Vision of the Eucharist in the Seventeenth Century*. London: Darton Longman and Todd, 1994.

Stopes-Roe, Harry. "Principles and Life Stances: A Humanist View." In *Principles of Health Care Ethics*, edited by Raanan Gillon, 117–33. New York: Wiley, 1994.

Stout, Jeffrey. "Comments of Jeffrey Stout." *Journal of the Society of Christian Ethics* 24 (2004) 187–91.

———. *Ethics after Babel: The Language of Morals and Their Discontents*. Boston: Beacon, 1988.

Bibliography

Strauss, Danie F. M. *Philosophy: Discipline of the Disciplines.* Grand Rapids: Paideia, 2009.

Strong, Carson. "Specified Principlism: What Is It, and Does It Really Resolve Cases Better than Casuistry?" *Journal of Medicine and Philosophy* 25 (2000) 323–41.

Sturm, Douglas. "Contextual and Covenant: The Pertinence of Social Theory and Theology to Bioethics." In *Theology and Bioethics*, edited by Earl E. Shelp, 135–61. Boston: Reidel, 1985.

Suchman, Anthony L. "A Model of Empathic Communication in the Medical Interview." *Journal of the American Medical Association* 277 (1997) 678–82.

Sullivan, Dennis M. "Defending Human Personhood: Some Insights from Natural Law." *Christian Scholar's Review* 37 (2008) 289–302.

Sulmasy, Daniel P. "The Essentialist Medical Ethics of Edmund Pellegrino: Analysis and Critique." In *Physician Philosopher: The Philosophical Foundation of Medicine: Essays by Dr. Edmund Pellegrino*, edited by Roger J. Bulger and John P. McGovern, xvii–xxx. Charlottesville, VA: Carden Jennings, 2001.

———. *The Rebirth of the Clinic: An Introduction to Spirituality in Health Care.* Washington, DC: Georgetown University Press, 2006.

Sumner, Leonard W. "Does Medical Ethics Have Its Own Theory." *Hastings Center Report* 12 (1982) 38–39.

Tatian. *The Writings of Tatian and Theophilus.* London: T. & T. Clark, 1867.

Taylor, Charles. "Justice After Virtue." In *After MacIntyre*, edited by John Horton and Susan Mendus. Cambridge: Polity, 1994.

———. *The Malaise of Modernity.* Concord, ON: Anansi, 1991.

———. *Sources of the Self.* Cambridge: Harvard University Press, 1989.

Thomasma, David C. "Choices, Autonomy, and Moral Capacity." In *The Variables of Moral Capacity*, edited by David C. Thomasma and David N. Weisstub, 9–22. International Library of Ethics, Law, and the New Medicine 21. Dordtrecht: Kluwer Academic, 2004.

Trinterud, Leonard J. "The Origins of Puritanism." *Church History* 20 (1951) 37–57.

Troost, Andree. *The Christian Ethos.* Bloemfontein: Patmos, 1983.

Tubbs, J. B, Jr. "Theology and the Invitation of the Stranger." In *Duties to Others*, edited by Courtney S. Campbell and B. Andrew Lustig, 39–53. Theology and Medicine 4. Dordrecht: Kluwer Academic, 1994.

Tversky, Amos, and Daniel Kahneman. "Judgment under Uncertainty: Heuristics and Biases." *Science* 185 (1974) 1124–31.

Van Gelder, Craig. "The Covenant's Missiological Character." *Calvin Theological Journal* 29 (1994) 190–97.

Van Leeuwen, Evert, and Gerrit K. Kimsma. "Philosophy of Medical Practice: A Discursive Approach." In *The Influence of Edmund D. Pellegrino's Philosophy of Medicine*, edited by David C. Thomasma, 99–112. Dordrecht: Kluwer, 1997.

Vaux, Kenneth L. *Health and Medicine in the Reformed Tradition.* New York: Crossroad, 1984.

Veatch, Robert M. *Gifford Lecture: Hippocratic, Religious and Secular Medical Ethics: The Points of Conflict.* No pages. Online: http://www.ed.ac.uk/schools-departments/humanities-soc-sci/news-events/lectures/gifford-lectures/archive/archive-2007-2008/prof-robert-veatch.

———. "Models for Ethical Medicine in a Revolutionary Age." *Hastings Center Report* 2 (1972) 5–7.

———. *A Theory of Medical Ethics*. New York: Basic, 1981.
Verhey, Allen. "The Hippocratic Oath—and a Christian Swearing It." In *On Moral Medicine: Theological Perspectives in Medical Ethics*, edited by Stephen E. Lammers and Allen Verhey, 108-19. 2nd ed. Grand Rapids: Eerdmans, 1998.
———. "On James Gustafson: Can Medical Ethics Be Christian?" In *Theological Voices in Medical Ethics*, edited by Allen Verhey and Stephen E. Lammers, 30-56. Grand Rapids: Eerdmans, 1993.
Verhey, Allen, and Stephen E. Lammers. "Introduction: Rediscovering Religious Traditions in Medical Ethics." In *Theological Voices in Medical Ethics*, edited by Allen Verhey and Stephen E. Lammers. Grand Rapids: Eerdmans, 1993.
Vlastos, Gregory. "Justice and Equality." In *Social Justice*, edited by Richard B. Brandt. Englewood Cliffs, NJ: Prentice-Hall, 1962.
Vollenhoven, D. H. T. *Introduction to Philosophy*. Sioux Center, IA: Sioux Center, 2005.
von Balthasar, Hans Urs. "Nine Propositions on Christian Ethics." In *Principles of Christian Morality*, edited by Joseph Ratzinger et al. San Francisco: Ignatius, 1986.
Vorgrimler, Herbert. *Sacramental Theology*. Collegeville, MN: Liturgical, 1992.
Vos, Gerhardus. *Biblical Theology*. Grand Rapids: Eerdmans, 1948.
———. "The Doctrine of the Covenant in Reformed Theology." In *Redemptive History and Biblical Interpretation: The Shorter Writings of Geerhardus Vos*, edited by R. B. Gaffin, 234-67. Phillipsburg, NJ: Presbyterian and Reformed, 1980.
Walker, A. D. M., and G. Wallace. "Introduction." In *The Definition of Morality*, edited by A. D. M. Walker and G. Wallace. London: Methuen, 1970.
Walsh, Brian J., and J. Richard Middleton. *The Transforming Vision: Shaping a Christian World View*. Downers Grove, IL: InterVarsity, 1984.
Walters, LeRoy. "Religion and the Renaissance of Medical Ethics in the United States: 1965-1975." In *Theology and Bioethics: Exploring the Foundation and Frontiers*, edited by Earl E. Shelp, 3-16. Philosophy and Medicine 20. Dordrecht: Reidel, 1985.
Ware, Timothy. *The Orthodox Church*. Harmondsworth: Penguin, 1964.
Warnock, Mary. *A Question of Life*. Oxford: Blackwell, 1985.
Weir, David A. *The Origins of the Federal Theology in the Sixteenth-Century Reformation Thought*. Oxford, UK: Clarendon, 1990.
Weithman, Paul J. *Religion and the Obligations of Citizenship*. Cambridge: Cambridge University Press, 2002.
Welch, Sharon. *A Feminist Ethic of Risk*. Minneapolis: Fortress, 1990.
Wenham, Gordon J. "Sanctuary Symbolism in the Garden of Eden Story." *Proceedings of the World Congress of Jewish Studies* 9 (1986) 19-25.
Whitbeck, Caroline. "A Theory of Health." In *Concepts of Health and Disease*, edited by Arthur Caplan et al., 611-26. Reading, MA: Addison-Wesley, 1981.
Whitehead, Alfred N. *Religion in the Making*. New York: McMillan, 1962.
Wildes, Kevin W. *Moral Acquaintances*. Notre Dame, IN: University of Notre Dame Press, 2000.
Williams, George H. *The Radical Reformation*. Philadelphia: Westminster, 1962.
Winkler, Earl. "Moral Philosophy and Bioethics: Contexualism versus the Paradigm Theory." In *Philosophical Perspectives in Bioethics*, edited by L. W. Sumner and Joseph Boyle, 50-78. Toronto: University of Toronto Press, 1996.
Witvliet, John D. *Worship Seeking Understanding*. Grand Rapids: Baker Academic, 2003.

Bibliography

Wolters, Albert M. "Christianity and the Classics: A Typology of Attitude." In *Christianity and the Classics: The Acceptance of a Heritage*, edited by Wendy Helleman, 189–210. Lanham, MD: University Press of America, 1990.

———. *Creation Regained: Biblical Basics For a Reformational Worldview*. 2nd ed. Grand Rapids: Eerdmans, 2005.

———. "On the Idea of Worldview and Its Relation to Philosophy." In *Stained Glass Worldview and Social Science*, edited by Paul Marshall et al., 14–25. Christian Studies Today. Lanham, MD: University Press of America, 1989.

———. "No Longer Queen: The Theological Disciplines and Their Sisters." In *The Bible and the University*, edited by David L. Jeffrey and C. Stephen Evans, 59–79. Scripture and Hermeneutics 8. Grand Rapids: Zondervan, 2007.

Wolterstorff, Nicholas. "Can Belief in God Be Rational If It Has No Foundations?" In *Faith and Rationality: Reason and Belief in God*, edited by Alvin Plantinga and Nicholas Wolterstorff, 135–86. Notre Dame, IN: University of Notre Dame Press, 1983.

———. *Justice: Rights and Wrongs*. Princeton: Princeton University Press, 2008.

———. *Reason Within the Bounds of Religion*. Grand Rapids: Eerdmans, 1984.

———. *Until Justice and Peace Embrace*. Grand Rapids: Eerdmans, 1983.

———. "Why We Should Reject What Liberalism Tells Us About Speaking and Acting in Public for Religious Reasons." In *Religions and Contemporary Liberalism*, edited by Paul J. Weithman, 162–81. Notre Dame, IN: University of Notre Dame Press, 1997.

Woodward, P. A. *The Doctrine of Double Effect: Philosophers Debate a Controversial Moral Principle*. Notre Dame, IN: University of Notre Dame Press, 2001.

Wright, N. T. *The Climax of the Covenant: Christ and the Law in Pauline Theology*. Minneapolis: Fortress Press, 1992.

———. *Jesus and the Victory of God*. London: SPCK, 1996.

———. *Surprised by Hope*. London: Society for Promoting Christian Knowledge, 2007.

Wulff, Henrik. R. "Against the Four Principles: A Nordic View." In *Principles of Health Care Ethics*, edited by Raanan Gillon, 277–86. New York: Wiley, 1994.

Zaki Hasan, K. "Islam and the Four Principles: a Pakistani View." In *Principles of Health Care Ethics*, edited by Raanan Gillon, 93–103. New York: Wiley, 1994.

Zaner, Richard M. "Encountering the Other." In *Duties to Others*, edited by Courtney S. Campbell and B. Andrew Lustig, 17–38. Theology and Medicine 4. Dordrecht: Kluwer Academic, 1994.

———. "Illness and the Other." In *Theological Analyses of the Clinical Encounter*, edited by Gerald P. McKenny and Jonathan R. Sande, 85–202. Dordrecht: Kluwer Academic, 1993.

Zuidervaart, Lambert. "Good Cities or Cities of the Good?" In *Radical Orthodoxy and the Reformed Tradition*, edited by James K. A. Smith and James H. Olthuis, 135–49. Grand Rapids: Baker Academic, 2005.

Index

abortion, 257, 259, 261
accountability to God, 205
Adam, 140, 142–43, 176, 205, 206–7
Adelman, Ronald D., 237
advisory commissions, 65
After Virtue (MacIntyre), ix
agape love, 62, 85n79, 227, 231, 242, 247–48
   atheistic, 268
   Beauchamp and Childress on, 267
   and justice, 266
   Ramsey on, 89
Albert the Great, 17
Allen, Joseph, 146–47, 151, 175, 176, 229
analytical method, preoccupation with, 22
ancient times, philosophy relationship to medicine, 257–58
Anglican bioethicists, diversity among, 98–103
antifoundationalism, 19–20
applied ethics, vs. theoretical, 21
Aquinas, Thomas, 14–15, 17, 77, 144, 209
Arras, John, 232
Asklepeions, 234
atheistic *agape*, 268
Audi, Robert, 269
Augustine, 141
authority, 84
autonomous choice, 36

autonomy, 8–9, 74, 243, 250
   analysis, 49
   dominance in principlism, 75
   Engelhardt and, 83
   Finnis on, 102
   of patient decision making, 160, 162
   Steinberg on, 96
   tyranny of, 250

Bacon, Roger, 13–14
Baier, Kurt, 29
Bartholomew, Craig, 150, 153, 162, 197, 199
Bavinck, Herman, 140–41, 143, 145, 181, 195, 206
Beauchamp, Tom, 4, 33–34, 98–99, 183
   Principles of Biomedical Ethics, 1, 40–47, 127, 201–2, 244
Beecher, Henry, 28
belief in God, 19
Belmont Commission, 4, 27–35, 65, 241, 243
   nonmaleficence and beneficence, 245
   Pellegrino on, 71
   report, 1, 35–37, 44
Benedict XVI (pope), 148–49
beneficence, 36, 37, 75, 105, 243, 252–55
   analysis, 49
   in balance, 256–62
   Childress's principles of, 61

Index

beneficence (*cont.*)
  Finnis on, 102
  Hume on, 45
  vs. nonmaleficence, 253
  Pellegrino on, 9, 76
  Ramsey on, 93, 108
  role of, 41
  Sharia law on, 95
benevolence, 100, 167
berith (covenant), 140
Berkhof, Louis, 141
Berkouwer, G. C., 142
Bible
  Genesis, 205
  Deuteronomy, 265
  Jeremiah, 143
  Hosea 6:6, 255
  John 8:32, 248n21
  Acts, 16
  Romans 2:11–16, 245
  Romans 2:16, 17
  Romans 8:18–21, 248n21
  1 Corinthians, 16
  1 Corinthians 2:4, 5, 277
  2 Corinthians 3:12–18, 248n21
  covenant theme, 150
  Good Samaritan, 253–54
  Old Testament covenant relationships, 145
  Ten Commandments, 14
biblical anthropology, building covenantal relationality on, 170–77
biblical covenantal ethics, 129
  for biomedical ethics, 184–213
  God's love as core, 179–82
  history in, 274
  importance of personhood, 201–13
  justice within, 269–71
  normative expression of, 188
  and principlism, 241–48, 250
  response to covenantal relationship development, 247

biblical theology, vs. systematic theology, 199
bioethical thinking
  insufficiencies in contemporary, 24
  loss of expression of religious reasons for, 3
  personal moral beliefs affecting decisions, 23
bioethics
  inadequacies of contemporary, 117
  justifying moral decisions, 24–25
biomedical ethics, 10
  biblical covenantal ethic for, 184–213
  covenantal relationships as focus, 108
  reclaiming relational core for, 127–29
  secularization of, 59–67
body of Christ, church as, 188
Boersma, Hans, 233
Bok, Sissela, 20, 27
Botha, Elaine, 179
Bouma, Hessel III, 168–69
Breck, John, 84
Brock, Brian, 215–16
Brody, Baruch, 56–57
Brothers, Kyle, 134
Brunner, Emil, 266
Buddhist ethics, 265
Bullinger, Heindrich, 138
Butler, Joseph, 100

Cahill, Lisa, 65, 190–91, 274–76
Callahan, Daniel, 38–39, 60
Calvin, John, 139–40
Camenisch, Paul, 87, 161
Campbell, Courtney, 61–62, 230
care, responsibility for, 238
caregivers, 135–36, 214, 256
caring about persons, 38

Index

Carrick, Paul, 257
Cassel, Christine, 134
casuistry, 15, 17, 18, 53–54, 81
Chaplin, Jonathan, 217–18, 224–25
children
  participation in nonbeneficial experimentation, 91
  sacrifice, 259
  terminally ill, 241
Childress, James, 4, 29, 32–33, 61, 98–99, 183
  Principles of Biomedical Ethics, 1, 40–47, 127, 201–2, 244
Christian bioethicists, 59
Christian covenantal ethical framework, developing, 176
Christian ethics, Hauerwas on, 63
Christian freedom, 151
Christian life, 59
Christian philosophy
  of medical practice, 220–25
  merging with covenantal ethics, 210–13
Christian physicians, Pellegrino on, 71
Christian Scriptures, covenantal relationships in, 137–55. *See also* Bible
Christian worldview, 185–93, 245–46
Christians
  belief in God as final authority, 60
  diversity, 68–94
  Eastern Orthodox, 80, 84, 106, 191
  ethical worldview for, 218
  mission in society, 189
  response to covenantal relationship development, 137
  scientists as, 197
church, as body of Christ, 188
Clarke, W. Norris, 212
classical liberalism, 20

Clouser, K. Danner, 1–2, 40, 49–52
Clouser, Roy, 112
code of conduct, in Hippocratic Oath, 131
Coffey, Sue, 135
coherence theory, 43
commercial exploitation, protecting human subjects from, 94
common good, 44
common moral ground, 20
common moral law, 235
common morality, 8, 121–22, 272, 273, 277
  belief in, 178
  Engelhardt on, 82
  modernist hopes of achieving, 128
  Preston on movement, 43n111
  and private moralities, 243–44
  Veatch proposal on, 157
communicative ethic, 235–36
Communion, as covenant renewal, 193
community, 73, 166
compromise, 217
conceit of philanthropy, 231
confessional pluralism, 177
conscience, 17, 100, 103, 192
consensus, 2, 33, 262, 275–76
consent, Ramsey's emphasis on, 91
context for justice, 264
contingent process framework, 121
contraception, 257
contracts, vs. covenants, 165, 181
covenant, 129–30, 150
  biblical theology, Christian worldview and, 185–89
  Calvin on, 139–40
  Christian notions of, 203–6
  as conscious relationship with God, 78, 161
  vs. contracts, 165, 181
  of creation, 141, 142, 153, 154

303

Index

covenant (*cont.*)
  divine-human and human-human, 145–47
  between God and Jewish patient, 96
  of grace, 137, 138
  inclusive, 146–47, 168, 169, 175
  of the kingdom, 153
  as mission, 152
  with Noah, 140
  Ramsey's use of terminology, 88
  of redemption, 153
  redemptive, 146
  of trust, 133–34
  Veatch on, 49
  of works, 137, 141
covenant fidelity, 163
covenant love, 231
covenantal ethic, 4, 6, 210–13, 248–51, 272. *See also* biblical covenantal ethics
covenantal love, Ramsey's emphasis on, 87
covenantal relational network, medical practice as, 225–30
covenantal relationships
  between caregiver and patient, 108
  in Christian scriptures, 137–55
  and medicine, 137
covenantal theme, comprehensiveness of, 149–50
covenantal voluntarism, 224–25
Cranfield, C. E. B., 245
creation, covenant of, 141, 142, 153, 154, 236
creation theme, 162
creative discernment, 151
crisis casuistry, 81
Cunningham, Laurence, 103
Cyprian, 16

Dallmayr, Fred, 115
Daniels, Norman, 46

Decalogue, 151
deception, 106
DeGrazia, David, 53
deliberative democracy, 275
demoralization by example, 134n31
Dengerink, Jan, 219
Derrida, Jacques, 118, 194–95, 247
Devettere, Raymond, 57–58
Didache (Teaching of the Twelve Apostles), 69
Diderot, Denis, 20
dignity, 209–10, 258
Dilthey, Wilhelm, 110, 193–94
disinterested reflection, 34
disinterestedness, 165
distributive justice, 33–34, 83, 93, 262
divine-human relationship, biblical concept of, 160
Donagan, Alan, 56
Dooyeweerd, Herman, 172–74, 177, 196, 210, 217–20, 222
double covenant idea, 139
double relationship of humans with God, 144
doubt, 18
Dumbrell, William, 153
Dunn, James, 246

Eastern Orthodox Christian tradition, 80, 84, 106, 191
Edelstein, Ludwig, 131
Edwards, Jonathan, 91–92
egalitarian justice, 267
egalitarianism, 9
ekklesia, 166
elderly patients, 237
Ellul, Jacques, 210, 216
emotivists, 29
Engelhardt, H. Tristan, 33, 69, 80–85, 105–6, 184
  The Foundations of Bioethics, 80
  The Foundations of Christian Bioethics, 80, 81, 82, 106

Index

Engelhardt, H. Tristan (*cont.*)
  on moral strangers, 232
  on philosophical vs. theological ethics, 34
  on religious nature of secular morality, 81–82
enkaptic function, 223
enkaptic structural whole, 173, 210
enlightened unselfishness, 160
Enlightenment, x, 43, 45, 59, 99, 154
essential triad, 237
ethical considerations, iterative process, 57
ethical crisis, in human research, 27–37
ethical norms, 53
ethics, xi, 13–14, 21, 194. *See also* covenantal ethic; *entries beginning with* moral
evaluative expressions, 30
Evans, John H., 5, 64
evil, 175
expression, ethics as functions of, 29

fairness, 46
faith, 180
  expressing influence of, 3
  as gift of God, 77
  in rationality, 58, 113, 122
faithfulness, 86, 147
faithlessness, common morality of, 122
false claims, Beauchamp and Childress on, 42
fidelity, 108
Finnis, John, 101–2
Fletcher, Joseph, 85, 266
Florida, R. E., 265
foundation for principles, 56
foundationalism, 19, 24
The Foundations of Bioethics (Engelhardt), 80

The Foundations of Christian Bioethics (Engelhardt), 80, 81, 82, 106
four principles. *See* principlism
fragmentation in modern society, 128
fragmenting care, 236
Frankena, William, 37–38
free agents, respect for persons as, 80
freedom, 80, 95, 248n21
freedom of subjectivity principle, 114

Galen (physician), 130, 264
Gardner, Clinton, 138, 145
gender, discrimination based on, 264
generosity, 50n9
Georgetown University, Center for Bioethics, 71
Gert, Bernard, 1–2, 49–52
gift-giving, and expectant reciprocation, 231
Gilleman, Gerard, 266
Gillon, Raanan, 98–99
  Principles of Health Care Ethics, 98
Glas, Gerrit, 174–75
global health care, 226
God
  belief in, 19
  covenant with, 78, 96, 137–43, 184
  creational covenant with, 141, 142, 153, 154, 236
  emphasis on care for needy, 165
  faithfulness of, 260
  as final authority, 60
  humanity created in image of, 141, 206
  personal accountability to, 8
  in reformed subjectivist principle, 158

305

Index

God (cont.)
   relationship of individual person to, 16
   relationship with worldview, 205
Goheen, Michael, 197, 199
Golden Rule approach, 73
good for man, concept of, 31
good of the patient, 72, 77, 78
Good Samaritan, 253–54
goods, hierarchy of, 76
grace, 104, 137, 138
Grant, George, 216
gratuitousness, 164
Greaves, Richard, 138
Greco-Roman culture, 234, 260
Green, Ronald M., 24–27
Griffioen, Sander, 111, 116
groundless nature, Clouser and Gert on, 51
grounds, 20, 78
Guardini, Romano, 190
Gustafson, James M., 63–64

Habermas, Jurgen, 114–16, 239, 267
Habgood, John, 100–101, 103
Halakhah, 96
Hare, Richard M., 22, 29, 56, 118
Hasan, Zaki, 264
Hasting Center Studies, 38
Hauerwas, Stanley, 3, 87, 185
   comparison with Childress, 61
   on Ramsey, 68, 90
   rejection of natural law, 63
healing relationship, Pellegrino on, 228
health care inequalities in U.S., 262
Hegel, Georg, 113–14
helpfulness, obligation of, 36
heuristic devices, principles as, 54
Hippocratic Oath, 74, 129–32, 172, 279–80
Hippocratic tradition, Veatch's criticism of, 156

historical differentiation, Parsons's concept of, 32
historicism, 119
Hittinger, Russell, 144
Hoeksema, Anthony A., 142
Holmes, Arthur, 188
Holmes, Robert, 21–23
Holy Spirit, 84, 151, 179, 277
Hoose, Bernard, 102–3, 104
hope, as gift of God, 77
Horton, Michael, 230
hospitality to stranger, 233–34
human embryos, 121, 212
human fetuses in research, policy development for use, 202
human research, ethical crisis in, 27–37
human righteousness, 205
human rights, 31, 270
human subjects in research, 28, 94
human worth, 258, 259–60
human-assisted reproduction, Royal Commission (UK) on implications, 118–19
humanists, on health care allocation, 46–47
humans
   created in God's image, 141, 206
   as enkaptic structural whole, 173
   inherent value of each person, 239
   priestly perception of, 191
   relationship to God of the covenant, 200
   structural principle of being, 204
   vulnerability of, 277
Hume, David, 37–38, 45
Husserl, Edmund, 195

ICCR (Interfaith Center on Corporate Responsibility), 226

Iltis, Ana Smith, 56, 122
imago Dei, 61n57, 143–45, 208
  Bavinck on, 206
  creation covenant linked to, 153
  and embryo as human, 212
  Jewish interpretation, 207
  Wolterstorff on, 270
inclusive covenant, 146–47, 168, 169, 175
individualism, 31, 86, 232, 248
individuality, 170
infanticide, 257, 259
infirmed and disabled, mercy killing of, 102
informed consent, 28, 35, 91, 108, 160
instrumental reason, x
Interfaith Center on Corporate Responsibility (ICCR), 226
intuitionism, 23
intuitive inductions, 37
Irenaeus, 151
I-self relationship, 174
Islamic perspectives, 94–96, 264–65
Israel
  law given to, 246
  as priestly royalty, 204
  prohibition of infanticide, child sacrifice, abortion, 259

Jefferson, Thomas, 31
Jerome, Saint, 17
Jesus Christ
  believer's relationship with, 162–63
  as center of Reformed ethics, 168
  and change in relationships, 260
  covenant in, 151
  and covenant redemption, 186
  covenant restoration, 176, 247
  expectation for followers, 268–69

Good Samaritan parable, 254
  love for humanity, 92
  moral paradoxes of ethical teachings, 15–16
  righteousness from faith in, 246
  Sermon on the Mount, 151
  summary of law, 14–15
Jewish perspectives, 64, 94–97, 207, 265
Jochemsen, Henk, 220–21, 224
John Chrysostom, 84
Jones, David Albert, 131
Jones, W. H. S., 130
Jonsen, Albert, 39, 53, 66, 80, 117–23
Journal of Medicine and Philosophy, 71
justice, 10, 36, 37, 83, 101, 262–69
  and *agape* love, 266
  analysis, 49
  context for, 264
  egalitarian, 267
  Islamic perspectives, 95
  Jewish perspectives, 265
  Pellegrino on, 76–77
  perception within biblical covenantal ethic, 269–71
  Ramsey on, 93
  theory of, 46
justification
  in law, 139
  metaethical, 22
just-war debate, 30

Kant, Immanuel, 110
Kasenene, Peter, 264
Kass, Leon, 3, 64, 132
Kelly, David, 70
Kennedy Institute of Ethics, 71
Kerner, George, 39
Kierkegaard, Søren, 195
Klapwijk, Jacob, 189, 196
Kline, Meredith, 141, 146, 152–53
koinonia, 166, 173

Index

Kopelman, Loretta, 23
Kuyper, Abraham, 192, 195

Landis, David, 135–36, 171–72
language, 118
law
    as given to Israel, 246
    justification in, 139
    scriptural idea of, 144
Levinas, Emmanuel, 194
liberalism, classical, 20
life support, for critically ill, 261–62
Lillback, Peter, 139–40
linguistic reductionism, 236
Little, David, 32
liturgical living, role of, 107
Locke, John, 20
Lord's Supper, as covenant renewal, 193
love, 9, 73–74, 167, 243, 262–69, 276. See also *agape* love
    as gift of God, 77
    of God, 181
    of neighbor, 87, 92, 211
    Ramsey's views, 86
love-command, 152, 227, 249, 255
loyalty, 86, 108
Lustig, B. Andrew, 230
Lutheran perspectives, 141, 205–6
lying, 106

MacIntyre, Alasdair, 29, 30–31, 43
    After Virtue, ix
The Malaise of Modernity (Taylor), x
maleficence, constraints on, 167
Marshall, Paul, 197
May, William F., 46, 69, 108, 127, 135, 162–65, 176
    on covenant as relationship, 169–70, 256
    focus on healing act, 228–29
    on gift-giving, 231
    on Hippocratic Oath, 132
    on individual responsibility, 243
    Sturm on, 159
McArdle, Patrick, 191, 214
McCarthy, Dennis, 130, 148
McCarthy, Rockne, 177
McCormick, Richard, 2, 62–63, 70, 112, 234–35
McFadyen, Alistair, 212
medical ethics, Veatch's efforts to develop theory, 25–26. *See also* biomedical ethics
medical oaths
    Hippocratic Oath, 74, 129–32, 172, 279–80
    in Islamic countries, 95
medical practice
    administrative and corporate participants, 226
    Christian philosophy of, 220–25
    as covenantal relational network, 225–30
    and principlism, 214–17
    relational network in, 223
medicine
    covenantal model for, 162
    ethic for, 155, 181
    need for better relationship models, 133–37
    relationship to philosophy in ancient times, 257–58
Medina, Bartholomew, 17
Meilaender, Gilbert, 5, 64, 65
Meland, Bernard, 159
mercy, 102
mercy killing of infirmed and disabled, 102
Meslin, Eric, 54–55
metaethical justification, 22
metaethics, 117–18
metaphilosophy of worldview, 194
modernity, 112–14, 116
monotheism, historical transitions from, 110–11

Moore, G. E., 22, 29, 117
Moore, Peter, 173
moral, meanings of, 30
moral agent, 73, 176, 247
moral communities, 81–82
moral conduct, 221
moral decisions
   analytical process, 57–58
   in bioethics, justifying, 24–25
   certainty in, 18, 27
   consensus in, 33
   justification of, 52
   natural law as justification for, 14
moral Esperanto, 64
moral grounding, 55–57
moral isolation, 232
moral philosophy, 2
moral principles, 120
moral probablism, 17
moral reasoning, x, 29, 89
moral reflection, 250
moral relativism, 72
moral responsibilities, 147
moral sharing, 181
moral status, 201–203
moral strangers, 81, 230–40
moral victims, 57
morality. *See also* common morality
   origin of norms, 42
   Preston on, 99
   principles-based ethics, 40–47
   private vs. particular, 272–73
   private-versus-public split in, 31
   religious viewpoints as qualifiers, 32
   society creation of, 30
Mount, Eric, 178
Mouw, Richard, 170, 190
multiple care relationships, communication role in, 236–37
Murray, John, 142
mutual respect, 34

National Commission on the Protection of Human Subjects, 29
natural law, 14, 70, 104, 268
   common-morality roots in, 42–43
   in covenant thinking, 143–45
   McCormick's views on, 62–63
   reinterpretations of, 234–35
natural virtues, 77
Naugle, David, 110–11, 188
need, principle of, 262
needy, God's emphasis on care for, 165
neighbor love, 87, 92, 211
Nelson, James, 215
neutral analysis, problems from, 22
neutralizing of positions, 65
new covenant, 167
New England Journal of Medicine, 28
Newbigin, Lesslie, 185
Nicholson, R. H., 264
Niebuhr, H. Richard, 189n24, 266
Nielsen, Kai, 268
Nietzsche, Friedrich, x
Nisker, Jeff, 134–35
Noah, 140, 154
noetic structures, 19
non-believers, 207
nonbeneficial experimentation, child participation in, 91
nonindifference, 38
nonmaleficence, 1, 4, 9, 44, 245, 252–55
   vs. beneficence, 253
   Childress's principles of, 61
   Ramsey on, 91
   role of, 41
   Sharia law on, 95
normative individualism, 144n77
Normative Reflective Practitioner model, 221, 224, 229
norms, 41n104

Index

Norris, Christopher, 113
Novak, David, 207, 259–60
Nozick, Robert, 72
nurse practitioners, 222, 224
nurse-patient relationship, 135
Nygren, Anders, 266

obedient love, 161
O'Donovan, Oliver, 150, 151, 152, 187, 249
Oecolampadius, Johann, 138
Olthuis, James, 188
ontic evils, 102
openness, 116, 180
opinion, doubt and, 18
order, principles of, 152, 188, 255
ordering-principle, 152, 181, 255
Oregon health care system, communitarian model, 101n8
Orr, Robert, 132
otherness, 134
others, 195
Outka, Gene, 268

Parsons, Talcott, 32
particular moralities, 272–73
part-time medical practice, 227
Pascal, Blaise, 18
paternalism, 73, 76, 84, 136, 250
The Patient as Person (Ramsey), 91
patient consent, 44
patient-physician covenant, 133
patients
    autonomy of decision making, 160
    and physicians, 223
    relationships with caregivers, 214
Paul (apostle), 245–46, 277
Pellegrino, Edmund, 7, 8, 69–80, 128, 184
    on beneficence, 9
    on beneficence and paternalism, 76
    criticism of, 79
    on healing relationship, 133, 228
    on love, 255
    on principlism, 74, 104–5, 241, 242
permission, principle of, 83, 253
person, Beauchamp on, 203
personal accountability to God, 8
personal preference, expressions of, 30
personhood, 8, 16, 170, 174, 201–13, 248
persuasion, 274–75, 277
Philip the Chancellor, 17
Philo, 207
philosophical ethics, 34, 211
philosophy
    relationship to medicine in ancient times, 257–58
    relationship to theology, 198
    relationship with worldview, 193–98
    top priority of, 194
    transcendental hermeneutical idea of, 196
physician assistants, 224
physicians
    fear of supply crisis, 226–27
    indebtedness of, 256
    medical self-development, 171
    and patients, 223
    Pellegrino on autonomy of, 75
    role as primarily moral agents, 164
    separation of personal moral values from societal values, 216
Pius XII (pope), 70
Plantinga, Alvin, 19, 20, 115, 190
pluralism, 177, 232
pluriform codes, vs. principles of order, 152
Porter, Jean, 14, 143
postmodernism, 113, 114–17

power of physician, 75
practical moral reasoning, 29
preferred triad, 237
prescriptivists, 29
Preston, Ronald, 99, 103
pre-theoretical common sense moral judgments, 41
priestly royalty, Israel as, 204
principles, 10, 41n104, 54, 89
Principles of Biomedical Ethics (Childress and Beauchamp), 1, 40–47, 127, 201–2, 244
Principles of Health Care Ethics (Gillon), 98
principles of order, 152, 188, 255
principles-based ethics, 1, 40–47
principlism, 272. *See also* beneficence; justice; nonmaleficence; respect for persons
   absence of unifying principle, 276
   alternative ethical covenantal framework needed, 109
   analysis of Christian responses to, 103–9
   and biblical covenantal ethics, 241–48, 250
   Clouser and Gert alternative, 52
   critique of, 183, 215
   efforts to improve, 53–55
   ethical vacuum in, xi
   faith in reason as anchor, 122
   historical backdrop, 13–28
   inadequacies of, 3, 247, 278
   key assumptions, 41
   as means to union with God, 84
   and medical practice, 214–17
   as particular morality, 273
   personhood and, 201–3
   postmodern worldview elements, 119
   presuppositional roots of, 109–23
   response to, 48–67
   revisiting, 200–201
   term coined, 2
   ultimate objective, 217
priorities for limited resources, 262
private moralities, 8, 41, 243–44, 272–73
probable certitude, 17
process theology, 158
proportionalism, 70
Protestant Reformation, 59, 138
Protestant theologians, 59–60
prudence, 53
public allowability, 52
public policy debates, 65
public pressure, for policy development, 27

Ramsey, Paul, 2, 3, 60, 69, 85–94, 160–63, 184
   ethic of, 107–8
   Hauerwas on, 68
   organization for medical ethics, 90
   The Patient as Person, 91
   on value of covenantal thinking, 169
rational reflection, 26
rationality, 58, 113, 190, 274
Ratzinger, Joseph, 148–49
Rawls, John, 39, 46, 156
reality, inherent value of, 221
reason, 273
   conflict on relative importance, 15
   faithful vs. unfaithful, 190
   God's command in relation to, 249
   guidance of, 101
   instrumental, x
   moral guidance through faith in, 72
   and worldview of modernity, 112–14

Index

reconciling nature of God's love, 181
redemptive covenant, 146
reflective equilibrium, 43n112, 57, 120
reformed subjectivist principle, 158
Reformed tradition, 160–70, 192, 198–200
relational structures, 180
relational theory, 202
relational triads, 237
relationships
  individual person to God, 16
  in medicine, covenantal models for, 155–57
  personhood and, 8
religion. See also *specific traditions and denominations*
  academic role of belief, 20
  atheistic moral equivalent of, 21
  belief's influence on moral position, 25
  Habermas on, 115
  and worldviews, 110–11
repentance, 181
research
  best interests of subjects, considering, 34
  fairness in subject selection for, 36
  maximization of societal benefits, 34
research ethics boards, 54
respect, 205
respect for persons, 35–36, 44, 66
  as children of God, 101
  within covenantal ethic, 248–51
  as free agents, 80
  principle of, 34
rhetoric, 13
Richardson, Henry, 53
Ridderbos, Herman N., 146
Rieff, Philip, *Sacred Order/Social Order*, xi

rightness
  concern about calling a decision right, 22
  by human convention, vs. naturally right, 150
Robertson, O. Palmer, 141
Robinson, John A. T., 245–46
Roman Catholic theologians, 59
Roman Catholic tradition, 27, 69–70, 83, 98–103, 190–91
Rorty, Richard, 20–21, 82
Ross, W. D., 29, 37, 45
rules, 41n104, 52

Sabbath, 148
sacred grounding for ethics, xi
Sacred Order/Social Order (Rieff), xi
sacredness, Childress on, 32
sanctity of life, 160, 163
Schmemann, Alexander, 106, 191
Scripture, narrative study of, 185. See also Bible
secular morality, Engelhardt on religious nature of, 81–82
secular worldview, need for term redefinition, 196
secularization, 59–67
self
  Christian concept of, 170
  medical vs. personal, 171–72
self-evident principle, 15
self-evident propositions, 19, 158
selfhood, 173, 175
sentimentalization, 164
Sermon on the Mount, 151
Serour, G. I., 94, 265
Sharia law, 94–95
Siegler, Mark, 250–51
sin, 145, 147, 176, 178, 204, 209, 228
  Habermas on, 239
  law and, 246

Index

situationalism, Ramsey's opposition to, 85
Smith, David H., 161, 169
Smith, James K. A., 107, 185
social consensus, 262
social contract theory, 26, 154, 156, 157–58
social justice. *See* justice
social philosophy, Dooyeweerd's, 217–20
social relationships
    Christian pluralist notion of, 177
    Dooyeweerd's typology of, 219–20
social structures
    in medical practice, 221–22
    Western philosophies influencing, 177
societal benefits of research, maximization of, 34
societal pluralism, Engelhardt on, 105
Somerville, Margaret, 203
soul, 258
special covenants, 147
specification, 53
specified principlism, 53
Spirit. *See* Holy Spirit
Spykman, Gordon, 148, 149, 155, 199
Steer, Simon, 233
Steinberg, Avraham, 95, 265
stem-cell research, 121
Stoics, 14
Stopes-Roe, Harry, 46
Stout, Jeffrey, 64, 65
strangers
    alienation vs. hospitality, 31
    care for, 164
    vs. moral strangers, 233
Strauss, Danie F. M., 204, 210
Strong, Carson, 54

structure and direction, neo-Calvinist language of, 105
Sturm, Douglas, 157–60
subjectivism, 116n75
subsidiarity, principle of, 102
suffering, 9, 166, 250
Sulmasy, Daniel, 79, 209
summary principles, Ramsey on, 89n101
supreme ordering-principle, 152
surrogate decision makers, 75–76
synderesis, 17
systematic theology, vs. biblical theology, 199

Taylor, Charles, 9, 45, 203–4, 250
The Malaise of Modernity, x
technicism, 210–11
Ten Commandments, 14
terminally ill children, 241
terminological redemption, 196
theological ethics, vs. philosophical, 34
theological language, 39
theology
    biblical vs. systematic, 199
    diminuation of influence, 5
theoretical ethics, vs. applied, 21
theory, moral ethicists' use of term, 39
Thomist virtue ethics, 75
Torah, moral essence of, 96
transcendent concept of healing art, 136
Trinterud, Leonard, 137
Troost, Andre, 211
true spirit, 111
trust, covenant of, 133–34, 162n156
truth
    in Christian worldview, 111
    by consensus, and postmodern worldview, 114–17
    diversity of private views of, 128

Index

Tubbs, James, 233
Tutu, Desmond, 173
Twiss, Sumner, 32

ubuntu, 173, 248
unborn
    status of, 162, 257
    value and worth of, 261
unethical practices, report on, 28
universalism, discontent with, 65–66
universalizability, principle of, 22, 56
unselfishness, enlightened, 160

values, 42n104
Vaux, Kenneth, 166–68, 169, 180
Veatch, Robert, 25–26, 49, 155–57, 178
Verhey, Allen, 132
vertical in authority (VIA), xi
virtue ethics, 77, 174–75, 242
virtues of moral agent, 73
Vlastos, Gregory, 267
Vollenhoven, D. H. T., 200
von Balthasar, Hans Urs, 144, 154
Vos, Geerhardus, 141
vulnerable others, 178

Walters, LeRoy, 33, 60
Ware, Timothy, 106
Warnock, Mary, 118
Weir, David, 137, 138
Weithman, Paul, 116
Welch, Sharon, 235
Weltanschauung, 110
Western society, diversity of beliefs in, 2

Whitehead, Alfred, 158
wisdom tradition, 148n88
Witvliet, John, 193
Wolters, Albert, 103–4, 112, 192, 195–96
Wolterstorff, Nicholas, 20, 116, 269, 270
women physicians, 226–27
Word of God, 243
works, covenant of, 137, 141
worldview, 188
    Christian and non-Christian distinction, 111–12
    definition from Goheen and Bartholomew, 111
    metaphilosophy of, 194
    notion of, 109–12
    postmodern, and truth by consensus, 114–17
    relationship with philosophy, 193–98
worldview-yields-philosophy model, 196
worship, 149
Wulff, Hendrik, 73
Wyatt, John, 215–16

Yahweh, prohibition on pictorial images, 259. *See also* God

Zaner, Richard, 214–15, 234
Zuidervaart, Lambert, 116
Zwingli, Huldrych, 138

www.ingramcontent.com/pod-product-compliance
Lightning Source LLC
Chambersburg PA
CBHW050617300426
44112CB00012B/1547